W9-ARI-931

THE PSYCHOLOGY OF COUPLES AND ILLNESS

THE PSYCHOLOGY OF COUPLES AND ILLNESS: THEORY, RESEARCH, & PRACTICE

Edited by

Karen B. Schmaling

and

Tamara Goldman Sher

American Psychological Association, Washington, DC

BS

Published by
American Psychological Association
750 First Street, NE
Washington, DC 20002

Copies may be ordered from
APA Order Department
P.O. Box 92984
Washington, DC 20090-2984

In the U.K., Europe, Africa, and the Middle East, copies may be ordered from
American Psychological Association
3 Henrietta Street
Covent Garden, London
WC2E 8LU England

Typeset in Goudy by Monotype Composition

Printer: Data Reproductions Corporation, Auburn Hills, MI
Cover Designer: Anne Masters, Washington, DC
Production Editor: Kristine Enderle

The opinions and statements published are the responsibility of the authors, and such opinions and statements do not necessarily represent the policies of the APA.

Library of Congress Cataloging-in-Publication Data

The psychology of couples and illness : theory, research, and practice / [edited by] Karen B. Schmaling, Tamara Goldman Sher.—1st ed.
    p. cm.
    Includes bibliographical references and index.
    ISBN 1-55798-649-5 (cloth)
    1. Married people—Health and hygiene. 2. Unmarried couples—Health and hygiene. 3. Intimacy (Psychology)—Health aspects. 4. Sick—Family relationships. I. Schmaling, Karen B. II. Sher, Tamara Goldman.

R726.5 .P785 2000
155.6'45—dc21   99-059782

British Library Cataloguing-in-Publication Data
A CIP record is available from the British Library.

Printed in the United States of America
First Edition

To Art, Brian, Emily, and Hannah

CONTENTS

CONTRIBUTORS

Niloofar Afari, PhD, Department of Medicine, University of Washington, Seattle

Donald H. Baucom, PhD, Department of Psychology, University of North Carolina, Chapel Hill

Kristin Bingen, BA, Institute of Psychology, Illinois Institute of Technology, Chicago

W. Jeffrey Canar, MA, Institute of Psychology, Illinois Institute of Technology, Chicago

Andrew Christensen, PhD, Department of Psychology, University of California, Los Angeles

Sharon Danoff-Burg, PhD, Department of Psychology, University at Albany, State University of New York

Allison Deeter, MA, Behavioral Medicine Program, Stanford University Medical School, Standford, CA

Dawn M. Ehde, PhD, Department of Rehabilitation Medicine, University of Washington, Seattle

Gabriele Fehm-Wolfsdorf, Dr. Rer. Soc., Institut für Psychologie, Universität Kiel, Kiel, Germany

Rebecca Gaither, MA, Institute of Psychology, Illinois Institute of Technology, Chicago

Thomas Groth, Dr. Phil., Institute für Psychologie, Universität Kiel, Kiel, Germany

Kurt Hahlweg, Dr. Phil., Institute für Psychologie, Technische Universität Braunschweig, Braunschweig, Germany

W. Kim Halford, PhD, School of Applied Psychology, Griffith University, Nathan, Queensland, Australia

Joyce Hopkins, PhD, Institute of Psychology, Illinois Institute of Technology, Chicago

Andrew Jones, MS, Institute of Psychology, Illinois Institute of Technology, Chicago

Seth C. Kalichman, PhD, Center for AIDS Intervention Research, Medical College of Wisconsin, Milwaukee

Kirsten D. Linney, MS, Department of Child and Family Studies, University of Wisconsin—Madison

Colleen M. McBride, PhD, Department of Community and Family Medicine, Duke University, Durham, NC

Carleton A. Palmer, MA, Department of Psychology, University of North Carolina, Chapel Hill

Lauri A. Pasch, PhD, Department of Pediatrics, University of California, San Francisco

Lynn A. Rankin-Esquer, PhD, Graduate School of Education and Psychology, Pepperdine University, Culver City, CA

Tracey A. Revenson, PhD, Department of Psychology, City University of New York Graduate Center, New York

Linda J. Roberts, PhD, Department of Child and Family Studies, University of Wisconsin—Madison

Karen B. Schmaling, PhD, Department of Psychiatry and Behavioral Sciences, University of Washington, Seattle

Lauren Schwartz, PhD, Department of Rehabilitation Medicine, University of Washington, Seattle

Jennifer L. Scott, MCP, School of Applied Psychology, Griffith University, Nathan, Queensland, Australia

Tamara Goldman Sher, PhD, Institute of Psychology, Illinois Institute of Technology, Chicago

Jill Smythe, BPsych (Honors), School of Applied Psychology, Griffith University, Nathan, Queensland, Australia

C. Barr Taylor, MD, Behavioral Medicine Program, Stanford University Medical School, Stanford, CA

Violet Theodos, MA, Institute of Psychology, Illinois Institute of Technology, Chicago

Dennis C. Turk, PhD, Department of Anesthesiology, University of Washington, Seattle

Michael Young, PhD, Institute of Psychology, Illinois Institute of Technology, Chicago

FOREWORD

DENNIS C. TURK

People live for the most part in social contexts, not in isolation. The most intimate relationships are between couples (spouses, significant others, or partners) who live together. Couples have a structure, functions and assigned roles, modes of interaction, resources, a life cycle, a history, and two individual members each with her or his own unique history. Each of these components and the dynamic interactions that extend and change over time need to be considered when discussing health, illness, and couples.

The *structure*, or *configuration*, of a couple refers to characteristics of the individual members, including age, educational level, and ethnicity. *Function* refers to the tasks the couple performs for society and for each other (e.g., educational, economic, and reproductive).

The assigned *roles* of couples encompass the division of responsibilities, expectations, and rights of each partner and the boundaries established. Thus, one partner may be designated the role of breadwinner and another the overseer of health care. Roles do not have to be mutually exclusive, and they seldom are. Roles always have responsibilities with behavioral referents.

Modes of interaction are related to the style adopted by the couple to deal with the environment and with one another and in decision making. *Resources* include general health of the partners, social support and skills, personality characteristics, and financial support. These resources influence the way that the couple interprets events. *Couple history* refers to sociocultural factors as well as prior history of illness and modes of coping with stress. As was the case for resources, the history of the couple will affect the way in which the couple interprets and responds to various events.

Couples also have a life cycle, which changes and evolves over time. The couple progresses through a reasonably well defined set of phases of development, beginning with courtship and ending with death. Each phase is associated with certain developmental tasks, the successful completion of which leads to different levels of couple functioning.

Finally, couples comprise two individual members who have unique experiences, prior learning histories, and personalities that preexisted their status as a couple. People have their own unique conceptions and behavioral repertoires, which account for a substantial portion of what is observed within the context of the couple. The unique characteristics of the two partners need to be considered when thinking about the couple itself.

All of the characteristics of the couple outlined above, including the unique contributions of the individuals, influence a variety of important health and illness issues throughout the life span. It is because of this complexity that studying couples is difficult, why such a paucity of research exists, and why so much of the available data are difficult to interpret. I am reminded of the entomologist who was retiring after a 50-year career that consisted of specialization in the anatomy and functioning of the hind legs of grasshoppers. When asked if, in retrospect, there was anything he would change about his career, on a moment's reflection, he indicated yes, he would change one thing. If he had to do it over again, he would study only one of the hind legs of the grasshopper because studying two was excessively complex. Indeed, studying a pair, a couple, is more complex than studying each one separately, and the whole is surely greater than the sum of its parts.

People live in social groups, beginning with their families and, as adults, progressing to significant relationships. These most intimate relationships may cease only after divorce or the death of one of the partners. Thus, health and illness do not occur in a social void; they are incorporated within and superimposed on the complexity of the relationship between the individuals making up the couple and the unique features of both partners. Although it may seem intuitively obvious, the majority of the research on health and illness focuses on a single individual when ill—the identified patient. However, people define their symptoms by consulting their partner. Even when professional help is sought and therapy prescribed, couples retain the responsibilities for making decisions about the management of therapies within the confines of their relationship. Partner attitudes play significant roles in the promotion and maintenance of health, adaptation to diseases and injuries, treatment decision making, participation in treatment, and compliance with treatment recommendations.

The presence of health-defeating behaviors (e.g., smoking or substance abuse) or an illness in a partner will place a significant burden on the healthy partner. Depending on the nature (e.g., specific symptoms, acute, progressive, chronic, life threatening) and severity of an illness—along with the extent of impairment and complexity of the home management requirements—its presence in one partner will pose a significant emotional and caregiving burden on the healthy partner. Well-established roles, responsibilities, and boundaries may have to change. Demands for both emotional and instrumental support may become excessive. Because many diseases are chronic, extending over time, the burden may have a cumulative effect. The caregiving partner may feel trapped in the relationship. He or she may feel tired and emotionally drained by the long duration of the illness, the extent of the caregiver workload, feelings of powerlessness, and the need to be emotionally strong. Healthy partners may have contradictory feelings: They have their own needs but are obligated to care for their partner, they have to balance dependence and autonomy of the patient with their own needs. The demands of the caregiver role may have a physiological impact on the caregiver, influencing his or her own health. When considered, the emphasis tends to be the impact of the healthy partner on the adaptation of the patient. However, burnout—physical and emotional distress—may be experienced by some caregivers. Yet rarely is treatment targeted on this member of the couple.

It is overly simplistic to consider the intimate relationship as simply providing beneficial social support. Not all support is positive, even if well intended. The line between support, smothering, and controlling is not clear. Not all people need or want the same type of support, and not every healthy partner knows what type of support is desired or is capable of providing that type of support. Moreover, demands may change with the course of the disease. What is helpful support during one stage of the disease or for one problem area may not be for another, and what is viewed positively by one person and one point in time may not be well received by a different person or at a different time along the course of an illness or during the process of changing health-damaging to health-promoting behavior.

In addition to coping with the illness, the partner who is ill may feel guilty about the demands his or her illness makes on the healthy partner. He or she may resent the change in roles and responsibilities caused by the limitations imposed by the illness and must deal with the threat to his or her autonomy and the need to depend on the healthy partner. Conversely, the healthy partner will have concerns not only about the identified patient but also about the consequences of the disease for his or her life and, depending on the couple's developmental stage, the consequences for children.

All chronic conditions include a number of common features that each represent an assault on multiple areas of functioning and not just on the body. Couples with various chronic illnesses may face changes in their roles, responsibilities, and boundaries; separation from family, friends, and other sources of gratification; disruption of plans for the future; assaults on the self-image and self-esteem of each partner; uncertain and unpredictable futures; and distressing emotions (e.g., anxiety, depression, resentment, and feelings of helplessness), as well as such illness-related factors in the patient as permanent changes in physical appearance or bodily functioning.

On the basis of such an extensive set of adjustive demands, one might expect that the presence of a chronic illness will, inevitably, result in significant emotional difficulties and breakdown in integrated functioning. Perhaps because of this assumption, the emphasis of the literature in this area has been on impact, distress, and incapacity resulting from the illness. Much less attention has been afforded to effective ways of responding and meeting challenges and the satisfactory restructuring of relationships and lives. Nevertheless, despite the presence of conditions and situations that are clearly traumatic and disruptive, a substantial proportion of couples make satisfactory if not magnificent adjustments. This observation attests to the remarkable human capacity to transcend pain and suffering with adjustment to a whole set of new circumstances and demands.

Most of what is known about coping and adapting by couples is based on those who are having difficulty and seek treatment for emotional problems and other difficulties. There is much that can be learned by studying those who adjust well to significant threats, demands, and burdens posed by chronic illnesses. There is tremendous individual variation among couples in how they navigate the demands. Assessment needs to seek out such differences, and appropriate treatments need to be matched to these unique response patterns.

Recall the entomologist studying the hind legs of grasshoppers, who felt the complexity of studying both was limiting. It cannot be contested that studying couples is complex—and not merely twice as complex as studying the individual patient. The authors of this volume have accepted the challenge. Each chapter focuses on the intimate relationship characterizing a couple as partners confront problems of promoting health and adapting to the presence of an illness. The authors not only address the complexities inherent in couple adaptation by providing general observations but also make the situations real by including case examples. The authors identify the many issues involved in studying couples in the context of particular health or illness circumstances and also provide recommendations for assessment methods.

As noted earlier, people live primarily in intimate relationships with a partner. Failure to recognize this fundamental point will impede understanding of adaptation of problems of health and illness. Without understanding the influence of caregivers, we will not be able to provide optimal treatment when it is required. The authors of this volume present insights into treatment approaches that address specific issues of the disease or maladaptive health behavior viewed by both partners, not solely the identified patient or target of health behavior change. It is particularly noteworthy that in a number of instances the authors describe research demonstrating that the functioning of the couple may have a direct effect on the disease process. This, then, is a unique book in that it goes beyond the individual or identified patient, addressing the challenge of understanding, assessment, and treatment from the perspective of the intimate relationship of the couple.

PREFACE

This volume was conceptualized following many long conversations between the editors and among the editors and other colleagues who were looking for source for the emerging literature on couples and illness. A few years ago, such a book would not have been possible. There was not enough empirical work being conducted in the area of couples and illness, nor was there enough interest in the topic to warrant such a volume. However, the enthusiasm of our colleagues to share their expertise of working with and studying couples coping with illness and of the American Psychological Association (APA) Books Program to publish such a volume made this book possible and convinced us that it would be beneficial to a wide audience. We envision this book as a resource to health professionals from a variety of disciplines, such as psychologists, physicians, nurses, clergy, and academic researchers interested in couples. In addition, we hope to capture the attention of others in the health professions, so that the body of literature in this area continues to grow. More focused attention to this area will benefit those of us already in the field, those of us interested in applying results to our clinical populations, and those of us who are part of the growing number of couples coping with illness.

Our experience includes training by eminent scientist–practitioners of couples therapy, who continue to encourage our interest in research on couples. We both have worked in medical settings, in clinical practice, and in research laboratories, studying how patients and their partners affect and are affected by medical problems. Together, we have spoken to hundreds of couples willing to share their experiences dealing with illness within the confines of their relationship. The book was a collaborative venture: The order of editorship was determined by coin flip. Editing this book has been exciting and instructive. We appreciate the encouragement, efforts, and thoughtfulness of our mentors, colleagues, and contributors, as well as the support of the editors at APA Books. In particular, we are indebted to our partners; their support was instrumental in allowing us to complete this work and to give it meaning on many different levels.

Finally, Dr. Neil S. Jacobson was planning to coauthor the foreword of this book with Dr. Turk and served as a mentor to us. We regret his untimely death.

THE PSYCHOLOGY OF COUPLES AND ILLNESS

INTRODUCTION

KAREN B. SCHMALING AND TAMARA GOLDMAN SHER

Many relationship commitment ceremonies include vows for partners to be steadfast together in the face of adversity. To be partners "in sickness" is noted as a particularly stressful event that challenges the integrity of the couple. This volume was inspired by the increasing number of behavioral scientists interested in the influence of illness on intimate relationships and of intimate relationships on illness and the promise of couple-involved interventions to enhance health, health behavior, and functional status. This book fulfills a unique niche: Although a few volumes have addressed the effects of illness on the larger family unit from a family systems perspective (Akamatsu, Stephens, Hobfall, & Crowther, 1992; Lyons, Sullivan, & Coyne, 1995; Ramsey, 1989; Rolland, 1994), none have focused specifically on the reciprocal impact of intimate relationships on illness from a behavioral perspective. Furthermore, comprehensive reviews of the associations of intimate relationship factors with specific illnesses or conditions are lacking, probably because of a paucity of research data for any given condition.

An exception is a literature review by Burman and Margolin (1992) on couples and illness, which moved the field forward in several ways. First, it demonstrated the usefulness of focusing on the couple, rather than on the family, to understand health status. Second, it identified three types or levels of couple variables that could have an impact on health variables: (a) relationship status (whether or not one is in a significant relationship), (b) relationship quality (satisfied vs. dissatisfied), and (c) couple interaction, as assessed by the observation of specific behaviors.[1] Third, Burman and Margolin proposed a model of the associations between intimate relationships and health status, which include interpersonal, intraindividual, psychological, and physiological variables. These researchers concluded that "marital variables affect health status but the effect is indirect and nonspecific" (Burman & Margolin, 1992, p. 39), suggesting both the importance and innovation of future research in the area. In recent years, sufficient data have accumulated in an emerging field of couples-focused behavioral medicine that allowed the current volume to be assembled.

Before considering further the importance of the interaction of couple variables and illness, let us review briefly the significance of each factor. In population-based surveys, most adults report at least one significant intimate relationship. For example, among persons age 65 and over in the United States, only 4% report never having been married (U.S. Bureau of the Census, 1998). An additional portion of the adult population are involved in same-gender relationships or other types of committed relationships, suggesting that almost all of us are part of a couple for a portion of our life. Similarly, the incidence of chronic illness is high and rising. It has been estimated that by 2030, 150 million Americans will have a chronic illness, and although the likelihood of acquiring a chronic illness increases with age, the majority of persons with a chronic illness are under the age of 65 (Hoffman, Rice, & Sung, 1996). Taken together, these statistics suggest that our relationships are likely to affect and be affected by illness.

The book contains chapters that address couple variables across five levels of physical conditions. The first chapter reviews the basic psychophysiological consequences of couple interaction. It contains a unique, comprehensive review of the immunology, endocrinology, and cardiovascular effects of couple interaction. The next five chapters review the association of couple variables (i.e., relationship status, quality, and specific behaviors) among couples in which one person has an illness with well-characterized pathophysiology, such as coronary heart disease (CHD), respiratory and rheumatic illnesses, cancer, or HIV. These chapters present comprehensive, systematic reviews of the associations between illness and couple factors and posit innovative, integrative models of interpersonal and physiological factors. The next three chapters address conditions in which the pathophysiol-

---

[1]Burman and Margolin (1992) used the term *marital* rather than *couple* or *relationship*. Throughout this volume, we have attempted to use these latter terms whenever possible because of their inclusiveness of varied sexual orientations. Although we recognize that most of the research referenced in this volume used heterosexual couples, it is our hope that future research efforts will be more inclusive of same-gender couples.

ogy is less understood, less easily documented, and more difficult to diagnose, such as chronic pain, premenstrual syndrome, or fertility problems. The health status for patients with these conditions may be strongly influenced by couple variables, perhaps because the ambiguity associated with these conditions increases the potency of the effects of the environment—more than for patients with conditions involving well-characterized pathophysiology. Next, two chapters address couple factors and behaviors that have direct implications for health and illness: alcohol and tobacco use. Relatively more research and interventions involving couples exist for these health behaviors. The final chapter examines how chronic illness in children affects the parents' intimate relationship. This chapter contributes a unique developmental perspective to understanding the effects of children's illness on parental couple functioning.

All of the chapters review the current state of the literature addressing couple factors and the specific population as well as make suggestions for future research endeavors. In addition, they all address how couple variables affect and are affected by the illness and review couple-involved assessment and intervention strategies. In each chapter, a clinical scenario is presented to illustrate the concepts that are addressed. Furthermore, several chapters outline comprehensive intervention programs for couples coping with illnesses: chapter 2, for CHD; chapter 5, for early-stage breast and gynecologic cancers; chapter 7, for chronic pain; chapter 10, for alcohol problems; and chapter 11, for smoking cessation. Other chapters depict the treatment of illness issues in the context of couples therapy or partner-involved therapy using idiographic treatment plans based on the specific needs of each case. Illness-specific couples-focused treatment development work is likely to be one line of work that we will see in the future. An overview of each chapter is provided below.

Chapter 1, "Basic Research on the Psychobiology of Intimate Relationships," by Thomas Groth, Gabriele Fehm-Wolfsdorf, and Kurt Hahlweg, reviews existing and new data, addresses common methodological issues in this area, and summarizes the status of the field. The authors review the growing body of research that indicates that negative interactions in intimate relationships are stressful, as reflected by a variety of physiological measures, and are linked to long-term deleterious health outcomes. It has long been noted that women are more emotionally sensitive to conflict than men (Barry, 1970) and that intimate relationships benefit men more than women (Schumm, Webb, & Bollman, 1998). The integration of these two observations suggests that for men, a female partner helps with instrumental functions (men neither are so sensitive to nor need help with emotional functions). However, women tend to ask for but not receive emotional help (e.g., in a demand–withdraw pattern; see chapter 9 for further discussion of this dyadic interaction pattern), leading to negative health outcomes that in the short term can be observed in certain physiological measures. Women tend to show more cardiovascular and immunological reactivity to negative intimate interactions, although men show deleterious cardiovascular effects in some situations (e.g., situations involving achievement expectations). Cardiovascular disease is relatively more common among men. Will emerging gender differences in physiological reactivity to negative interactions parallel gender differences in disease expression? There are a few studies that support this potential long-term causal connection (e.g., Kiecolt-Glaser et al., 1991) that warrants future research efforts. The information reviewed in this chapter also is helpful for understanding the pathophysiology referenced in later chapters regarding CHD, respiratory illnesses, cancer, and so forth.

Chapter 2, "Coronary Heart Disease and Couples," by Lynn A. Rankin-Esquer, Allison Deeter, and C. Barr Taylor, highlights the significance of CHD as the leading cause of death for men and women. The authors link being part of a couple with a variety of positive health outcomes, including less mortality after a myocardial infarction (MI) and better adherence to post-MI rehabilitation programs. The intimate relationship may be a common pathway by which known behavioral and psychosocial risk factors, such as hostility and cardiovascular reactivity, and protective factors, such as social support, affect CHD. To this end, the authors present a comprehensive intervention, the Relationship Support Program, to help couples cope with the consequences of a cardiac event and to examine how relationship issues are related to the event and cardiac health, in general, and enhance general relationship skills. Outcome data from a clinical trial are forthcoming.

Karen B. Schmaling and Niloofar Afari review how respiratory diseases affect and are affected by intimate relationships in chapter 3, "Couples Coping With Respiratory Disorders." Negative or stressful relationship events may prompt illness among persons with intermittent respiratory conditions such as asthma and upper respiratory illness. Chronic and severe respiratory conditions, such as cystic fibrosis, chronic obstructive pulmonary disease, and obstructive sleep apnea, appear to be associated with relatively decreased relationship satisfaction, in particular, sexual difficulties. Intimate relationship factors are important for medical treatment and, therefore, medical outcomes. For example, being in a relationship has been associated with better adherence with medication regimens among patients with asthma. The authors suggest that many couples living with a respiratory illness would benefit from educational (to enhance medical and relevant psychosocial information), change-based (communication and problem solving), and acceptance-based interventions chosen on the idiographic needs of the couple. The authors conclude their chapter by presenting a new model of premorbid, interpersonal, and physiological factors and posit mechanisms through which the interaction of these factors is associated with respiratory illness.

In chapter 4, "Rheumatic Illness and Relationships: Coping as a Joint Venture," Sharon Danoff-Burg and Tracey A. Revenson describe the impact that rheumatic diseases have on couples. In a thorough description of various rheumatic diseases and the impact of these diseases on the individual, the relationship, and society, they offer assessment and treatment suggestions based on their extensive clinical and research experience. Uniquely, this chapter offers a model from which to conceptualize the effect of a chronic illness such as a rheumatic disease on a relationship. Using an "illness in context," or ecological, perspective, the authors note the importance of understanding illness as a function not only of individual characteristics but also of the broader interpersonal, social, political, and cultural context. In addition, they describe the effect of an illness on a relationship as a reciprocal one, whereby both the patient's and the partner's distress and coping strategies are affected by each other. This conceptualization leads to the authors' suggestions for future directions with these couples, in both the clinical and research arenas organized around questions they anticipate from the readers of this volume.

In chapter 5, W. Kim Halford, Jennifer L. Scott, and Jill Smythe first put cancer morbidity in perspective in "Couples and Coping With Cancer: Helping Each Other Through the Night." Although cancer is a frightening diagnosis and the second most frequent cause of death in the United States, the majority of people recover from it. Whereas cancer should not be equated with a death sentence, adaptation to it can be challenging. As Halford, Scott, and Smythe show, the most significant distress is observed in relatively younger patients with advanced cancers, and patient adjustment and partner adjustment are highly correlated: Distressed patients with poor adjustment tend to have distressed partners with poor adjustment. Certain forms of coping and social support can assuage distress. The authors outline a six-session cognitive–behavioral program for women with early-stage breast or gynecological cancer and their partner. The program is based on empirically supported strategies to reduce distress (e.g., controlling arousal through relaxation training) and enhance support, communication, and coping (e.g., through tasks such as formulating a list of questions the couple wants to ask the physician). Strategies to address existential issues, sexuality concerns, and relapse prevention are included. The results from the authors' randomized, controlled trial of 90 women suggest that program participation is associated with improved mood and less psychological morbidity than is the case with standard care. The authors' systematic approach to the formulation of a new treatment program for couples coping with cancer is a model for others seeking to formulate relevant treatment protocols.

In chapter 6, "Couples With HIV/AIDS," Seth C. Kalichman conceptualizes HIV and AIDS as "a disease of couple relationships" (p. 171). He notes that in the United States today, the large majority of HIV infection occurs in the context of an intimate relationship, and hence, people infected with HIV are often in the dual roles of being both patient and partner. After describing HIV disease trajectories and the most common routes of infection, Kalichman notes that due to medical advances, today people are living longer with HIV/AIDS and that this presents a special challenge to those patients within committed relationships. Unlike with other chronic or terminal illnesses, Kalichman notes, people infected with HIV are often hesitant to disclose their diagnoses to people outside of their intimate relationship, placing the burden of emotional and medical care solely on their intimate partner. The author notes that couples living with HIV/AIDS are either seroconcordant or serodiscordant, with regard to who in the relationship is affected, and that health professionals need to understand the differences in these types of couples if their needs are to be adequately addressed. He also notes the difficulty of assessing and working with these couples because of both the characteristics of the populations most affected by HIV/AIDS and the uncertain course of HIV disease. Despite these caveats, Kalichman provides focused guidance for the practitioner in the assessment and treatment of couples living with HIV/AIDS, with an emphasis on the need to assess for the presence of substance abuse or trauma; the difficult nature of a healthy and satisfying sexual relationship; and other areas of unique concern for these couples. Future directions are presented for both the practitioner and the researcher.

In chapter 7, "Couples and Chronic Pain" Lauren Schwartz and Dawn M. Ehde highlight the important contributions to the literature dealing with chronic pain and couples. They provide a succinct overview of what is understood about the etiology of chronic pain as well as models for understanding pain that are widely acknowledged by those working with patients with chronic pain. They also discuss the unique impact of chronic pain on couple functioning and the high incidence of relationship and sexual dissatisfaction among couples dealing with chronic pain. Unlike with other conditions in this volume, Schwartz and Ehde observe the consistent findings in the literature that how a partner responds to chronic pain within the context of a relationship affects the nature and course of the condition. With this background, the authors then apply a common intervention with couples without a medical condition, integrative behavioral couples therapy, to a hypothetical couple in which one partner has chronic pain. They detail the assessment and intervention strategies that should be included in working with similar couples and suggest directions for future clinical and research work, with an emphasis on the need for more work focusing on couple or relationship issues.

In chapter 8, "Couples and Premenstrual Syndrome: Partners as Moderators of Symptoms?" Andrew Jones, Violet Theodos, Tamara Goldman Sher, and Michael Young present an alternative model for the traditional way of looking at premenstrual syndrome (PMS). Instead of considering PMS dichotomously (i.e., that women either have or do not have PMS), the authors suggest that PMS be conceptualized as existing on a continuum. That is, similar to an illness behavior model, they propose that all menstruating women fall somewhere on a continuum of menstrually related symptoms ranging from minimal symptoms unlikely to interfere with daily functioning to severe symptoms likely to be accompanied by significant distress and impairment. Despite the authors' caveat that little research has been conducted on the association between relationships and PMS, a number of controlled studies are reviewed. Overall, several studies suggest that greater relationship satisfaction predicts lower PMS symptom severity scores. In addition, the authors discuss how a diagnosis of PMS, as it has traditionally been viewed, can impact a relationship and how the proposed model of PMS can allow a woman or a couple to view a PMS symptom severity score in terms of all the medical and psychosocial contributing variables. Suggestions for assessment and intervention are made, with specific inventories reviewed, and an intervention approach is offered that includes a biopsychosocial approach to PMS symptomatology.

In chapter 9, "Couples Facing Fertility Problems," Lauri A. Pasch and Andrew Christensen present an introduction to the psychology of couples and infertility. Similar to HIV/AIDS, infertility is a condition couples face that is defined at the couple level. As a result, there is a body of literature from which to draw in making suggestions for assessment and intervention for couples experiencing fertility problems. The authors of this chapter note the difficulty of the treatment for infertility and the concomitant psychological, sexual, financial, and social ramifications of this diagnosis. They also note the challenge of working with couples who may interpret and cope with the diagnosis differently from each other. Pasch and Christensen offer recommendations for intervention for medical professionals and mental health professionals in separate sections. In addition, using integrative couples therapy as a model, they delineate a treatment program for couples facing infertility that is comprehensive and focused. Suggestions for future directions are made for both clinical and research purposes.

In chapter 10, "Alcohol Problems and Couples: Drinking in an Intimate Relational Context," Linda J. Roberts and Kirsten D. Linney describe the unique challenges couples face in dealing with alcohol within their relationship. Throughout the chapter, the authors note the heterogeneity of couples with alcohol problems and that alcohol can enhance or damage relationships. The authors carefully review the literature on the interpersonal effects of alcohol. They note that the impact of alcohol on a person or on a relationship is shaped by the alcohol but just as much by nonalcohol factors such as the genetic makeup and personality of the individual, her or his drinking motives and expectancies, her or his immediate social environment, and the broader social, cultural, and historical context of drinking. They also cite a broad literature focusing on the connections between relationship disruption and drinking and between relationship quality and drinking and the impact of problem drinking on a relationship, as well as problem drinking as a consequence of intimate relationship problems.

Citing an increase in violence, sexual difficulties, and communication difficulties associated with drinking, the authors carefully examine the mechanisms behind the association between relationship problems and drinking problems. They offer specific advice regarding assessment instruments and intervention strategies that include a partner and suggest future directions for both clinical and research goals.

In chapter 11, "Couple Approaches to Smoking Cessation," Carleton A. Palmer, Donald H. Baucom, and Colleen M. McBride review couple approaches to smoking cessation. They review the significant concordance in smoking behavior among couples: Smokers' partners tend to be smokers, and smoking cessation is unlikely if only one partner in a smoking dyad tries to quit. These data argue for a couple approach to smoking cessation. However, partner smoking status has not been routinely assessed and addressed in previous studies. Assessing couples' motivation to quit smoking also has not been done routinely. The authors indicate several types of events that could be points of enhanced motivation for individuals and couples considering smoking cessation, such as pregnancy or a threatening illness. Quitting smoking is a challenging and aversive process. Certain negative behaviors by nonsmoking partners (e.g., nagging or criticizing) have been associated with the decreased likelihood of smoking cessation by the smoking partner. Smoking cessation has been associated with decreased relationship satisfaction; quitting smoking may introduce stress into the relationship. Palmer, Baucom, and McBride pose a series of excellent and heretofore unanswered questions about the function of smoking in intimate relationships that would be extremely useful queries for future research. Finally, they outline specific interventions that would be indicated in partner-assisted treatment, in which the partner's role is that of coach or assistant therapist, and in disorder-specific treatment, in which general relationship issues are the focus of treatment.

In chapter 12, "When the Bough Breaks: The Relationship Between Chronic Illness in Children and Couple Functioning," Rebecca Gaither, Kristen Bingen, and Joyce Hopkins find that childhood chronic illness is common. They review the literature on the effects on couples of having a child with a common childhood illness or condition (e.g., cancer, spina bifida, or diabetes). In general, the literature suggests that having a child with an illness or medical condition is stressful but that the increased stress does not necessarily decrease couples' relationship satisfaction or put their relationship status at risk. Indeed, the authors' review includes reports of positive effects on couples' relationships, such as increased closeness. Some areas of the existing literature suffer from methodological limitations such as not using standardized assessment instruments or appropriate control groups; the observations offered by the authors will be helpful for researchers interested in similar topics. Few studies have addressed the effects of couples' relationship satisfaction and other couple variables on child health, despite a well-documented association between couple distress and child distress. Such issues require longitudinal studies because the direction of effects in the association of couple satisfaction and child health cannot be determined in cross-sectional designs. The authors suggest useful areas of focus for assessment, such as couple responsibilities and tasks, to identify possible role strain, which is one common area of dysfunction in couples with a chronically ill child. They also summarize possible couple, child, and family intervention strategies. Across these modalities, the authors remind us that ill children need to be treated as children, with appropriate discipline and attention to developmental milestones, and with sensitivity to the developmentally appropriate needs of an ill child.

The individual chapters will be of interest to clinicians working with ill patients and their partners. Additionally, researchers will find the chapter authors committed to the empirical basis of their topics. We hope this volume will encourage more scientist–practitioners to pursue work with couples coping with illnesses.

REFERENCES

Akamatsu, T. J., Stephens, M. A. P., Hobfall, S. E., & Crowther, J. H. (Eds.). (1992). *Family health psychology*. Washington, DC: Taylor & Francis.

Barry, W. (1970). Marriage research and conflict: An integrative review. *Psychological Bulletin, 73*, 41–54.

Burman, B., & Margolin, G. (1992). Analysis of the association between marital relationship and health problems: An interactional perspective. *Psychological Bulletin, 112*, 39–63.

Hoffman, C., Rice, D., & Sung, H. Y. (1996). Persons with chronic conditions: Their prevalence and costs. *Journal of the American Medical Association, 276*, 1473–1479.

Kiecolt-Glaser, J. K., Dura, J. R., Speicher, C. E., Trask, O. J., & Glaser, R. (1991). Spousal caregivers of dementia victims: Longitudinal changes in immunity and health. *Psychosomatic Medicine, 53*, 345–362.

Lyons, R. F., Sullivan, M. J., & Coyne, J. C. (1995). *Relationships, chronic illness, and disability*. New York: Sage.

Ramsey, C. N. (Ed.). (1989). *Family systems in medicine*. New York: Guilford Press.

Rolland, J. S. (1994). *Families, illness, and disability: An integrative treatment model*. New York: Basic Books.

Schumm, W. R., Webb, F. J., & Bollman, S. R. (1998). Gender and marital satisfaction: Data for the National Survey of Families and Households. *Psychological Reports, 83*, 319–327.

U.S. Bureau of the Census. (1998). *PPL-100 Marital status and living arrangements; March 1998 [Update]*.

1

BASIC RESEARCH ON THE PSYCHOBIOLOGY OF INTIMATE RELATIONSHIPS

THOMAS GROTH, GABRIELE FEHM-WOLFSDORF, AND KURT HAHLWEG

This chapter provides an overview of basic psychobiological processes related to intimate relationships, with an emphasis on couples in unsatisfactory relationships. From a biobehavioral perspective, prolonged or repeated activation of the sympathetic–adrenal–medullary (SAM) system and the hypothalamic–pituitary–adrenal (HPA) axis, as well as long-lasting immunological alterations, is thought to have adverse consequences for physical and psychological health and well-being. Each system is discussed, to provide a basic understanding of its biological functions, appropriate measures, and methods of measurement. We also review studies that provide preliminary evidence that tensions in intimate relationships and negative couple interactions are associated with increased cardiovascular and endocrine reactivity and immunological down regulation (decreased reactivity of the immune system). Finally, we attempt to integrate these empirical findings. Possible pathways through which troubled intimate relationships can affect health and their clinical implications are discussed.

PSYCHOBIOBEHAVIORAL PERSPECTIVES OF STRESS IN COUPLES

There is growing evidence that the lack of an intimate relationship or the presence of a troubled relationship is likely to be associated with health problems. For example, a review of six large, prospective studies that examined the relationship between health outcomes and the quality and quantity of social relationships provided evidence that mortality is higher among more socially isolated individuals (House, Landis, & Umberson, 1988). Furthermore, social isolation appears to be a major psychosocial risk factor for the development of cardiovascular disease (for a review, see Krantz, Contrada, Hill, & Friedler, 1988). Despite the well-documented supportive and stress-buffering function of close relationships, a troubled intimate relationship itself can be a significant source of stress. First, relationship problems and tensions can lead to a higher frequency of negative interactions between partners, which can be the most distressing events in the couple's day-to-day life (Bolger, DeLongis, Kessler, & Schilling, 1989). Relationship problems can also increase the impact of environmental stressors (e.g., work stress, interpersonal conflicts), because the partner's support is not available. Moreover, a troubled relationship seems to be associated with over involvement in relationship problems which can have adverse effects on social contacts outside the partnership and reduce the partners ability to seek social support from others (Coyne & DeLongis, 1986). Thus, a troubled relationship can directly or indirectly increase the level of stress experienced by the partners. In a recent review, Burman and Margolin (1992) presented a hypothetical model of the association between relationship factors (marital status, relationship quality, and dyadic interaction) and health outcomes. Data from more than 40 reviewed studies suggest that the effect of relationship variables on health seems to be indirect and nonspecific. For example, negative dyadic interaction can affect relationship quality and reduce the support one receives from the partner. Moreover, low relationship quality can change one's affect and perception of the relationship and lead to poorer health-related behaviors, such as less exercise or substance abuse.

For a better understanding of possible causal pathways leading from dyadic distress in couples to health problems, it seems necessary to address more specific hypotheses about the associations between different aspects of the hypothetical model. According to Burman and Margolin (1992), the most conclusive way to demonstrate specific associations between relationship variables and the development of health problems would be to show that dyadic interaction directly affects physiological responses in couples. Figure 1.1 shows a heuristic model of the psychophysiology of dyadic interaction in close relationships.

Negative dyadic interaction can be regarded as a significant stressor that may directly result in acute physiological changes. From a psy-

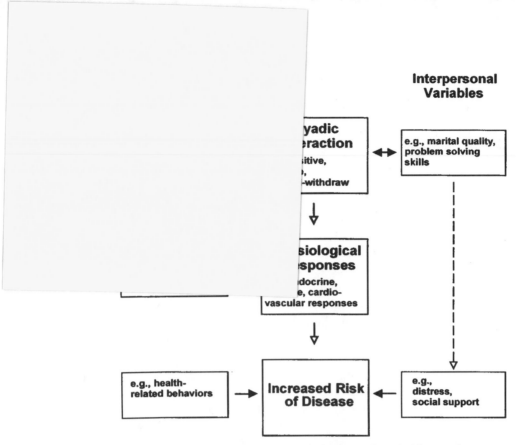

Interpersonal Variables

yadic eraction itive, , -withdraw	**e.g., marital quality, problem solving skills**
siological sponses docrine, e, cardio- vascular responses	
e.g., health- related behaviors → **Increased Risk of Disease** ←	**e.g., distress, social support**

Figure 1.1. A heuristic model of the psychobiology of marital interaction.

chobiobehavioral perspective of human health and well-being, investigators have long been interested in the role of physiological responses to everyday stress in the development of physical and psychiatric illness. However, in stress research, most laboratory tasks are asocial (e.g., reaction time tasks, mental arithmetic tasks). For example, Lassner, Matthews, and Stoney (1994) reported that more than 95% of cardiovascular reactivity studies published in 1988 and 1989 in *Psychosomatic Medicine* used tasks performed alone. Results of these studies may have limited impact on the understanding of psychophysiological responses to social stress. For example, Van Doornen and van Blokland (1989) reported that in a sample of 49 male students, the correlation between the mean heart rate reactivity to three reaction time tasks and two interpersonal tasks was .22, suggesting that heart rate reactivity to an asocial stressor may account for less than 5% of the variance in the reactivity to a social stressor. We agree with Lassner et al. that the use of laboratory analogues of interpersonal conflict represents an excellent approach to examining the role of a naturally occurring social stressor in the development of health problems.

In our model, we included factors that are known to affect both dyadic interaction and physiological stress responses. Substantial differences between the dyadic interaction behavior of distressed and nondistressed couples have been well described in the marital literature. Distressed couples can be characterized by a higher rate of negative interaction behaviors (e.g., complaining or criticizing) and a specific destructive interaction pattern, the *demand–withdraw* interaction sequence (for reviews, see Christensen, 1987; Weiss & Heyman, 1990), in which one partner, typically the woman in heterosexual dyads, makes demands on the other partner, who subsequently withdraws. Thus, distressed partners may be more negatively affected by a conflictual discussion.

Gender can play a major role in the degree of psychophysiological responses to acute stressors. Differences between men and women in cardiovascular, endocrine, and immune responses have been addressed in a series of studies. For example, Kirschbaum, Wüst, and Hellhammer (1992) reported consistent differences in the adrenocortical stress response, with men showing a 1.5- to 2-fold higher secretion of cortisol than women after psychological stress. Gender differences in psychophysiological stress reactivity may even account for differences between men and women in relationship problem behavior and health outcomes after chronic relationship distress (Gottman & Levenson, 1988; Kiecolt-Glaser, Malarkey, Cacioppo, & Glaser, 1994; Kiecolt-Glaser et al., 1996). We address this topic in depth in the following sections. In addition, this chapter provides a general overview of dyadic interaction and its relation to psychophysiological stress responses (the most central aspects of the model presented in Figure 1.1). An exhaustive analysis of all possible interactions of the different factors in the model is beyond the scope of this chapter.

PSYCHOPHYSIOLOGICAL ASSESSMENT

An understanding of the basic physiological processes and methodological aspects related to biological measures is essential when studying the psychophysiological correlates of dyadic interaction in couples. A central issue is the choice of an appropriate stress measure of relevance for the particular disease being investigated. Other significant issues concern measurement techniques (e.g., noninvasive, invasive, blood, saliva, urine) and procedures (e.g., sampling rate, timing of samples, diurnal rhythms). For example, the secretion of cortisol, one of the most prominent stress hormones, shows a clear diurnal rhythm with a morning peak at about 30 minutes after awakening, a sharp decline during the day, and the lowest values at around midnight. Therefore, the time of cortisol sampling must be considered when interpreting cortisol responses to psychological stress (Kirschbaum & Hellhammer, 1994; Prüßner et al., 1997).

The following section provides a more detailed overview of the most commonly investigated endocrine, cardiovascular, and immune measures in psychophysiological stress research. Because of limitations of space and our intent to provide a basic understanding of psychobiological processes related to dyadic interaction for a broad audience, we excluded some other biological indicators of psychological stress (e.g., muscle tension, skin conductance, or gastrointestinal peptides). For each biological measure described, there exist a number of sources that provide a comprehensive review of basic physiological functions, measurement procedures, and the rationale for their use. The interested reader may seek further details in the given literature.

Neuroendocrine Measures of Stress

Psychosocial stress is associated with a cascade of neuroendocrine changes. Activation of the HPA axis, with a subsequent release of cortisol, the primary glucocorticoid for humans, and the release of catecholamines (epinephrine and norepinephrine) from the adrenal medullas and sympathetic neurons during sympathetic nervous system (SNS) activity are of considerable importance in the neuroendocrine stress response. We focus on these neuroendocrine factors because catecholamines and glucocorticoids are the most common endocrine measures in stress research and are thought to play a significant role in the development of disease under chronic stress conditions (Cohen, Kessler, & Gordon, 1995).

Other neuroendocrine factors that are associated with stress include prolactin, growth hormone, insulin, thyroid hormones, gonadal hormones, endogenous opioid peptides (e.g., beta-endorphin), and serotonin. The meaning of changes of these measures during stress is only partially understood. For example, increases of prolactin and growth hormone during stress seem to enhance immune function (Kelley & Dantzer, 1991).

Neuroendocrine Function

The SAM and HPA systems are the primary mechanisms that maintain homeostasis during stress. Both catecholamines and glucocorticoids have a wide range of metabolic effects that are part of the initiation and regulation of the stress response and help mobilize the body's energy resources. For example, during stress, the release of catecholamines increases the availability of glucose and affects heart rate and cardiac contractility, which increase blood pressure and blood flow to skeletal muscles. Moreover, catecholamines can mediate immune function (see e.g., Ader, Felten, & Cohen, 1991; Baum & Grunberg, 1995).

The secretion of glucocorticoids is controlled by a complex feedback mechanism at different levels of the HPA axis and shows a clear diurnal rhythm (Kaplan, 1992). Glucocorticoid functions include metabolic (e.g., increased gluconeogenesis), circulatory, and SNS effects. Almost every cell in the body contains glucocorticoid receptors and can be affected by these hormones. Thus, glucocorticoids hold an exceptional position within the endocrine stress response system. One of the most important functions of glucocorticoids is the regulation of immune function. Glucocorticoids have anti-inflammatory effects and can suppress immune function through the inhibition of the production and release of cytokines (Munck & Guyre, 1991; Munck, Guyre, & Holbrook, 1984).

Measurement of Neuroendocrine Activity

Levels of catecholamines can be estimated by assaying blood samples or measuring free epinephrine and norepinephrine or metabolites of epinephrine and norepinephrine in the urine. Blood samples are more appropriate in measuring short-term changes in catecholamine levels during acute stress, whereas urine samples provide more information about SNS activity over a period of hours (Baum & Grunberg, 1995). Thus, urine samples are typically used in studies on chronic stress (e.g., 24-hour urine samples). There are two biochemical techniques available to assay catecholamines: radioenzymatic assay and high-performance liquid chromatography. Both techniques require trained technicians and equipment, which can be cost intensive and may confront a social scientist with logistic constraints. With regard to sampling and assay procedures, a number of important issues should be considered when using blood or urine samples to determine neuroendocrine activity (e.g., sample collection, processing, storage; for reviews, see Baum & Grunberg, 1995; Grunberg & Singer, 1990). Levels of cortisol can be estimated by assaying a blood, urine, or saliva sample. The use of blood and urine samples is a more common but even a more expensive and reactive method of measuring HPA function than the use of saliva samples. For example, venipuncture itself is a significant stimulus for cortisol secretion from the adrenal glands.

The development of new techniques to measure cortisol in saliva (e.g., radioimmunoassay) has provided scientists with the opportunity to examine HPA function and stress reactivity in a more natural setting. The use of salivary cortisol measurement has been established as a reliable method in stress research (for reviews, see Kirschbaum & Hellhammer, 1989, 1994). One important advantage of salivary cortisol measurement is that samples of saliva can be easily obtained with a special cotton swab in a small plastic tube by the participants themselves, e.g. Salivette (Sarstedt, Rommelsdorf, Germany). Thus, salivary cortisol levels can be estimated continuously (e.g., per 2-hour interval) in participants' day-to-day life, to provide information about associations between chronic stress levels and diurnal cortisol profiles (e.g., Ockenfels et al., 1995). With regard to cortisol reactivity, the HPA axis is not as rapidly responsive as is the SNS. Salivary cortisol increases about 20 to 30 minutes after stress exposure (Kirschbaum & Hellhammer, 1994) and therefore is most appropriate for measuring stress responses hypothesized to occur within this time frame.

Both catecholamines and glucocorticoids have been repeatedly shown to increase during acute psychological stress. Since the early work of Hans Selye on hormonal responses of the HPA axis (e.g., Selye, 1974) and Walter Cannon's studies on SAM activation during emergency situations (fight-or-flight response; Cannon, 1932), a growing number of studies have been published on hormonal stress responses to acute stress exposure. Social, cognitive, and genetic factors influence the endocrine stress reactivity (Hellhammer & Wade, 1993). Gender may be another important factor that accounts for differences in neuroendocrine stress responses (e.g., Kirschbaum et al., 1992). Chronic exposure to stressors results overall in significant changes in neuroendocrine reactivity (Sapolsky, Krey, & McEwen, 1986). For example, higher diurnal cortisol levels and a dampened cortisol response could be observed in animals exposed to chronic social stress (Sapolsky, 1989). Moreover, recently dampened HPA axis function (hypocortisolism) has been observed in humans under conditions of chronic stress exposure and in patients with posttraumatic stress disorder (e.g., Demitrack, 1993; Yehuda, Giller, & Mason, 1993). According to Hellhammer and Wade (1993), disturbed HPA axis function can be a significant mediator of stress vulnerability.

Cardiovascular Measures of Stress

The measurement of cardiovascular stress reactivity has become a major variable in recent psychophysiological stress research. The most widely used indicators of the activation of the cardiovascular system are blood pressure (BP) and heart rate (HR). We limit our discussion to these measures because BP and HR increases to acute stressors are considered important indicators of cardiovascular reactivity in the research regarding coronary heart disease (CHD) and essential hypertension. A detailed summary of the fundamental aspects of the physiology and function of the cardiovascular system can be found in Papillo and Shapiro (1990) or Krantz and Falconer (1995).

Cardiovascular Function and Measurement of Cardiovascular Reactivity

Briefly, the cardiovascular system consists of the heart and blood vessels. In the circulatory system, blood flows through various body tissues to transfer oxygen and other nutrients from the blood to the tissues (Papillo & Shapiro, 1990). During situations with different psychological or behavioral demands, BP and HR levels can rise rapidly. For example, in our laboratory, we observed systolic BP (SBP) changes of more than 30 mmHg above baseline levels after a brief dyadic conflict discussion in some participants.

However, BP and HR responses vary to a great extent among individuals and situations with different psychological or behavioral demands. BP and HR alterations are controlled by a complex feedback system. Both sympathetic and parasympathetic influences can be observed at different sites of the cardiovascular system (Papillo & Shapiro, 1990).

Due to the development of commercially available and user-friendly instruments for the noninvasive measurement of BP and HR, cardiovascular stress responses can be obtained in natural settings. Most of the studies published on cardiovascular responses to psychological stressors have used the auscultatory method of BP determination (typically, BP measured in the upper arm by means of a pressure cuff). HR can be easily measured through electrocardiography or by using automatic techniques that directly palpate the pulse.

Note that despite the availability of reliable noninvasive instruments for BP and HR measurement, some significant issues regarding measurement procedures must be considered when a scientist wants to obtain BP or HR responses (Frohlich et al., 1988; Papillo & Shapiro, 1990). These include acute factors affecting BP and HR such as medications, recent food or fluid intake, and smoking. Guidelines for the experimental study of BP have been summarized in an article by Shapiro et al. (1996).

Cardiovascular Reactivity and Health

The difference between the BP or HR measured after stressor exposure and a baseline measurement usually serves as a measure of reactivity (for problems involved in baseline measurements, see, e.g., Shapiro et al., 1996). An issue in cardiovascular stress research is the considerable heterogeneity of the used stressors (e.g., cold pressor test, reaction time tasks, mental arithmetic), measurement techniques (e.g., invasive vs. noninvasive), and measurement methods (continuous vs. intermittent). An unequivocal interpretation of the vast number of studies published in this field seems hardly possible, and so far, many important questions regarding the relation between cardiovascular reactivity and the development of cardiovascular disease remain unanswered. Support for an association between increased cardiovascular reactivity and CHD or essential hypertension has been derived mostly from animal studies, retrospective case studies, and high-risk-group analyses, but there are few prospective studies (for a review, see Manuck & Krantz, 1986). According to different models developed on the basis of the results of these studies, individuals are at a long-term risk of developing CHD or hypertension when they show stronger, more frequent, or prolonged reactions of the cardiovascular system to acute stressors (Clarkson, Manuck, & Kaplan, 1986; Obrist, 1981).

In addition to traditional cardiovascular risk factors (e.g., salt consumption and smoking), anger, coping with anger, hostility, and the type A behavior pattern are important psychological risk factors for the development of cardiovascular diseases (Cohen et al., 1995). Positive correlations between frequent or intense anger expression and increased cardiovascular reactivity to different stressors have been repeatedly postulated. In a recent meta-analysis, Myrtek (1998) concluded that the correlations reported in the literature are only modest. A similar lack of large effect sizes has been found for the correlation of cardiovascular reactivity with type A behavior or with hostility. Of the different cardiovascular measures examined, SBP was the most likely to yield effects consistent with the postulated relationship (Myrtek, 1998).

The social support a person receives in a stressful situation is considered to be another modifier of acute cardiovascular reactivity. Uchino, Cacioppo, and Kiecolt-Glaser (1996) analyzed 15 experimental studies published between 1974 and 1995. They concluded that especially in the studies that experimentally manipulated social support, the presence of an emotionally supportive other was associated with reduced BP and HR responses.

Gender differences in cardiovascular reactivity have been discussed as the possible cause for the considerably higher prevalence of cardiovascular diseases among men. In the majority of studies published on this issue, men were found to show larger BP and HR responses to experimentally induced stress than women (for a comprehensive overview, see Stoney, Davis, & Matthews, 1987). Yet, in some cases, stronger cardiovascular stress responses in women or no gender differences were found (Myrtek, Hilgenberg, Brügner, & Müller, 1997). These results raise the question of whether gender differences in cardiovascular reactivity actually reflect habitual differences. Results reported by Lash, Gillespie, Eisler, and Southard (1991) suggest that the sex-specific relevance of the stressor or involvement can play an important part in determining cardiovascular response. They found that men showed larger BP and HR responses to the cold pressor test than women only under "masculine" achievement-oriented instruction conditions.

Immunological Measures of Stress

Since the early 1980s, considerable attention has been paid to psychosocial or behavioral modulation of the immune function. There is growing evidence that stressful life events and chronic stress are associated with longer term down regulation of immune function (Kiecolt-Glaser & Glaser, 1991, 1995). Thus, people who are exposed to chronic stress may be at greater long-term risk for health problems (Kiecolt-Glaser & Glaser, 1995).

This section addresses some important issues regarding immunological function and measurement to provide a basic understanding of psychoneuroimmunological correlates of social stress. More comprehensive reviews of psychoneuroimmunology can be found in several sources (e.g., Ader et al., 1991; Kiecolt-Glaser & Glaser, 1995).

Immunological Function

The central function of the immune system is to protect the body from infections. Organs of the immune system are the thymus, bone marrow, lymph nodes, spleen, tonsils, appendix, and Peyer's patches (immune tissue located in the small intestine). Immune responses are triggered by invading substances (antigens), which are identified by the immune system as "nonself" (e.g., viruses, bacteria). Two defense systems can be distinguished: the humoral immune system and the cellular immune system. Both include specific and nonspecific immune responses.

Humoral mediated immune responses involve the release of immunoglobulins by B lymphocytes into the circulatory system. Immunoglobulins are specific antibodies that react with antigens and are involved in the defense against bacteria and viruses. Cellular-mediated immune responses comprise T lymphocytes and natural killer (NK) cells. T lymphocytes are important for the defense against fungi, viruses, and multicellular parasites. In contrast to T lymphocytes, NK cell activity is nonspecific. NK cells play an important role in protecting the body against cancer and virus-infected cells. Different parts of the immune system communicate through lymphokines (also called *cytokines*), which are synthesized by lymphocytes. Several studies indicate that immune function can be mediated by hormones and through direct SNS input (Baum & Grunberg, 1995). For example, glucocorticoids are known to suppress immune function (Ader et al., 1991). With regard to SNS–immune system interactions, stress-induced secretion of catecholamines can also affect immune responses (Kiecolt-Glaser & Glaser, 1995).

Blood samples must be drawn to assess immune function. There are a number of significant logistic issues involved in the measurement of immune responses (e.g., sample procedures, storage, control for intervening variables) beyond the scope of this chapter. For further information, see the comprehensive review by Kiecolt-Glaser and Glaser (1995) on the measurement of immune responses.

There are two principal ways to measure immune function: enumerative assays and functional assays. Enumerative assays involve simple counts of the number of lymphocyte subpopulations. Although enumerative assays provide information about the number of different kinds of immune cells in peripheral blood, they do not necessarily give information about immune capacity. Functional assays are more strongly and reliably related to psychological stressors than are enumerative assays (Kiecolt-Glaser & Glaser, 1995). In most of the studies on stress and immunity in humans, lymphocyte proliferation response and NK cell cytotoxic activity are the primary functional assays (Herbert & Cohen, 1993). Other common assays are latent herpes virus antibody titers (e.g., Epstein–Barr virus).

Chronic Stress and Immune Changes

Psychoneuroendocrinological studies have shown repeatedly that immunological alteration follows naturally occurring stressful social situations (for a review, see, e.g., Herbert & Cohen, 1993). For example, lower immune function has been observed in medical students who feel isolated (Kiecolt-Glaser, Garner, & Speicher, 1984). Moreover, divorce or bereavement seems to be closely related to immunological down regulation in men and women (Kiecolt-Glaser et al., 1987, 1988; Schleifer, Keller, Camerino, Thornton, & Stein, 1983). Immunological impairment has been associated with chronic relationship stress: Kiecolt-Glaser, Dura, Speicher, Trask, and Glaser (1991) assessed immunity in 69 spousal caregivers of patients with dementia. Participants provided care for an average of 5 years. Changes in immune function over a 13-month period suggested that more distressed caregivers had a greater decline in immunocompetence from pre- to posttest and a higher rate of infectious illnesses. Overall, these results suggest that individuals undergoing chronic stress may show significant decrements in immunocompetence and may have an elevated risk for health problems.

EMPIRICAL FINDINGS

In contrast to the growing literature on psychophysiological stress research, relatively few studies have investigated autonomic, endocrine, and immune responses of couples to disagreements. We expect that distressed partners and couples who engage in conflictual discussions would show greater physiological responsiveness than nondistressed couples. In this section, we provide empirical evidence that there is indeed a close relationship among interaction behavior, relationship quality, and psychophysiological reactivity. Table 1.1 summarizes studies on dyadic interaction behavior and psychophysiological reactivity in couples. Concerning the main empirical emphasis, these studies can be placed into three categories: (a) acute psychophysiological reactivity during dyadic interaction, (b) effects of communication skills training on psychophysiological reactivity during interpersonal conflict, and (c) psychophysiological predictors of decline in relationship quality. In this section, some examples of studies on the effect of a dyadic conflict task on psychophysiological reactivity are elaborated to provide practical information on the typical experimental procedures used in psychophysiological relationship research.

TABLE 1.1

Studies of the Psychophysiology of Spousal Interaction

Authors	Sample	Task	Design; statistical analyses	Measures	Relevant findings, comments
Psychophysiological reactivity to spousal conflict interactions					
Brown and Smith (1992)	45 married couples (age range 20–40), average level of marital quality (MAT)	Preparation (4 min), structured interaction (8 min), free interaction (4 min), topic was assigned to couples	Cross-sectional, experimental manipulation of interaction style; comparison of D vs. I	Physiology: SBP, DBP, HR Behavior: SASB Subjective stress: anger, anxiety	SBP: I husbands +13.1 mmHg, I wives +7.0 mmHg, D husbands +6.4 mmHg, wives +5.3 mmHg; husbands had stronger SBP responses in I; no information on BP or HR
Ewart, Taylor, Kraemer, and Agras (1991)	24 women and 19 men with essential hypertension (age range 32–73) and their spouses; 75% of the participants happily married (MAS greater than 100)	Discussion of neutral topic (10 min) plus controversial topic currently relevant to couple (10 min)	Cross-sectional, correlations, multiple regressions; comparison of conflict discussion vs. neutral conversation (= baseline)	Physiology: SBP, DBP Behavior: MICS Marital satisfaction: MAS	SBP (conflict minus baseline): male patients +3.1 mmHg, female patients +7.8 mmHg, DBP (conflict minus baseline): male patients +2.8 mmHg, female patients +2.1 mmHg; women showed stronger SBP responses; SBP changes correlated with behavior and marital satisfaction only in women; no data reported for spouses

GROTH ET AL.

Study	Sample	Design/Procedure	Measures	Results
Fehm-Wolfsdorf, Groth, Kaiser, and Hahlweg (in press)	80 couples (age range 23–64), average duration of partnership 11.5 years, 70% maritally distressed	Marital conflict discussion (15 min); selection of conflictual topic was based on a problem inventory	Cross-sectional; comparison of positive vs. negative vs. asymmetrical interaction behavior (grouped according to the trend analyses of the couple's KPI data)	Physiology: SBP, DBP, HR, endocrine parameters (cortisol) Marital satisfaction: partnership questionnaire, PFB Behavior: KPI	BP and HR: only modest changes in BP (less than 3 mmHg) and no changes in HR (no group differences); Endocrine data: more pronounced increases of cortisol in women after conflict discussion, cortisol nonresponse in negative-interacting women
Kiecolt-Glaser et al. (1993), Malarkey, Kiecolt-Glaser, Pearl, and Glaser (1994)	90 newlywed couples (age range 20–37), high marital satisfaction (MAT)	Discussion (30 min) of two to three couple-specific conflictual issues (RPI); mental stress (mental arithmetic)	Cross-sectional; comparison of high-negative and low-negative couples (interaction behavior, median split of MICS coding)	Physiology: SBP, DBP, HR, immune parameters (e.g., NK activity), endocrine parameters (e.g., epinephrine, norepinephrine, cortisol) Marital satisfaction: MAT Subjective stress	Larger SBP and DBP responses to conflict interaction in high-negative group (SBP +1.6 mmHg, DBP +4.87 mmHg); no group differences in responses to mental arithmetic; higher endocrine reactivity and immunological down regulation in the high-negative group; higher stress reactivity in women; no increases in cortisol levels after conflict discussion

(table continued)

TABLE 1.1 (continued)

Studies of the Psychophysiology of Spousal Interaction

Authors	Sample	Task	Design; statistical analyses	Measures	Relevant findings, comments
Kiecolt-Glaser et al. (1996)	62 newlywed couples (age range 20–37), high marital satisfaction (MAT); subsample of Kiecolt-Glaser et al. (1993)	Discussion (30 min) of two to three couple-specific conflictual issues (RPI); mental stress (mental arithmetic)	Correlations, multiple regressions; interrelations between behavior patterns (MICS coding) and hormone levels during hospital admission	Physiology: endocrine parameters (e.g., epinephrine, norepinephrine, ACTH, cortisol, prolactin, and GH) Behavior: MICS	Extent of negative conflict behavior (e.g., the demand–withdraw pattern) correlated with hormone levels in female participants
Lassner, Matthews, and Stoney (1994)	51 couples (mean age: men, 43; women, 41) and their sons	Two mental stress tasks, physical exertion, family interaction task (10-min conflict discussion between parents), ACQ	Correlations; interrelation between cardiovascular reactivity to social (family interaction) and nonsocial stress (mental stress, physical exertion)	Physiology: SBP, DBP, HR	Parental conflict interaction—women: SBP +8.5 mmHg, DBP +5.8 mmHg, HR +1.1 bpm; men: SBP +7.0 mmHg, DBP +2.8 mmHg, HR +6.2 bpm; correlations between reactions to social and nonsocial stressors only in women
Levenson and Gottman (1983)	30 married couples, no sociodemographic data reported	Discussion of neutral (15 min) plus controversial (15 min) topics; selection of conflictual topic based on problem inventory	Correlations, multiple regressions; interrelations between physiological reactivity–covariation and retrospective assessment of affective state obtained in a video-recall session 3 to 5 days after interaction session	Physiology: HR (interbeat interval; IBI), pulse transmission time to the finger (PTT) Marital satisfaction	Physiological covariation between spouses correlated significantly negatively with marital satisfaction; gender differences in stress reactions were not examined

Study	Sample	Design	Task	Measures	Results
Morrell and Apple (1990)	24 women (age range 40–60), and their husbands	Cross-sectional; comparison of high-negative vs. low-negative affect (median split using FAMISS-II coding)	Marital conflict discussion (10 min); selection of conflictual topic based on problem inventory	Physiology: SBP, HR; Behavior: affect expression (FAMISS–II); Marital satisfaction: MSI	Mean cardiovascular responses: SBP +7.32 mmHG, HR +6.58 bpm; greater SBP responses in high-negative than low-negative affect; no correlation between affect expression and marital satisfaction; no data of spouses reported
Notarius and Johnson (1982)	6 couples (mean age: men, 34.3; women, 31.7), high marital quality	Cross-sectional; assessment of gender differences in psychophysiological reactivity	Discussion of couple-specific conflict issue (30 min)	Physiology: skin resistance response; Behavior: CISS, assessment of affective state	Men tended to show higher physiological responses during conflict discussion ($.10 > p > .05$)

Effects of communication training

Study	Sample	Design	Task	Measures	Results
Ewart, Burnett, and Taylor (1983)	2 male patients with essential hypertension (age 44 and approximately 50), low marital quality	Longitudinal; Treatment weeks vs. control weeks (ABAB design), no control group	Problem-solving discussion of given topic (vignette, 10 min) and couple-specific conflict topic (10 min), ACQ	Physiology: SBP, DBP; Behavior: MICS	Smaller blood pressure increments during problem solving during treatment weeks than during control weeks; reduction of negative and increase of positive conflict behavior in treatment weeks; no data of wives reported

(table continued)

TABLE 1.1 (continued)

Studies of the Psychophysiology of Spousal Interaction

Authors	Sample	Task	Design; statistical analyses	Measures	Relevant findings, comments
Ewart, Taylor, Kraemer, and Agras (1984)	20 patients with essential hypertension (7 men, 13 women; age range 48–70); subsample from Ewart, Taylor, Kraemer, and Agras (1991)	Discussion of neutral (10 min) plus current conflictual topic (10 min discussion of a significant marital conflict); two laboratory sessions 9 weeks apart	Preintervention–postintervention comparison; treatment group ($n = 10$) vs. control group ($n = 10$)	Physiology: SBP, DBP Behavior: MICS Marital satisfaction: MAS	Treatment group: SBP–pre = 11.4 mmHg, SBP–post = 2.6 mmHg; DBP–pre = 4.0 mmHg, DBP–post = 1.0 mmHg; control group: SBP–pre = 10.0 mmHg, SBP–post = 7.6 mmHg; DBP–pre = 4.2 mmHg, DBP–post = 3.5 mmHg; reduction of the extent of negative behavior in the treatment group; no data of spouses reported

Predictors of decline in relationship quality

| Levenson and Gottman (1985) | 19 married couples, no sociodemographic data reported, subsample of Levenson and Gottman (1983) | Discussion of neutral (15 min) plus controversial (15 min) topics; selection of conflictual topic based on problem inventory | Prospective, correlations, multiple regressions; interrelation between physiological reactivity–covariation and marital satisfaction after 3 years | Physiology: HR (interbeat interval; IBI), pulse transmission time to the finger (PTT), skin conductance level (SCL) and general somatic activity Marital quality | Greater physiological reactivity to the problem discussion was associated with higher declines in marital satisfaction after 3 years |

| Gottman and Levenson (1992) | 73 married couples (mean age: men, 31.8; women, 29.0) | Discussion of neutral (15 min) plus controversial (15 min) topics; selection of conflictual topic based on problem inventory | Prospective, correlations, multiple regressions; interrelation between physiological reactivity–covariation during discussion and marital satisfaction 4 years later; comparison of couples with high vs. low risk for separation | Physiology: HR (interbeat interval; IBI), pulse transmission time to the finger (PTT), skin conductance level (SCL) and general somatic activity; Marital quality | Women from couples with high risk for separation showed on average higher HR and finger pulse amplitude during conflict discussion |

Note. Another study on the psychophysiological reactivity to acute marital conflicts (Levenson, Carstensen, & Gottman, 1994) was not included in this overview, because it does not address gender differences in the absolute extent of the physiological stress reaction or the interrelations between behavior and physiological parameters. Age is in years. ACQ = Areas of Change Questionnaire (Weiss, 1980); CISS = Couples Interaction Scoring System (Notarius & Markman, 1981); D = discussion; DBP = diastolic blood pressure; FAMISS–II = Family and Marital Interaction Scoring System (Margolin & Basco, 1983); GH = growth hormone; HR = heart rate; I = interaction; KPI = coding system for marital and family interaction (Hahlweg et al., 1984); MAS = Marital Adjustment Scale (Locke & Wallace, 1959); MAT = Marital Adjustment Test (Locke & Wallace, 1959); MICS = Marital Interaction Coding System (Weiss & Summers, 1983); MSI = Marital Satisfaction Inventory (Snyder, 1985); + = increase; RPI = Relationship Problem Inventory (Knox, 1971); SASB = Structural Analysis of Social Behavior (Benjamin, 1974); SBP = systolic blood pressure.

Acute Psychophysiological Reactivity During Dyadic Interaction

Cardiovascular parameters are the most commonly examined biological measures in dyadic interaction research. Ewart, Taylor, Kraemer, and Agras (1991) studied BP responses during a conflict task in a sample of 43 patients (24 women, 19 men) with essential hypertension. Patients and partners were instructed to discuss a significant relationship conflict for 10 minutes and try to resolve it. BP was measured at 1-minute intervals during neutral baseline discussions and during the conflict task. Reactivity scores were defined as the difference between the mean BP level during the conflict task and the mean BP level during the baseline. The conflict task produced significant increases in BP. However, SBP increases were greater in women (women: +7.8 mmHg, men: +3.1 mmHg). Moreover, Ewart et al. (1991) examined correlations between dyadic interaction behavior and BP changes during the conflict discussion. Audiotapes of the conflict discussions were analyzed using a marital interaction coding system (Hops, Wills, Patterson, & Weiss, 1972; modified version of the Martial Interaction Coding System; MICS; Weiss & Summers, 1983). Only in women were dyadic interaction behaviors (hostile, supportive) and relationship quality significantly associated with BP changes. Intraindividual comparisons of the episodes of the two highest and the two lowest BP readings during the conflict discussion revealed a significant increase in the frequency of hostile behaviors during episodes of high BP; in contrast, there was no effect of supportive or neutral behaviors on BP changes. BP increases after a dyadic conflict task were found in patients with chronic back pain and healthy participants (Brown & Smith, 1992; Flor, Breitenstein, Birbaumer, & Fürst, 1995; Kiecolt-Glaser et al., 1993; Lassner et al., 1994, Morell & Apple, 1990). In keeping with the results of Ewart et al. (1991), Morell and Apple (1990) reported an association among active negative affect, self-reported relationship happiness, and cardiovascular reactivity in women. However, in this study, men's BP was not measured.

Empirical evidence that acute dyadic conflict discussions also are associated with endocrine and immunological changes is supported by a series of studies by Kiecolt-Glaser et al. (1993, 1996) and Malarkey, Kiecolt-Glaser, Pearl, and Glaser (1994). Ninety healthy newlywed couples were selected on the basis of stringent exclusion criteria and were admitted to a hospital research unit for 24 hours. A conflict task that was performed in the morning after admission consisted of a 30-minute discussion about disagreements. All discussions were videotaped, and interaction behaviors were scored using the MICS (Weiss & Summers, 1983). To examine differences in endocrine and immunological parameters dependent on the relationship interaction quality, couples were divided into low-negative and high-negative groups using the couples' total negative behavior frequencies based on a median split of negative MICS behavior. Blood samples were collected at several time points before, during, and after the conflict task to provide information on short- and long-term endocrine changes and immunological changes over the 24-hour period. With regard to short-term effects of the conflict task on endocrine function, five of the six hormones assayed before, during, and 15 minutes after the conflict task changed significantly (Kiecolt-Glaser et al., 1996; Malarkey et al., 1994). High-negative individuals showed greater decreases of prolactin levels and greater and more persistent increases of epinephrine, norepinephrine, growth hormone, and adrenocorticotropic hormone during the conflict task when compared with low-negative partners. These differences were more pronounced in women. Moreover, only in women were conflict behavior and demand–withdraw interaction sequences significantly associated with long-term endocrine changes over 24 hours. Baseline levels of cortisol and norepinephrine were higher in women whose husbands were more likely to withdraw after the women's negative behavior during the conflict discussion. Negative interaction behavior also led to impressive immunological down regulation (Kiecolt-Glaser et al., 1993). High-negative individuals showed greater decrements in NK cell activity and higher antibody titers to latent Epstein–Barr virus on exit from their 24-hour admission when compared with immunological assays obtained on entry. Again, immunological decrements were more pronounced in women.

As Kiecolt-Glaser et al. (1996) pointed out, observed gender differences in endocrine and immunological responses are in accordance with the results of the aforementioned studies on cardiovascular reactivity during dyadic conflict discussions. Thus, women seem more physiologically affected than men by negative couple interactions. These empirical findings are in contrast to the escape-conditioning model proposed by Gottman and Levenson (1988), which suggests that men's avoidance and withdrawal from dyadic conflict may be attributed to greater physiological arousal. Gottman and Levenson (1988) have speculated that men's withdrawal is a protective mechanism. However, only one study with a small sample of six couples seems to support the escape-conditioning model (Notarius & Johnson, 1982). Note that the samples studied were highly selected (e.g., patients with hypertension or couples who are healthier than the average couple). Moreover, the couples investigated in the Kiecolt-Glaser et al. (1993, 1996) and Malarkey et al. (1994) study were in the early stage of their marriage and reported overall a very high relationship satisfaction. Therefore, even high-negative couples showed a small frequency of negative interaction behaviors during the dyadic interaction. Thus, the impact of negative interaction behavior on physiological responses in distressed couples may be underestimated (Kiecolt-Glaser et al., 1996).

Following this line of argument, we decided to study psychophysiological stress responses during a 15-minute conflict task in couples who were not newlyweds (Fehm-Wolfsdorf, Groth, Kaiser, & Hahlweg, in press). A total of 78 couples participated in this study. The average duration of the relationship was 11.5 years; 65 couples were married, and 13 couples were cohabitating. Concerning self-reported relationship quality (Partnership Questionnaire; Hahlweg, 1996), 70% of the couples were distressed. All couples participated in a 2-hour-long study. To provide information about cardiovascular and endocrine responses, BP, HR, and saliva samples for cortisol assays were obtained at five times before (50 minutes before, 20 minutes before, and immediately before) and after (immediately after and 30 minutes after) the 15-minute conflict task. All discussions were videotaped. The analysis of dyadic interaction behavior with a coding system for couple and family interaction comparable to the MICS (Kategoriensystem für partnerschaftliche Interaktion; Hahlweg et al., 1984) revealed three interaction groups. In 16 couples, both partners showed more positive (e.g., self-disclosure, acceptance) than negative interaction behavior. In 36 couples, both partners were highly negative; negative interaction behavior (e.g., criticism, negative solution) comprised more than 40% of all behaviors. The remaining 26 couples were assigned to an asymmetrical group. In this group, one partner displayed predominantly positive behavior whereas the other partner displayed predominantly negative behavior during the conflict discussion.

Overall BP and HR changes during the evening sessions were moderate. There were no gender or group effects on cardiovascular responses to the conflict discussion, which may have been due to the use of simple change scores. Therefore, it seems to be more appropriate to measure BP and HR continuously before, during, and after the conflict discussion (e.g., Ewart et al., 1991). With regard to cortisol responses after the dyadic conflict discussion, we found a significant increase of salivary cortisol levels in women 30 minutes after the conflict task compared with a decrease in cortisol levels in men during the evening session (see Figure 1.2). Moreover, only in women were cortisol responses related to the dyadic interaction behavior. Women in the positive and the asymmetrical groups showed a significant increase in cortisol levels, whereas for women in the negative group, cortisol levels decreased after the discussion (see Figure 1.3). Note that the couples in the negative group rated the conflict discussions just as stressful as did the couples in the other groups. Thus, the endocrine nonresponse may indicate dampened HPA axis function due to chronically abrasive relationships. In conclusion, these couples may be at greater risk for health problems. However, further clarification is needed about the endocrine nonresponse among these couples characterized by extremely negative interactions. Cortisol responses in women interacting positively with their partners were unexpected but can be explained with the relatively high frequency of negative behaviors in these couples. Our couples' frequency of negative behavior seemed comparable to the negative group in the Kiecolt-Glaser et al. (1993, 1996; Malarkey et al., 1994) study. To summarize, this study provides additional empirical evidence that relationship distress can have deleterious consequence for women's health status over the short term; longer term effects require further investigation.

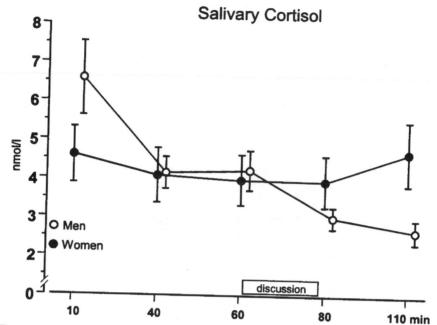

Figure 1.2. Gender differences in salivary cortisol response after a 15-minute conflict discussion.

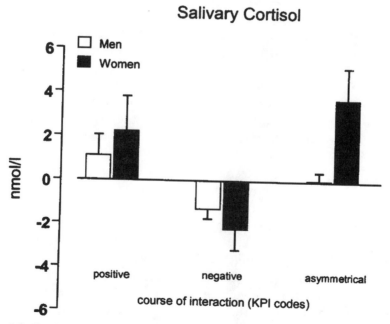

Figure 1.3. Cortisol responses (changes from baseline) after a 15-minute conflict. KPI = coding system for marital and family interaction.

Effects of Communication Training on Psychophysiological Reactivity During Interpersonal Conflict

The first empirical evidence that communication training is effective in reducing cardiovascular responses during a relationship problem discussion was based on two case studies reported by Ewart, Burnett, and Taylor (1983). In this study the effects of communication training on BP and HR were analyzed using an ABAB experimental design. During a treatment phase of 2 weeks, two male patients with hypertension and their female partners were exposed to the communication skills training. Conflict discussions were conducted several times a week and were analyzed with a modified version of the MICS (Hops et al., 1972). BP and HR were recorded continuously during the experimental sessions. In both participants, the relative frequency of negative interaction behavior was lower during the treatment phases (Weeks 2 and 4) than during the baseline phases (Weeks 1 and 3). Overall, BP increases during the conflict discussions were positively related to the frequency of negative interaction behaviors. Thus, communication training seems to affect cardiovascular stress responses during a couple's argument. However, no relationship was found between communication patterns and HR responses.

In a second study, Ewart, Taylor, Kraemer, and Agras (1984) analyzed the effect of a nine-session communication skills training intervention on cardiovascular stress responses during a dyadic conflict task using a preintervention–postintervention control group design. Twenty patients with hypertension and their partners (a subsample of the aforementioned Ewart et al., 1991, study) were assigned randomly to the intervention group (3 men, 7 women) or to an assessment-only control group (4 men, 6 women). Again, 10-minute conflict discussions were audiotaped pre- and postintervention and analyzed using the MICS (Hops et al., 1972). For each experimental session, BP reactivity scores were computed. Preintervention–postintervention comparisons revealed a significant decrease in the frequency of hostile behavior and reduced systolic reactivity in the training group at posttest (preintervention = 11.4 mmHg; postintervention = 2.6 mmHg). In contrast to these results, the control group displayed a smaller but noteworthy reduction in systolic reactivity (preintervention = 10.6 mmHg; postintervention = 7.2 mmHg), although the relative frequency of hostile behavior increased from pre- to posttest. In both groups, there were no significant changes in the frequency of positive remarks. Thus, the total frequency of negative communication behavior during a conflict discussion seems to be a significant predictor of cardiovascular stress reactivity. With regard to the unexpected decrease of systolic reactivity in the control group at posttest, more information is needed about the course of the couples' conflict discussions, to understand the appearance of a psychophysiological stress response during a distressing dyadic interaction. Results of the studies of Fehm-Wolfsdorf et al. (in press) and Kiecolt-Glaser et al. (1996) suggest that a specific interaction style (e.g., asymmetrical or demand–withdraw pattern) can account for differences in psychophysiological reactivity, independent of the couple's total amount of negative interaction behaviors.

Psychophysiological Prediction of Decline in Relationship Quality

At least two studies have examined correlations between psychophysiological variables and long-term change in relationship quality (Gottman & Levenson, 1992; Levenson & Gottman, 1985). In these studies, physiological data were obtained during an experimental session that included a quiet baseline period, a 15-minute "events of the day" discussion, and a 20-minute relationship problem discussion. In the latter discussion, couples were instructed to identify a salient problem and try to resolve it. To provide information about a broad range of physiological changes, four physiological parameters were sampled: HR (interbeat interval), pulse transmission time to the finger, skin conductance level, and general somatic activity. The hypothesis that the partners' psychophysiological reactivity would predict declines in self-reported relationship satisfaction was confirmed both for men and women. In one study of 19 couples (Levenson & Gottman, 1985), men's HR during the 5-minute baseline period before the conflict task and men's HR during the conflict discussion were correlated with the change in the couple's relationship satisfaction over a 3-year period ($r = .92$). In women, a similar pattern was found for skin conductance (baseline: $r = -.58$, conflict discussion $r = -.76$). Given these results, increased arousal before and during a relationship problem discussion seems to predict a decline in the couple's relationship satisfaction. The results of a second study (Gottman & Levenson, 1992) suggested that correlations between physiological responses to a relationship problem discussion and the decline in a couple's relationship satisfaction may be more pronounced in women than in men: Women at high risk for subsequent relationship dissolution had faster HR and greater peripheral vasoconstriction during the conflict discussion than low-risk women. High- and low-risk men did not differ. However, the results must be interpreted carefully. A critical issue concerns the data reduction and analysis (for a critical comment, see Woody & Costanzo, 1990). Moreover, Gottman and Levenson (1992) reported no data on psychophysiological responses during the conflict task. Thus, a comparison with the aforementioned studies on psychophysiological reactivity during a relationship problem discussion is not possible.

CONCLUSIONS AND FUTURE DIRECTIONS

In this chapter, we have reviewed studies on the psychophysiology of dyadic interaction in intimate relationships. With regard to a heuristic model of the association between relationship factors and health outcomes, we expected that a relationship problem discussion would directly affect physiological responses in couples, which in the long-term would expose distressed couples to a greater risk for health problems. We have provided empirical evidence that prolonged or repeated activation of the SAM system and the HPA axis, as well as long-lasting immunological alterations, can have adverse consequences for physical and psychological health and well-being.

Although results are still preliminary, the stress responses in couples discussing a disagreement have strong endocrine, cardiovascular, and immunological impact. Empirical evidence suggests that the associations between dyadic behavior in couples and psychophysiological function may be an important factor in understanding why partners in distressed relationships are more susceptible to disease (Glenn & Weaver, 1981; Weissman, 1987). Note that we excluded some other important factors (e.g., social support, environmental distress, health-related behaviors) that also can have a strong impact on health. However, conflict discussions are frequent in distressed couples and can be regarded as a significant contributor to chronic stress in these couples. Different dyadic interaction behavior variables that have been studied in relation to psychophysiological changes tend to have effects in the same direction. Overall negativity as well as specific destructive interaction patterns (demand–withdraw or asymmetrical interaction pattern) are associated with stronger hormonal and cardiovascular reactivity and immunological down regulation. Moreover, the magnitude of physiological stress responses depends mainly on the frequency of negative behaviors (e.g., criticizing or blocking), whereas positive behaviors and physiological stress responses after a dyadic conflict task seem to be uncorrelated with physiological stress measures.

Gender is another important modifier of stress responses in couples. Differences between men and women in psychophysiological responses after a relationship problem discussion were examined in most of the studies reviewed above. With one exception, associations between psychophysiological stress responses and relationship variables (conflict behavior, relationship satisfaction) were more pronounced in women than in men. Thus, women appear to differ from men in their stress-related psychophysiological activity in terms of the type of the social stressor. Women seem to be more engaged during conflict discussions than their partner. Moreover, there is empirical evidence that women are more emotionally sensitive to negative aspects of dyadic interaction and are better at decoding their partner's emotional messages than are men (Fehm-Wolfsdorf et al., in press; Noller & Fitzpatrick, 1988). In accordance with these results, intimate relationships appear to be more beneficial for men's health than for women's (Burman & Margolin, 1992; House et al., 1988). Given the observation that many couples live in stable but unhappy relationships (Markman & Hahlweg, 1993), one possible way to improve relationship quality and health may be to provide communication training to these couples (Kaiser, Hahlweg, Fehm-Wolfsdorf, & Groth, 1998). There is limited empirical evidence that a brief communication skills training intervention reduces BP responses in couples (Ewart et al., 1983, 1984). However, more research is needed to explore the effects of dyadic communication training on endocrine, immunological, and cardiovascular measures.

To understand better the impact of stressors on health-related processes, the study of more naturalistic stressors in psychophysiological stress research is needed (e.g., Lassner et al., 1994). The use of laboratory analogues of dyadic conflict allows the examination of stressful interaction patterns and psychophysiological stress responses in couples in a more natural setting. It can be argued that couples are constrained to discuss an unpleasant topic and therefore suppress socially undesirable behaviors (e.g., aggression). However, although there are some limitations due to the experimental procedure (e.g., laboratory setting, physiological measurement), laboratory analogue techniques have been shown to be valid. For example, couples participating in the Fehm-Wolfsdorf et al. (in press) study reported a high correspondence between their interaction behavior in the laboratory and in their day-to-day life. However, a single laboratory session provides no information about the stability of psychophysiological response patterns. In a recent review, Karney and Bradbury (1995) reported a lack of longitudinal studies on relationships and marriage that included psychophysiological measures. Thus, perhaps the most important conclusion is that there is a strong need for longitudinal research on psychophysiological stress responses in couples to track the development of health problems in psychophysiologically reactive people.

REFERENCES

Ader, R., Felten, D. L., & Cohen, N. (Eds.). (1991). *Psychoneuroimmunology* (2nd ed.). San Diego, CA: Academic Press.

Baum, A., & Grunberg, N. E. (1995). Measurement of stress hormones. In S. Cohen, R. C. Kessler, & L. U. Gordon (Eds.), *Measuring stress: A guide for health and social scientists* (pp. 175–192). New York: Oxford University Press.

Benjamin, L. S. (1974). Structural analysis of social behavior. *Psychological Review, 81*, 392–425.

Bolger, N., DeLongis, A., Kessler, R. C., & Schilling, E. A. (1989). Effects of daily stress on negative mood. *Journal of Personality and Social Psychology, 6*, 111–129.

Brown, P. C., & Smith, T. W. (1992). Social influence, marriage, and the heart: Cardiovascular consequences of interpersonal control in husbands and wives. *Health Psychology, 11*, 88–96.

Burman, B., & Margolin, G. (1992). Analysis of the association between marital relationships and health problems: An international perspective. *Psychological Bulletin, 112*, 39–63.

Cannon, W. B. (1932). *The wisdom of the body.* New York: Norton.

Christensen, A. (1987). Assessment of behavior. In K. D. O'Leary (Ed.), *Assessment of marital discord* (pp. 13–57). Hillsdale, NJ: Erlbaum.

Clarkson, T. B., Manuck, S. B., & Kaplan, J. R. (1986). Potential role of cardiovascular reactivity in atherogenesis. In K. A. Matthews, S. M. Weiss, T. Detre, T. M. Dembroski, B. Falkner, S. B. Manuck, & R. B. Williams, Jr. (Eds.), *Handbook of stress, reactivity, and cardiovascular disease* (pp. 35–47). New York: Wiley.

Cohen, S., Kessler, R. C., & Gordon, L. U. (Eds.). (1995). *Measuring stress: A guide for health and social scientists.* New York: Oxford University Press.

Coyne, J. C., & DeLongis, A. (1986). The role of social relationship in adaptation. *Journal of Consulting and Clinical Psychology, 54,* 454–460.

Demitrack, M. A. (1993). Neuroendocrine research strategies in chronic fatigue syndrome. In P. J. Goodnick & N. G. Klimas (Eds.), *Chronic fatigue and related immune deficiency syndromes.* Progress in Psychiatry, No. 40 (pp. 45–66). Washington, DC: American Psychiatric Press.

Ewart, C. K., Burnett, K. F., & Taylor, C. B. (1983). Communication behaviors that affect blood pressure. *Behavior Modification, 7,* 331–344.

Ewart, C. K., Taylor, C. B., Kraemer, H. C., & Agras, W. S. (1984). Reducing blood pressure reactivity during interpersonal conflict: Effects of marital communication training. *Behavior Therapy, 15,* 473–484.

Ewart, C. K., Taylor, C. B., Kraemer, H. C., & Agras, W. S. (1991). High blood pressure and marital discord: Not being nasty matters more than being nice. *Health Psychology, 10,* 155–163.

Fehm-Wolfsdorf, G., Groth, T., Kaiser, A., & Hahlweg, K. (in press). Cortisol responses to marital conflict depend on marital interaction quality. *International Journal of Behavioral Medicine.*

Flor, H., Breitenstein, C., Birbaumer, N., & Fürst, M. (1995). A psychophysiological analysis of spouse solicitousness towards pain behaviors, spouse interaction and pain perception. *Behavior Therapy, 26,* 255–272.

Frohlich, E. D., Grim, C., Labarthe, D. R., Maxwell, M. H., Perloff, D., & Weidmann, W. H. (1988). Recommendations for human blood pressure determination by sphygmomanometers: Report of special task force appointed by the steering committee, American Heart Association. *Hypertension, 11,* 210A–222A.

Glenn, N. D., & Weaver, C. N. (1981). The contribution of marital happiness to global happiness. *Journal of Marriage and the Family, 43,* 161–168.

Gottman, J. M., & Levenson, R. W. (1988). The social psychophysiology of marriage. In P. Noller & M. A. Fitzpatrick (Eds.), *Perspectives on marital interaction* (pp. 182–200). Clevedon, England: Multilingual Matters.

Gottman, J. M., & Levenson, R. W. (1992). Marital processes predictive of later dissolution: Behavior, physiology, and health. *Journal of Personality and Social Psychology, 63,* 221–233.

Grunberg, N. E., & Singer, J. E. (1990). Biochemical measurement. In J. T. Cacioppo & L. G. Tassinary (Eds.), *Principles of psychophysiology: Physical, social and inferential elements* (pp. 149–176). New York: Cambridge University Press.

Hahlweg, K. (1996). *Partnership questionnaire.* Göttingen, Germany: Hogrefe.

Hahlweg, K., Reisner, L., Kohli, G., Vollmer, M., Schindler, L., & Revensdorf, D. (1984). Development and validity of a new system to analyze interpersonal communication (KPI). In K. Hahlweg & N. Jacobson (Eds.), *Marital interaction: Analysis and modification* (pp. 182–198). New York: Guilford Press.

Hellhammer, D., & Wade, S. (1993). Endocrine correlates of stress vulnerability. *Psychotherapy and Psychosomatics, 60,* 8–17.

Herbert, T. B., & Cohen, S. (1993). Stress and immunity in humans: A meta-analytic review. *Psychosomatic Medicine, 55,* 364–379.

Hops, H., Wills, T. A., Patterson, G. R., & Weiss, R. L. (1972). *Marital interaction coding system.* Unpublished manuscript, University of Oregon, Eugene.

House, J. S., Landis, K. R., & Umberson, D. (1988). Social relationships and health. *Science, 24,* 540–545.

Kaiser, A., Hahlweg, K., Fehm-Wolfsdorf, G., & Groth, T. (1998). The efficacy of a compact psychoeducational group training program for married couples. *Journal of Consulting and Clinical Psychology, 5,* 753–760.

Kaplan, N. M. (1992). The adrenal glands. In J. E. Griffin & S. R. Ojeda (Eds.), *Textbook of endocrine physiology* (2nd ed., pp. 247–275). New York: Oxford University Press.

Karney, B. R., & Bradbury, T. N. (1995). The longitudinal course of marital quality and stability: A review of theory, methods, and research. *Psychological Bulletin, 118,* 3–24.

Kelley, K. W., & Dantzer, R. (1991). Growth hormone and prolactin as natural antagonists of glucocorticoids in immunoregulation. In N. Plotnikoff, A. Murgo, R. Faith, & J. Wybran (Eds.), *Stress and immunity* (pp. 433–453). Boca Raton, FL: CRC Press.

Kiecolt-Glaser, J. K., Dura, J. R., Speicher, C. E., Trask, O. J., & Glaser, R. (1991). Spousal caregivers of dementia victims: Longitudinal changes in immunity and health. *Psychosomatic Medicine, 53,* 345–362.

Kiecolt-Glaser, J. K., Fisher, L. D., Ogrocki, P., Stout, C. J., Speicher, C. E., & Glaser, R. (1987). Marital quality, marital disruption, and immune function. *Psychosomatic Medicine, 49,* 13–34.

Kiecolt-Glaser, J. K., Garner, W., & Speicher, C. E. (1984). Psychosocial modifiers in immunocompetence in medical students. *Psychosomatic Medicine, 46,* 7–14.

Kiecolt-Glaser, J. K., & Glaser, R. (1991). Stress and immune function in humans. In R. Ader, D. Felten, & N. Cohen (Eds.), *Psychoneuroimmunology* (pp. 849–867). San Diego, CA: Academic Press.

Kiecolt-Glaser, J. K., & Glaser, R. (1995). Measurement of immune response. In S. Cohen, R. C. Kessler, & L. U. Gordon (Eds.), *Measuring stress: A guide for health and social scientists* (pp. 213–229). New York: Oxford University Press.

Kiecolt-Glaser, J. K., Kennedy, S., Malkoff, S, Fisher, L., Speicher, C. E., & Glaser, R. (1988). Marital discord and immunity in males. *Psychosomatic Medicine, 50,* 213–229.

Kiecolt-Glaser, J. K., Malarkey, W. B., Cacioppo, J. T., & Glaser, R. (1994). Stressful personal relationships: Immune and endocrine function. In R. Glaser & J. K.

Kiecolt-Glaser (Eds.), *Handbook of stress and immunity* (pp. 321–339). San Diego, CA: Academic Press.

Kiecolt-Glaser, J. K., Malarkey, W. B., Chee, M., Newton, T., Cacioppo, J., Mao, H. Y., & Glaser, R. (1993). Negative behavior during marital conflict is associated with immunological down-regulation. *Psychosomatic Medicine, 55,* 395–409.

Kiecolt-Glaser, J. K., Newton, T., Cacioppo, J. T., MacCallum, R. C., Glaser, R., & Malarkey, W. B. (1996). Marital conflict and endocrine function: Are men really more physiologically affected than women? *Journal of Consulting and Clinical Psychology, 64,* 324–332.

Kirschbaum, C., & Hellhammer, D. H. (1989). Salivary cortisol in psychobiological research: An overview. *Neuropsychobiology, 3,* 150–169.

Kirschbaum, C., & Hellhammer, D. H. (1994). Salivary cortisol in psychoendocrine research: Recent developments and applications. *Psychoneuroendocrinology, 19,* 313–333.

Kirschbaum, C., Wüst, S., & Hellhammer, D. H. (1992). Consistent sex differences in cortisol to psychological stress. *Psychosomatic Medicine, 54,* 648–657.

Knox, D. (1971). *Marriage happiness.* Champaign, IL: Research Press.

Krantz, D. S., Contrada, R. J., Hill, R. O., & Friedler, E. (1988). Environmental stress and biobehavioral antecedents of coronary heart disease. *Journal of Consulting and Clinical Psychology, 56,* 333–341.

Krantz, D. S., & Falconer, J. J. (1995). Measurement of cardiovascular responses. In S. Cohen, R. C. Kessler, & L. U. Gordon (Eds.), *Measuring stress: A guide for health and social scientists* (pp. 193–212). New York: Oxford University Press.

Lash, S. J., Gillespie, B. L., Eisler, R. M., & Southard, D. R. (1991). Sex differences in cardiovascular reactivity: Effects of the gender relevance of the stressor. *Health Psychology, 10,* 392–398.

Lassner, J. B., Matthews, K. A., & Stoney, C. M. (1994). Are cardiovascular reactors to asocial stress also reactors to social stress? *Journal of Personality and Social Psychology, 66,* 69–77.

Levenson, R. W., Carstensen, L. L., & Gottman, J. M. (1994). Influence of age and gender on affect, physiology, and their interrelations: A study of long-term marriage. *Journal of Personality and Social Psychology, 67,* 56–68.

Levenson, R. W., & Gottman, J. M. (1983). Marital interaction: Physiological linkage and affective exchange. *Journal of Personality and Social Psychology, 45,* 587–597.

Levenson, R. W., & Gottman, J. M. (1985). Physiological and affective predictors of change in relationship satisfaction. *Journal of Personality and Social Psychology, 49,* 85–94.

Locke, H. J., & Wallace, K. M. (1959). Short-term marital adjustment and prediction tests: Their reliability and validity. *Journal of Marriage and Family Living, 21,* 251–255.

Malarkey, W. B., Kiecolt-Glaser, J. K., Pearl, D., & Glaser, R. (1994). Hostile behavior during marital conflict alters pituitary and adrenal hormones. *Psychosomatic Medicine, 56,* 41–51.

Manuck, S. B., & Krantz, D. S. (1986). Psychophysiological reactivity in coronary heart disease and essential hypertension. In K. A. Matthews, S. M. Weiss, T. Detre, T. M. Dembroski, B. Falkner, S. B. Manuck, & R. B. Williams, Jr. (Eds.), *Handbook of stress, reactivity and cardiovascular disease* (pp. 11–34). New York: Wiley.

Margolin, G., & Basco, M. (1983). *FAMISS–II: Interaction coding system.* Unpublished manuscript.

Markman, H. J., & Hahlweg, K. (1993). The prediction and prevention of marital distress: An international perspective. *Clinical Psychology Review, 13,* 29–43.

Morell, M. A., & Apple, R. F. (1990). Affect expression, marital satisfaction, and stress reactivity among premenopausal women during a conflictual marital discussion. *Psychology of Women Quarterly, 14,* 387–402.

Munck, A., & Guyre, P. M. (1991). Glucocorticoids and immune functions. In R. Ader, D. L. Felten, & N. Cohen (Eds.), *Psychoneuroimmunology* (2nd ed., pp. 456–474). San Diego, CA: Academic Press.

Munck, A., Guyre, P. M., & Holbrook, N. J. (1984). Physiological functions of glucocorticoids in stress and their relation to pharmacological action. *Endocrine Reviews, 5,* 25–44.

Myrtek, M. (1998). Metaanalysen zur psychophysiologischen Persönlichkeitsforschung [Meta-analyses on psychophysiological personality research]. In F. Rösler (Ed.), *Ergebnisse und Anwendungen der Psychophysiologie* (pp. 285–343). Göttingen, Germany: Hogrefe.

Myrtek, M., Hilgenberg, B., Brügner, G., & Müller, W. (1997). Influence of sex, college major, and chronic study stress on psychophysiological reactivity and behavior: Results of ambulatory monitoring in students. *Journal of Psychophysiology, 11,* 124–137.

Noller, P., & Fitzpatrick, M. A. (1988). Approaches to marital interaction. In: P. Noller & M. A. Fitzpatrick (Eds.), *Perspectives on marital interaction* (pp. 1–28). Clevedon, England: Multilingual Matters.

Notarius, C. I., & Johnson, J. S. (1982). Emotional expression in husbands and wives. *Journal of Marriage and the Family, 44,* 438–489.

Notarius, C. I., & Markman, H. J. (1981). The couples interaction scoring system. In E. E. Filsinger & R. A. Lewis (Eds.), *Observing marriage: New behavioral approaches.* Beverly Hills, CA: Sage.

Obrist, P. A. (1981). *Cardiovascular psychophysiology—A perspective.* New York: Plenum.

Ockenfels, M. C., Porter, L., Smyth, J., Kirschbaum, C., Hellhammer, D. H., & Stone, A. A. (1995). Effect of chronic stress associated with unemployment on salivary cortisol: Overall cortisol levels, diurnal rhythm, and acute stress reactivity. *Psychosomatic Medicine, 57,* 460–467.

Papillo, J. F., & Shapiro, D. (1990). In J. T. Cacioppo & L. G. Tassinary (Eds.), *Principles of psychophysiology: Physical, social and inferential elements* (pp. 456–512). New York: Cambridge University Press.

Prüßner, J. C., Wolf, O. T., von Auer, K., Jobst, S., Kaspers, F., Buske-Kirschbaum, A., Hellhammer, D. H., & Kirschbaum, C. (1997). *The cortisol response to awakening: Consistency, reliability, and individual differences.* Manuscript submitted for publication.

Sapolsky, R. M. (1989). Hypercortisolism among socially subordinate wild baboons originates at the CNS level. *Archives of General Psychiatry, 46*, 1047–1051.

Sapolsky, R. M., Krey, L. C., & McEwen, B. S. (1986). The neuroendocrinology of stress and aging: The glucocorticoid cascade hypothesis. *Endocrine Review, 7*, 284–301.

Schleifer, S. J, Keller, S. E., Camerino, M., Thornton, J. C., & Stein, M. (1983). Suppression of lymphocyte stimulation following bereavement. *Journal of the American Medical Association, 250*, 374–377.

Selye, H. (1974). *Stress without distress.* Philadelphia: Lippincott.

Shapiro, D., Jamner, L. D., Lane, J. D., Light, K. C., Myrtek, M., Sawada, Y., & Steptoe, A. (1996). Blood pressure publication guidelines. *Psychophysiology, 33*, 1–12.

Snyder, D. K. (1985). *Marital Satisfaction Inventory (MSI).* Los Angeles: Western Psychological Services.

Stoney, C. M., Davis, M. C., & Matthews, K. A. (1987). Sex differences in physiological responses to stress and in coronary heart disease: A causal link? *Psychophysiology, 24*, 127–131.

Uchino, B. N., Cacioppo, J. T., & Kiecolt-Glaser, J. K. (1996). The relationship between social support and physiological processes: A review with emphasis on underlying mechanisms and implications for health. *Psychological Bulletin, 119*, 488–531.

Van Doornen, L. J. P., & van Blokland, A. W. (1989). The relationship between cardiovascular and catecholamine reactions to laboratory and real-life stress. *Journal of Psychophysiology, 29*, 173–181.

Weiss, R. L. (1980). *The Area of Change Questionnaire.* Eugene: University of Oregon Marital Studies Program.

Weiss, R. L., & Heyman, R. E. (1990). Observation of marital interaction. In F. D. Fincham & T. N. Bradbury (Eds.), *The psychology of marriage* (pp 87–117). New York: Guilford Press.

Weiss, R. L., & Summers, K. (1983). The Marital Interaction Coding System III. In E. E. Filsinger (Ed.), *Marriage and family assessment* (pp. 85–115). Beverly Hills, CA: Sage.

Weissman, M. M. (1987). Advances in psychiatric epidemiology: Rates and risks for major depression. *American Journal of Public Health, 77*, 445–451.

Woody, E. Z., & Constanzo, P. R. (1990). Does marital agony precede marital ecstasy? A comment on Gottman and Krokoff's "Marital interaction and satisfaction: A longitudinal view." *Journal of Consulting and Clinical Psychology, 58*, 499–501.

Yehuda, R., Giller, E. L., & Mason, J. W. (1993). Psychoneuroendocrine assessment of posttraumatic stress disorder: Current progress and new directions. *Progress in Neuropsychopharmacology and Biological Psychiatry, 17*, 541–550.

2

CORONARY HEART DISEASE AND COUPLES

LYNN A. RANKIN-ESQUER, ALLISON DEETER, AND C. BARR TAYLOR

Coronary heart disease (CHD) is the leading cause of death and disability in the United States for both males and females (American Heart Association, 1995). There are approximately 14 million people currently living with CHD in this country, and nearly 1.5 million Americans have a heart attack (*myocardial infarction*; MI) each year (American Heart Association, 1987). After an MI, patients are commonly hospitalized for 3 to 10 days and may be in recovery for up to 6 weeks or longer (Ell & Dunkel-Schetter, 1994). In this chapter, we describe the physical expression of CHD, discuss nonmodifiable and modifiable risk factors, and focus on the role of couple functioning in both the development of CHD and the recovery from a cardiac event. In addition, we describe the effects of a cardiac event on the couple and family functioning. Finally, we address assessment and treatment of CHD as they relate to couple functioning, as well as discuss future directions in this field.

NATURE OF THE DISEASE

CHD is most often a manifestation of coronary artery atherosclerosis, which results in the development and continuous enlargement of atherosclerotic plaques (Cohen, Kaplan, & Manuck, 1994). The growth of these plaques narrows the arteries and eventually obstructs the normal flow of blood to the heart. MI occurs when the demand for oxygen in the heart muscle exceeds the supply. A decrease in the supply of oxygen occurs because of narrowing of the arteries, accentuated by blood clots or spasm in the coronary vessels. In clinical situations, CHD is most often expressed as angina pectoris (chest pain from insufficient coronary blood flow), acute MI (the death of the heart tissue due to interrupted coronary blood flow), cardiac arrhythmias (electrical instability), and sudden death (Sokolow & McIlroy, 1987).

RISK FACTORS IN THE DEVELOPMENT OF CHD

Both nonmodifiable and modifiable risk factors have been identified in the development of CHD, with the goal of preventing a cardiac event such as an MI or its recurrence. Although nonmodifiable factors, such as age or a family history of heart disease, can alert a person to the heightened possibility of developing CHD, there is little that can be done to directly alter these risk factors. However, behavioral and psychosocial risk factors can be modified to help avert an MI or to reduce the risk of subsequent cardiac events after an MI.

Behavior and Lifestyle

The major modifiable risk factors for CHD that have a behavioral component include cigarette smoking, high lipid serum levels (i.e., high blood cholesterol), a sedentary lifestyle, obesity, arterial hypertension, and chronic anger/hostility. Basic information on these risk factors is presented below; the relationship between these factors and couple variables is covered in detail in the next section.

Smoking

The evidence linking smoking with heart disease is substantial. In 14 studies involving over 3 million participants, smoking was consistently associated with disease. The U.S. surgeon general has estimated that about 30% of heart disease can be attributed to smoking. Overall, both male and female smokers have slightly more than twice the risk of dying from MI when compared with nonsmokers (Surgeon General, 1979). In addition, post-MI patients who continue to smoke have a significantly higher mortality rate than those who quit smoking. By some accounts (e.g., Wilhelmsson, Vedin, Elmfeldt, Tibblin, & Wilhelmsson, 1975), patients who continue to smoke after an MI experience twice the mortality compared with those who stop. Moreover, continued smoking after coronary angioplasty has been reported to be associated with increased restenosis (narrowing of arteries) rates (Galan, Deligonul, Kern, Chaitman, & Vandormael, 1988).

Serum Lipids

The Framingham risk factor trial (Kannel, Sorlie, Castelli, & McGee, 1980), which followed 2,336 men for over 20 years, demonstrated that elevated cholesterol levels were associated with significant increase in CHD risk. In recent decades, numerous studies have confirmed the overall association and have discovered that various types of serum lipoproteins (which constitute part of total cholesterol) differentially affect risk. The findings suggest that the low-density lipoproteins confer significant risk, whereas higher levels of another type of serum cholesterol, high-density lipoproteins, confer benefit.

Sedentary Living

Many studies have shown a strong inverse relationship between rates of CHD in a population and physical activity levels, whether measured as habitual occupational activity, leisure time physical activity, or physical fitness. Although this is still under debate, even moderate levels of physical activity appear to reduce CHD risk.

Hypertension

Elevated blood pressure is a significant predictor of heart disease and increases the risk of a subsequent heart attack after such an event. For instance, in the Framingham risk factor study, the men who remained hypertensive after a heart attack had a fivefold greater risk of mortality than did normotensive men (Kannel et al., 1980).

Psychosocial Variables

There is evidence that a number of psychosocial variables may increase the risk of the development of CHD as well as the risk of subsequent cardiac events after an MI. In addition, psychosocial variables such as social support are often interrelated with couple factors, as is discussed in a later section.

Type A Personality

Although the construct of type A behavior pattern has lost support in recent years, the hostility included in the pattern continues to be an active point of focus. For both males and females, hostility continues to be considered a significant risk factor for the development of CHD and a complicating factor in rehabilitation from a cardiac event (e.g., Barefoot, Dahlstrom, & Williams, 1983; Williams et al., 1980). Research has indicated that type A individuals often behave in a way that increases the frequency, duration, and intensity of stressors and seemingly affects cardiovascular reactivity (Rhodewalt & Smith, 1990).

Depression

There is growing evidence that negative emotions (e.g., sadness, hopelessness, anger, and anxiety) may represent risk factors for the development of CHD (e.g., Carney, Freedland, & Jaffe, 1990; Goldstein & Niaura, 1992). For example, a prospective analysis of 1,151 individuals initially free of heart trouble and assessed 15 years later provides direct evidence of depression as a risk factor for CHD (Pratt et al., 1996). Compared with respondents with no history of dysphoria, the odds ratio for MI associated with a history of dysphoria was 2.07 (95% confidence interval, 1.16 to 3.71), and the odds ratio associated with a history of major depressive episodes was 4.54 (95% confidence interval, 1.65 to 12.44), independent of coronary risk factors. These rates were not explained by the use of tricyclic antidepressant medications, which may increase the risk of sudden cardiac death.

The time after an MI also appears to be one of greater vulnerability to depression than that experienced by healthy individuals (e.g., Schleifer et al., 1989; Taylor, DeBusk, Davidson, Houston, & Burnett, 1981). This is particularly important given the research that suggests that depression at the time of or after a cardiac event has a major impact on mortality, morbidity, and functional recovery in patients (Carney et al., 1988; Garrity & Klein, 1975; Wells et al., 1989). Depressed patients have longer hospital stays after an MI than nondepressed patients and incur greater medical costs associated with CHD. For example, Wells et al. found that only 38% of patients with major depression had returned to work within 3 months of their MI, in contrast to 63% of the nondepressed patients.

In addition to depression, rates of anxiety in post-MI patients also are very high. During hospitalization for cardiac events, almost all patients experience significant levels of anxiety. Yet, even after the acute crisis resolves, significant levels of anxiety often remain. Furthermore, there is some evidence of an increased CHD mortality rate in anxious patients (Hayward, 1995).

Social Support

Social support has been found to relate significantly to a number of health benefits, including lower cardiovascular reactivity (Kamarck, Manuck, & Jennings, 1990), adjustment to and recovery from CHD-related events (e.g., heart surgery, MI; Mumford, Schlesinger, & Glass, 1982; Trelawny-Ross & Russell, 1987), and reduction in numerous causes of mortality including CHD (e.g., Berkman & Syme, 1979; Blazer, 1982; House, Robbins, & Metzner, 1982; Ruberman, Weinblatt, Goldberg, & Chaudhary, 1984). In fact, House, Landis, and Umberson (1988) determined that the magnitude of the risk for adverse health outcomes associated with lack of social support is comparable to that of the risk from smoking.

Many specific aspects of social support have been considered to help determine its role both in the development of CHD and in survival after a cardiac event. These include actual (observable) social support versus perceived support, instrumental versus expressive support, informational support (e.g., advice or guidance), quantity (e.g., total numbers of people available in support network), quality (e.g., emotional support), reciprocity (e.g., proportion of giving vs. receiving), who is named as closest confidant (e.g., partner vs. friend), and gender differences in the ways in which social support networks provide benefits. Despite the many operationalized definitions and some mixed findings, the social support literature shows impressive evidence of a relationship between lack of social support and increased mortality from CHD as well as other causes (e.g., Berkman & Syme, 1979; Blazer, 1982; House et al., 1982; Seeman et al., 1993).

ASSOCIATION OF ILLNESS AND COUPLE FACTORS

There are a number of ways that couple factors are related to the development and treatment of CHD. In this section, we consider more closely the relationship between couple factors and the development and treatment of CHD, as well as the mechanisms by which couple factors or couple status may be associated with CHD.

Separate from the general association between social support and health, a number of researchers have found evidence of a significant relationship between couple variables and the development of and recovery from CHD (Chandra, Szklo, Goldberg, & Tonascia, 1983; Orth-Gomer, Rosengren, & Wilhelmsen, 1993; Wiklund et al., 1988; Williams et al., 1992). For example, Orth-Gomer et al., in a prospective study of development of CHD, followed a random sample of 736 50-year-old men for 6 years. The researchers found that even when they controlled for other risk factors, attachment (emotional support from a very close person) and social integration (support from an extended network) were significant predictors of new CHD events. That is, in addition to emotional support from extended networks, emotional support from close others reduced incidence of new CHD events.

There is further evidence that couple status is significantly related to recovery from an MI. A number of studies indicate that married individuals show significantly fewer mortalities after an MI and that these favorable effects increase with time (Chandra et al., 1983; Wiklund et al., 1988; Williams et al., 1992). In addition, there is evidence that this positive effect of being married occurs for both men and women (Chandra et al., 1983). Case, Moss, Case, McDermott, and Eberly (1992) have suggested that rather than marital status, the crucial variable may be living alone. In their investigation of 1,234 mostly male post-MI patients, those who lived alone were at a significantly higher risk for future cardiac events. In addition, a comparison of only those patients from disrupted marriages indicated that those living alone compared with those who were living with someone other than their spouse were also at a higher risk of cardiac events and deaths.

Potential Couple Variables

Many have hypothesized that marriage or having an intimate partner serves a protective function against CHD (e.g., Fontana, Kerns, Rosenberg, & Colonese, 1989). There are a number of pathways through which marriage or having an intimate partner may affect the risk of CHD in both positive and negative directions.

Treatment-Seeking Behavior

Married or home-sharing individuals have been found to exhibit significantly lower medical utilization (for a variety of illnesses or symptoms) than nonmarried individuals (Morgan, 1980; Verbrugge, 1979). Some have suggested that spouses or partners may at times serve as a substitute for formal health care, and this interpretation helps explain the mixed findings when looking at the role of partners in treatment-seeking behavior as it applies to CHD symptoms. Chandra et al. (1983) have found that partners often help in the pursuit of treatment. In contrast, Hackett and Cassem (1969) have found that when a person is experiencing symptoms of a heart attack (e.g., chest pain), he or she is often less influenced to seek medical attention in response to a partner's urging than in response to friends' or colleagues' encouragement. Spouses themselves do not seem to know with any certainty how to react to CHD symptoms, vacillating between reassuring their partner and encouraging her or him to seek help (Skelton & Dominian, 1973). The role of partners in encouraging a partner to seek treatment is an important one, because most individuals who die from an MI do so through failure to seek treatment (e.g., Horwitz et al., 1990).

General Adherence to Treatment

Failure to adhere to treatment also has been found to increase risk of mortality (e.g., Horwitz et al., 1990), and there is evidence that being part of an intimate couple may affect adherence to treatment. Although one investigation failed to find a relationship between social or spousal support and adherence to treatment recommendations (Kulik & Mahler, 1993), several investigations provide evidence that marriage can increase adherence. Rankin-Esquer, Houston Miller, Myers, and Taylor (1997), in an investigation with 818 male and female post-MI patients, found a significantly greater tendency for nonmarried patients to drop out of a nurse-managed home-based multifactorial risk reduction program (MULTIFIT). Patients who were married may have had the encouragement or emotional support from an intimate other (e.g., spouse) to participate in the MULTIFIT program and thus were able to increase efforts toward improving health after a cardiac event. Overall, being married significantly increased the chances that a patient would participate in and complete the program; however, being married does not guarantee increased support for adherence. For example, among those married patients with spouses who were rated as high in spousal support, adherence was found to be significantly higher (Andrew et al., 1981; Doherty, Schrott, Metcalf, & Iasiello-Vailas, 1983).

Intimate-Relationship Social Support

Although the mechanisms by which the social support provided by an intimate relationship affects CHD development and recovery are not completely clear, there are numerous pathways by which the relationship could exert an effect on expression of CHD. It has been found that high levels of contact between the patient and his or her partner while the patient is in the hospital decrease pain medication use and decrease time in the intensive care unit compared with low levels of contact with the partner (Kulik & Mahler, 1989). Although Kulik and Mahler (1989) did not find a significant effect of marital quality, it seems likely that further studies that look more closely at the nature of the contact between partners could yield even more valuable associations.

Buffering Effect on Stress

The social support offered by an intimate relationship has been conceptualized as a buffer (or mediator) between life stressors and physical and psychological symptoms. Support for this hypothesis is found in a study of Fontana et al. (1989), in which 73 male cardiac patients were assessed at 3, 6, and 12 months after MI or bypass surgery. The researchers measured intimacy, stress, and psychological distress and used structural equation modeling to explore the causal relationships between intimacy and a number of

CHD-related variables. The factors related to CHD included stress or threat (e.g., likelihood of recurrence of symptoms or dying suddenly), distress, dyspnea (shortness of breath), and angina. In support of the buffering theory of intimate relationships, the researchers found that intimacy directly helped reduce the worry about recurrent symptoms or dying. In addition, this reduction helped reduce the effects that worry and distress can have on subsequent cardiac symptoms. The researchers also found that by decreasing threat and distress, intimacy indirectly decreased dyspnea and angina.

As further support of the buffering hypothesis, Waltz (1986) found that satisfying or close intimate relationships were related to decreased negative affect and increased coping ability (CHD risk factors). In addition, the provision of emotional support seems to be a pathway for the reduction of mortality risk. There is evidence that individuals with a low availability of emotional support are at an increased risk of dying (Hanson, Isacsson, Janzon, & Lindell, 1989). Medalie and Goldbourt (1976) have suggested that "a wife's love and support is an important balancing factor, which apparently reduces the risk of angina pectoris even in the presence of high risk factors" (p. 910). In addition, the extent to which individuals feel that they can have an open discussion with their intimate partner (*partner disclosure*) has been found to be significantly related to decreased chest pain following an MI and decreases in rehospitalization during the year after an MI (Helgeson, 1991). Whereas it is possible to receive emotional support from a range of people outside of the intimate relationship, it seems likely that being part of a couple increases the chances of receiving emotional support and may also increase specific kinds of support, such as intimacy.

Depression

Post-MI patients are at a greater risk of depression than healthy individuals (e.g., Schleifer et al., 1989; Taylor et al., 1981), and as mentioned earlier, depression during recovery from an MI increases the chance of a poor outcome (e.g., Carney et al., 1987). A depressed or dysphoric mood after an MI has been shown to have direct physiological effects and may interfere with recovery by affecting perceptions (Brown & Munford, 1983–1984), energy level, self-esteem, and motivation (Crawshaw, 1974). To the extent that an intimate relationship is characterized by partner disclosure and emotional support, it is likely that the risk of depression will be reduced. In support of this hypothesis, it has been found that spousal support enhances individuals' psychological functioning during recovery from an acute cardiac event (e.g., Ell & Haywood, 1984; Waltz, 1986; Winefield, 1982). Thus, one way that marriage or an intimate relationship can affect CHD outcomes is by preventing depressive or anxiety symptoms.

Likewise, a relationship that contributes to depressive symptoms is likely to increase the risk of future cardiac events. Dissatisfying relationships are likely to contribute to the stress of an MI and fail to provide the emotional and instrumental support that has been found to be effective in recovery from a cardiac event. In noncardiac populations, there is much evidence of a significant relationship between marital discord and depression (e.g., Beach, Whisman, & O'Leary, 1994; Coyne et al., 1987). There is evidence that either depression or marital discord can precede the other (thus, each could potentially be a cause of the other). Thus, it is possible that one pathway by which CHD patients become more vulnerable to depressive symptoms is through a discordant relationship. In addition, relationship problems that existed before the cardiac event tend to become worse after the episode (Wishnie, Hackett, & Cassem, 1971). Thus, it is likely that an individual who was distressed with the relationship before a cardiac event such as an MI would be at an even higher risk of exhibiting depressive symptoms during the recovery phase than if she or he had no preexisting relationship distress. As evidence, it has been found that post-MI patients in marriages with a combination of low intimacy and high conflict are more depressed and anxious compared with patients in supportive marriages (Waltz, 1986). Given the greater risk of mortality for depressed post-MI patients, this combination would seem to be particularly troublesome.

Couple Conflict and Cardiovascular Reactivity

One possible mechanism connecting relationship distress to an increase in risk of CHD is the effect that conflict between partners has on cardiovascular reactivity. There is some evidence, although it remains controversial, that increased cardiovascular reactivity leads to hypertension, which may in turn increase the risk of CHD (e.g., Pickering, 1996). Research on couples' communication has provided evidence that compared with happy couples, unhappy couples engage in a higher frequency and intensity of hostile exchanges and a lower frequency of supportive or affectional emotional exchanges (Margolin & Wampold, 1981; Notarius & Markman, 1989). In addition, those partners who experience greater arousal during conflicted interactions are at significantly greater risk of declines in relationship satisfaction and poorer health outcomes at a later date (Levenson & Gottman, 1983, 1985). It is likely that couples who are unable to resolve conflict are more likely to have numerous episodes of increased heart rate and blood pressure. As a result, "persisting failure to resolve marital or family conflicts thus might contribute to the enhanced sympathetic tone believed to play an early role in hypertension and atherogenesis" (Ewart, Taylor, Kraemer, & Agras, 1991, p. 155). In contrast, those couples who have skills for problem resolution are likely to have less episodes that raise blood pressure and heart rate. Ewart and colleagues (1991) found that for those couples who experience conflict in their relationship, communication skills training helped reduce blood pressure reactivity to the couples' arguments.

Hostility and Increased Blood Pressure

To the extent that cardiovascular reactivity leads to increased blood pressure, the hostility associated with relationship conflict is a risk factor for CHD. Hostile individuals are more likely to have unstable relationships and downplay the amount of social support that they receive from their environment (Eriksen, 1994). Although type A behavior pattern as a whole is no longer a focus of treatment, the hostility associated with it continues to be an important area of emphasis. In fact, in comparison with type Bs, type As have been found to show more frequent relationship conflicts or disagreements (Falger, 1983; Haynes, Feinleib, Levine, Scotch, & Kannel, 1978). Thus hostility, whether it is associated with type A behavior pattern or not, appears to be one pathway by which risk factors after an MI are increased. One pathway by which hostility affects CHD may be through relationship discord. The relationship discord may then lead to depressive symptoms, a lack of emotional support, a lack of instrumental support, and potential increases in blood pressure.

Negative Effects of Family or Partner

In considering the research reviewed above, it appears that the presence of relationship discord is likely to reduce a number of helpful partner behaviors, such as provision of emotional support and self-disclosure and provision of instrumental support to quit smoking and to exercise. In addition, the presence of relationship discord is likely to increase potentially harmful partner behaviors such as conflict or neglect. According to Croog, Levine, and Lurie (1968), up to 20% of men in the hospital with an MI attribute problems with their wife as an important cause. However, even for those partners and families who are satisfied with their relationships, there is evidence that both during and after hospitalization, some families or partners may make attempts at support that cause problems or anxiety for the patient (e.g., Coyne & DeLongis, 1986; Coyne, Wortman, & Lehman, 1988; Doerr & Jones, 1979). For example, partners may become overprotective toward the patient (Jenkins et al., 1983; Wishnie et al., 1971) or become emotionally overinvolved with the patient in a manner that is stressful to him or her even in an otherwise satisfying relationship (e.g., Coyne & DeLongis, 1986). It appears that receiving accurate information about the MI and the recovery process helps reduce some of these behaviors by educating the partner about the likely course of events after an MI (Doerr & Jones, 1979).

Couple Effects on Behavioral Risk Factors

It does appear that individuals in intimate relationships are more likely to receive support for reducing the modifiable risk factors associated with CHD, and in fact, those individuals in a supportive relationship are more likely to receive encouragement from their partner to quit smoking (or not to start), to exercise, and to lower cholesterol. Although Reed, McGee, Yano, and Feinleib (1983) found no relationship between social support and smoking prevalence, a number of other investigators have provided evidence that a high level of perceived support is significantly related to smoking cessation success rates (Billings & Moos, 1983; Hanson, Isacsson, & Janzon, 1990; Mermelstein, Lichtenstien, & McIntyre, 1983; Orth-Gomer et al., 1993; Westman, Eden, & Shirom, 1985). Orth-Gomer et al. also found a significant relationship between a lack of social support and failure to exercise. Although there are mixed findings with regard to cholesterol, Doherty et al. (1983) found that among healthy men with high cholesterol, adherence to lipid-lowering medication was significantly related to spousal support.

Effects of CHD on Relationships

Understandably, a person's hospitalization for a cardiac event is a frightening and upsetting experience for the partner and family. In fact, partners are often found to show more psychological distress than patients during the time of hospitalization (Mayou, Foster, & Williamson, 1978; Michela, 1987; Speedling, 1982), with symptoms including anxiety and depression (Stern & Pascale, 1979). There are a number of specific stressors that partners or family members tend to experience during a family member's hospitalization, including a sense of a lack of control over the events occurring in the hospital; failure to receive adequate information from hospital staff, in particular, a lack of information about sexual activity; few opportunities to express distress; a fear of loss of one's partner and of security; a fear of change in family roles; and a sense of self-blame for the partner's illness (Bedsworth & Molen, 1982; Bramwell, 1986; Gillis, 1984; Papadopoulos, Larrimore, Cardin, & Shelley, 1980; Skelton & Dominian, 1973; Thompson & Cordle, 1988). Once the patient returns home, significant distress often continues within the family, especially for partners (e.g., Bramwell, 1986; Skelton & Dominian, 1973). Conflict can arise over a number of issues, including the part a partner plays in a patient's resumption of roles in the house, as well as over differences between the partner and the patient in perceptions of the patient's health status (Bramwell, 1986; Finlayson & McEwen, 1977; Gillis, 1984).

In addition to reactions of anxiety and depression, some partners of CHD patients have also been found to exhibit overprotectiveness (e.g., Jenkins et al., 1983; Wishnie et al., 1971). Overprotective behavior is typically viewed as potentially harmful to the relationship and often produces distress in the patient. However, Fiske, Coyne, and Smith (1991) have suggested that the term *overprotectiveness* has been poorly defined and in fact includes both positive and negative aspects. They have found that the positive aspect of overprotectiveness (a warm protectiveness) was significantly related to the couple becoming closer after the MI, whereas the negative component, hostility, was associated with the couple's becoming more distant after the MI. Note that for most couples, the increase in negative emotions and relationship tensions appears to decrease within the first year of recovery. Also, it has been suggested that increased information and support from the hospital and physician can further ease the initial distress after an MI (e.g., Skelton & Dominian, 1973).

Another area of concern for a number of cardiac patients and their partners involves return to sexual activity after a cardiac event. A number of studies have indicated that after a cardiac event, patients and partners show concern about sexual activity, as well as a decrease in sexual activity (Bloch, Maeder, & Hassely, 1975; Hellerstein & Friedman, 1969; Mayou et al., 1978; Papadopoulos et al., 1980; Rudy, 1980). After an MI, 30% to 40% of male patients fail to return to the level of sexual activity to which they were accustomed before the MI (Trelawny-Ross & Russell, 1987; Weizman et al., 1991), and 44% of female patients report a decrease in their level of sexual activity (Papadopoulos, Beaumont, Shelley, & Larrimore, 1983). As a further complication, Folks, Blake, Freeman, Sokol, and Baker (1988) have found a high correlation between disturbances in sexual functioning and depressive symptoms after cardiac surgery. Compounding the sexual issue for a number of patients is the fact that few receive information about a return to sexual activity from health care workers. For example, one investigation reported that 33% of females had received information but only 3% had actually talked to a health care worker about returning to sexual activity (Baggs & Karch, 1987). An encouraging finding is that data gathered at 1 year after a cardiac event (MI or bypass surgery) suggest that interest in sexual activity and the actual level of sexual activity are both likely to increase during the year after the event (e.g., Langeluddecke, Fulcher, Baird, Hughes, & Tennant, 1989). In addition, there is some evidence to suggest that improvements in exercise that are part of a cardiac rehabilitation program are associated with increased sexual activity (Roviaro, Holmes, & Holmsten, 1984). Finally, treadmill exercise tests for eligible patients can help alleviate anxiety about sexual activity leading to a heart attack (Davidson, Houston, & DeBusk, 1978). In addition, when partners of patients have undergone treadmill tests themselves, they become significantly more confident about the capacity of their partner to resume their customary physical activities with safety. Thus, it is likely that the anxiety surrounding sexual activity is reduced by the ability of patients and partners to use the treadmill test baseline as a way to gauge the amount of safe sexual activity possible.

Role of Gender

Although a majority of the research on CHD has been conducted with men, in recent years there has been increasing attention to the need for research on CHD in women. Similar to that for men, CHD is the leading cause of death for women (Thom, 1987; World Health Organization, 1989). Although a number of investigations have looked at gender differences in morbidity and mortality in male versus female CHD patients, questions remain about true differences after adjusting for age. Some studies suggest that men and women show different mortality rates from CHD (e.g., Murabito, Evans, Larson, & Levy, 1993) and that mortality from CHD for women lags behind that for men by about 10 years (Lerner & Kannel, 1986). However, some report that age-adjusted CHD mortality rates are similar between men and women. There are some significant differences in the expression of CHD by gender, including the finding that women are more likely to die after an MI and are also more likely to reinfarct or die within the year after the MI than are men (Kuhn & Rackley, 1993). These findings may be due to the later age at which women tend to experience cardiac events. Given some of the differences found for men and woemn in the expression of CHD (for a detailed review of CHD and women, see Brezinka & Kittel, 1995), it is worth considering whether the relationship between relationship status and CHD is different for men and women. Although social isolation as a general phenomenon appears to be related to both the development of CHD and mortality from CHD in women as well as men (e.g., Chandra et al., 1983; Wingard & Cohn, 1987), there is some evidence that marriage, as a specific type of social support (and potential stressor), confers greater health benefits on men (Coombs, 1991; Shumaker & Hill, 1991). Clearly, more research on potential gender differences in the mechanisms of CHD development and rehabilitation would be useful, particularly in the way that the genders may benefit or be stressed by intimate relationships.

THE RELATIONSHIP SUPPORT PROGRAM

Although a number of investigations have shown clear correlations between cardiac and couple variables and several investigations have indicated the utility of including partners in treatment of the cardiac patient, few studies have explored truly couple-focused interventions. More commonly, the interventions that include the partner are focused either on providing information to both the patient and the partner or on helping the partner with her or his own distress about the patient's cardiac event. Thus, current interventions could be improved by targeting not just the needs of both partners but also the enhancement of couple functioning as a way to decrease CHD risk factors.

We have developed an intervention for cardiac patients and their partners to address this need. The Relationship Support Program (RSP) is designed to supplement concurrent medical interventions by focusing on enhancing the relationship between the patient and his or her partner. The intervention is designed to be presented to couples not as marital therapy but as a way to help them cope with the stress of a cardiac event as a couple. The RSP is an adaptation of cognitive–behavioral marital therapy (CBMT), a model that fits nicely with the needs of this population. CBMT has been found to be effective with maritally distressed as well as concordantly depressed and maritally distressed populations (e.g. Beach et al., 1994). CBMT offers couples a chance to cope with the cardiac event as a couple and improves the likelihood that the relationship will serve as a source of support rather than a stressor.

Assessment

Important areas of assessment in the RSP (see Exhibit 2.1) include gathering information on (a) recent history of MI and related medical care,

---

EXHIBIT 2.1
Relationship Support Program: Areas of Assessment

I. Recent history of cardiac event and related medical care (not from a doctor's perspective, but in terms of understanding the couple's experience and the effect on their lives)

II. Discussion of issues and problems created by the MI, for both the individuals and the couple

III. Individual functioning
   A. Physical—description of physical functioning
   B. Psychological—screen for anxiety and depressive symptoms
   C. Assessment of risk factors
      1. Exercise
      2. Smoking
      3. Cholesterol and diet
      4. Hypertension
      5. Psychosocial: Depression? Anxiety? Sense of support from partner and others? Conflicts or hostility that might contribute to cardiovascular reactivity?

IV. Couple functioning
   A. Pre- and post-MI, ask about or observe interaction in the following areas
      1. Relationship adjustment and satisfaction
      2. Communication styles
      3. Sexual interaction
      4. Level of protectiveness
      5. Cognitions about marriage

V. Current living situation
   A. Home environment—who lives in the home, roles and how these may have changed
   B. Occupational demands

VI. Coping styles and skills (as individuals and as a couple)
   A. Past (e.g., "How have you handled crises or problems in the past?")
   B. Present (e.g., "How do you feel you are handling this cardiac event?")

Note. Both members of the couple are asked about all areas. MI = myocardial infarction.

(b) issues and problems created by the MI, (c) individual functioning (including both physical and psychological, e.g., physical functioning, anxiety, and depressive symptoms), (d) couple functioning (pre- and post-MI, e.g., relationship adjustment, communication styles, cognitions about the relationship, sexual interaction, level of protectiveness, autonomy, and relatedness), (e) current living situation (e.g., who lives in the home or occupational demands), and (f) coping styles and skills (as individuals and as a couple).

More specifically, it is important to gather information about each partner's understanding of the events leading up to the cardiac event as well as the details surrounding the event. Were there signs before the event, or did it come as a surprise? What happened exactly from the time the patient first became aware of symptoms through the hospital experience? What did their physicians tell them about what happened and the risks still present? How long has it been since the event; since leaving the hospital if admitted? What have their lives been like (individually and as a couple) since the event?

It is also useful to gain an understanding of how the cardiac event has raised issues or problems for the individuals and the couple. How has this affected each person's life? How has this affected the couple's relationship? What issues do they anticipate continuing for a while?

A third important area of assessment is that of individual functioning, both physical and psychological. It is useful to gather information from both partners in these areas, because both may have physical problems (it is not uncommon, especially for those older in age, to have a partner with equal or more severe physical problems) and both are likely to have psychological reactions to the cardiac event. How are both currently functioning physically? Although it is not the purview of mental health professionals to make physical rehabilitation recommendations, it is useful to understand how much of a physical impact the cardiac event has had on the couple's life. What sort of emotional reactions have they had? In particular, research indicates that depression and anxiety are possibilities in both patients and partners; thus, assessment should include attention to these areas. In addition, it is clear that partners can help reduce modifiable risk factors; thus, the extent to which these risk factors are present should be assessed. Specifically, the extent to which the following factors are risks for this couple should be assessed: exercise, smoking, cholesterol and diet, hypertension, and psychosocial (e.g., social–partner support or existence of conflicts or hostility).

A fourth major area of assessment is that of couple functioning. Although in a more traditional marital therapy setting, a great deal of time would be spent in this area, it is important to recognize that cardiac couples do not necessarily view themselves as needing marital therapy. Therefore, the following areas may be assessed briefly or in more indirect ways than would be used in traditional couples therapy. It is helpful to get a sense of how satisfied the couple is with their relationship and the extent to which they have the ability to communicate their emotions as well as problems or decisions that need to be made. A topic that is especially relevant for cardiac couples is sexual interaction. Although this is often a difficult topic for mental health professionals to raise, research shows it is a concern of many cardiac patients, and thus it may be a relief for the couple to be asked if they have concerns about sexual functioning after the cardiac event. Questions about pre-event sexual functioning and current sexual functioning can naturally follow from this question about the couple's concerns. Several other issues particularly relevant to assess with cardiac patients are protectiveness of partner and, related to this, the balance of independence and closeness of the couple. Has the partner become overly protective of the cardiac patient? Has the balance of closeness and independence shifted in any distressing ways? Do they perceive these changes as temporary or more permanent? Finally, with regard to the couple's functioning, it is important to continue to assess the partners' beliefs about their relationship and relationships in general. There is research to suggest that the cognitions or thoughts that couples have about their relationship are significantly correlated with relationship satisfaction, communication, and depressive symptoms (e.g., Baucom, Epstein, Rankin, & Burnett, 1996; Rankin-Esquer, Baucom, Epstein, & Burnett, 1997). For example, if one partner thinks that "he must not care about me or he would be exercising," then it is likely to negatively affect the satisfaction with the relationship.

Finally, the last two areas of assessment include the couples' current living situation and their general coping skills. Who lives in the home? Who has been most affected by the cardiac event? How have things changed, or how do things need to change in the home? What are the occupational demands placed on both partners? How do those have to change, and how does that affect the relationship? With regard to coping skills, it is useful to find out how each partner has coped in the past with problems or crises as well as how each currently is coping. These same areas should also be assessed with regard to the couple, for example, "How do you feel that you have handled problems in the past as a couple?"

Intervention

There are three main phases of intervention to the RSP. The first maintains a specific focus on the cardiac event and helping the couple cope with the consequences of the event. The second phase continues to focus on the cardiac event but broadens the focus somewhat to look at how relationship issues affect and are affected by the cardiac event. The third phase broadens the intervention beyond the cardiac event to improve general relationship skills that can help the couple function beyond just coping with the cardiac event. Although all couples go through the three phases, the length of time needed can vary depending on the initial assessment of relationship functioning. For a couple who generally functioned well in their relationship before the cardiac event, the intervention should focus on coping with the event, making a transition to new roles if necessary (e.g., if the cardiac patient cannot perform physical labor around the house, the partners can switch roles), and giving the couple extra skills to continue to cope well (e.g., enhancing their communication skills). For couples who appear to have had relationship problems before the cardiac event, the same order of interventions would be used; however, a longer time would be taken on the third phase, generally improving relationship functioning beyond coping with the specific cardiac event. The goals of the second and third phases are to help shift a number of areas important to rehabilitation, including partner support for exercise, medication compliance, changes in diet, increases in emotional support, and decreases in conflict and hostility.

Whereas all risk factors are relevant to the RSP, they are addressed as they relate to the relationship. To fully address all of the patient's needs, the RSP would ideally be implemented in conjunction with a cardiac rehabilitation program or in collaboration with physicians and hospital staff. It is clear that providing information to partners and families decreases their anxiety and the patients' anxiety as well. An example of a cardiac rehabilitation program that works well with the RSP is MULTIFIT (DeBusk et al., 1994; Miller & Taylor, 1995), a multifactorial risk-reduction program developed from social learning theory and modified for medical problems. MULTIFIT includes smoking cessation, nutritional counseling, lipid-lowering drug therapy, and exercise training. Patients are administered a brief psychosocial screen in the hospital with further assessment as indicated. For example, patients reporting high levels of stress are given a workbook and relaxation tape to be used on their own. Patients are encouraged to monitor their stress levels in addition to monitoring their diet and exercise. After discharge, nurses conduct monthly follow-up telephone calls for the first 6 months after the cardiac event. These calls consist of a structured set of questions to assess the patient's mood and coping. The MULTIFIT program has shown significant changes in health outcome related to smoking cessation, exercise, and the lowering of lipids with both medication and diet changes. Although a number of cardiac rehabilitation programs were initially developed with specific CHD populations (e.g., post-MI), they have been expanded to include many ways that CHD is expressed, including patients experiencing MI, coronary artery bypass grafts, abnormal electrocardiograms, and angina.

Case Example

Larry, age 46, had an MI 4 weeks before beginning the RSP with his wife, Joan, age 48. The couple was referred to the RSP by cardiac rehabilitation program staff. The couple had been married for almost 21 years at the time of the MI, and both were taken by surprise, because Larry had shown no prior symptoms. The assessment interview revealed that although Joan was physically active in several sports, Larry had a history of minimal exercise. Both spouses reported that Joan was more interested in health generally and had become a vegetarian 10 years ago, whereas Larry continued to eat "whatever I want." Both spouses reported that the issue of healthy eating and exercise had been a significant area of conflict in the marriage for some time. At the time of intake, Joan reported a range of emotions, including fear related to Larry's brush with death, anger that he had failed to follow her health suggestions, and guilt over her anger. Larry reported strong feelings of guilt as well, in addition to anxiety and frustration because he believed that "now I will have to listen to her like she is my mother." He also rather reluctantly reported some anxiety and depressive symptoms, including sadness, lack of concentration, and a worry about the future ("I know I am going to die soon").

Other areas affected by the MI included the couple's living and working arrangements. Before the MI, Larry worked in a business that required him to travel a great deal while Joan ran a business out of their home. Although Larry planned to return to work shortly, he was negotiating with his company to switch to a position that did not require travel. These changes, in addition to the fact that Larry was currently still at home recuperating, meant that Joan had to adapt to having Larry at home much more frequently. Although she reported that she had been wishing for a long time to get more attention from him, Joan also reported that she found it difficult to concentrate on her business with Larry "always underfoot." Thus, the couple was faced with coping with a number of issues, including emotional reactions to the MI complicated by health conflicts before the MI, how to best effect changes in Larry's lifestyle (e.g., diet, exercise, and medication compliance) without pulling Joan into a "mother" role, and a transition to different patterns of living at home. Although the marriage had a number of strengths and both spouses described the marriage as fairly happy, as treatment progressed, several other problem areas became more obvious. The most distressing was the couple's inability to resolve problem discussions, leaving several areas of dissension unresolved for years.

Following the RSP model, the first couple of sessions after the intake session focused on discussing the MI and the reactions of the spouses to the MI. These sessions included an exploration of how they felt they were coping, as well as a discussion of strategies for increasing their coping. In addition, an assessment of the amount of educational information being provided by Larry's physician revealed that some areas of information had not been covered. Therefore, some time was spent covering normal reactions to a cardiac event. Both Larry and Joan reported that these early sessions were helpful and that they found it useful to learn what to expect in recovery and to express their feelings about the event.

Treatment then moved to focus on the ways in which the MI affected the couple's relationship and the ways in which their relationship was affecting recovery. Joan showed some reluctance to continue at this point, stating that "Larry has to diet and exercise; that has nothing to do with me. I have been trying to affect that process for years, and see where it got me?" This is an issue that is more likely to arise with cardiac couples than with couples who have self-identified as needing couples therapy. The therapist held a discussion about how interconnected spouses are and suggested that even when one person may not see something as a problem or feel a sense of control of the problem, it is helpful for both partners to be involved in the attempts to change. The couple was also given the rationale that it is helpful to include both partners in problem solving, even if it is focal to changing one person's behavior, because partners can help or distract from maintaining new behaviors, even unintentionally. Because neither spouse wanted Joan to be in role of supervising Larry's behavior changes, the therapist helped the couple set up individual behavioral contracts in which each planned an area of behavior change and rewarded himself or herself rather than depending on the partner for a reward. For example, Larry decided that he would start walking several times a week, and for this he would reward himself with the purchase of new books (reading was a hobby). Joan was encouraged to change a behavior as well "to keep him company," and she decided that she would decrease the number of times that she asked Larry how he was feeling (she admitted to "hovering" over him since the MI). She decided that asking him once a day but no more would be acceptable (and he agreed). When she asked him only once, she would reward herself with a half hour of television watching, which she enjoyed but did not do often. In addition, basic principles of behavior change (e.g., positive reinforcement and shaping) were covered with the couple to increase the chances that new behaviors would be maintained.

In the final phase of the treatment, the couple was taught communication skills to help them discuss feelings and resolve problems both related and unrelated to the cardiac event. Although the issue had been discussed at several points in the treatment, the conflict between Larry and Joan around healthy eating and exercise was reexamined. In earlier sessions, the therapist led the couple through these discussions; however, in this last phase, the emphasis was on the couple's learning to guide themselves through conflictual discussions. Thus, Larry and Joan practiced skills for expressing emotion about this issue and then used the same issue to learn and practice skills for solving problems. Although a number of other issues were covered during the course of treatment, these few examples provided give a sense of the order of events during the RSP. By the end of treatment, both spouses reported decreased distress over the MI, a change in health behaviors (Larry was exercising more, and after Joan stopped pressuring him to eat more healthy foods, he was able to show more appreciation for Joan's vegetarian cooking), and an increased belief in the ability of their relationship to sustain these changes. Although both spouses reported the belief that they had a good marriage before the MI, both also reported feeling a renewed sense of closeness and appreciation for each other after the MI and the RSP.

CONCLUSIONS AND FUTURE DIRECTIONS

The future of developing treatment of CHD looks promising for a number of reasons. One is that the overall mortality from heart disease has declined dramatically in the past 10–15 years (Hunink et al., 1997). In addition, there are many research investigations directing improvements in interventions, both physical and psychological. It is clear that inclusion of patients' significant relationships has the potential to increase both psychological and physical recovery after a cardiac event. However, there continue to be gaps in the research, and attention to these would improve intervention even further. It is likely that the field would benefit from further investigation of the gender differences in the relationship between intimate relationships and CHD risk factors. In addition, treatment-outcome studies focused on improving or supporting the role of an intimate relationship in recovery are much needed. Whereas it is clear that this type of relationship can play a crucial role in both the development and recovery from CHD, there are few data on the effects of interventions targeted to the couple. These interventions should go beyond the occasional inclusion of family members in dissemination of information. The interventions should focus on improving the quality of the intimate relationship, in particular, on increasing the ways in which both members of the couple are able to cope with the MI as individuals and as a couple. Whereas the medical field has shown remarkable improvements in the treatment of cardiac patients at the time of a cardiac event, interventions focused on the intimate relationships of patients hold the promise of improving both the quality and length of life in the months and years after discharge from the hospital.

REFERENCES

American Heart Association. (1987). *Heart facts*. Dallas, TX: Author.

American Heart Association. (1995). *Heart and stroke facts: 1996 statistical supplement*. Dallas, TX: Author.

Andrew, G. M., Oldridge, N. B., Parker, J. O., Cunningham, D. A., Reichnitzer, P. A., Jones, N. J., Buck, C., Kavanaugh, T., Shepard, R. J., Sutton, J. R., & McDonald, W. (1981). Reasons for dropout from coronary exercise programs in postcoronary patients. *Medicine and Science in Sports and Exercise, 13*, 164–168.

Baggs, J. G., & Karch, A. M. (1987). Sexual counseling of women with coronary heart disease. *Heart and Lung, 16*, 154–159.

Barefoot, J., Dahlstrom, W., & Williams, R. (1983). Hostility, CHD incidence, and total mortality: A 25 year follow-up of 255 physicians. *Psychosomatic Medicine, 45*, 59–63.

Baucom, D. H., Epstein, N., Rankin, L. A., & Burnett, C. K. (1996). Assessing relationship standards: The inventory of specific relationship standards. *Journal of Family Psychology, 10*, 72–88.

Beach, S. R. H., Whisman, M. A., & O'Leary, K. D. (1994). Marital therapy for depression: Theoretical foundation, current status, and future directions. *Behavior Therapy, 25*, 345–371.

Bedsworth, J. A., & Molen, M. T. (1982). Psychological stress in spouses of patients with myocardial infarction. *Heart and Lung, 11*, 450–456.

Berkman, L. F., & Syme, S. L. (1979). Social networks, host resistance, and mortality: A nine-year follow-up of Alameda County residents. *American Journal of Epidemiology, 109*, 186–204.

Billings, A. G., & Moos, R. H. (1983). Social–environmental factors among light and heavy cigarette smokers: A controlled comparison with nonsmokers. *Addictive Behavior, 8*, 381–391.

Blazer, D. (1982). Social support and mortality in an elderly community population. *American Journal of Epidemiology, 115*, 684–694.

Bloch, A., Maeder, J., & Hassely, J. (1975). Sexual problems after myocardial infarction. *American Heart Journal, 90*, 536–537.

Bramwell, L. (1986). Wives' experiences in the support role after husbands' first myocardial infarction. *Heart and Lung, 15*, 578–584.

Brezinka, V., & Kittel, F. (1995). Psychosocial factors of coronary heart disease in women: A review. *Social Science and Medicine, 42*, 1351–1365.

Brown, M. A., & Munford, A. (1983–1984). Rehabilitation of post-MI depression and psychological invalidism: A pilot study. *International Journal of Psychiatric Medicine, 13*, 291–298.

Carney, R. M., Freedland, K. E., & Jaffe, A. S. (1990). Insomnia and depression prior to myocardial infarction. *Psychosomatic Medicine, 52*, 603–609.

Carney, R. M., Rich, M. W., Freedland, K. E., Saini, J., TeVelde, A., Simeone, C., & Clark, K. (1988). Major depressive disorder predicts cardiac events in patients with coronary artery disease. *Psychosomatic Medicine, 50*, 627–633.

Carney, R. M., Rich, M. W., teVelde, A., Saini, J., Clark, K., & Jaffe, A. S. (1987). Major depressive disorder in coronary artery disease. *American Journal of Cardiology, 60*, 1273–1275.

Case, R. B., Moss, A. J., Case, N., McDermott, N., & Eberly, S. (1992). Living alone after myocardial infarction: Impact on prognosis. *Journal of the American Medical Association, 267*, 515–519.

Chandra, V., Szklo, M., Goldberg, R., & Tonascia, J. (1983). The impact of marital status on survival after an acute myocardial infarction: A population-based study. *American Journal of Epidemiology, 117*, 320–325.

Cohen, S., Kaplan, J. R., & Manuck, S. B. (1994). Social support and coronary heart disease: Underlying psychological and biological mechanisms. In S. A. Shumaker & S. M. Czajkowski (Eds.), *Social support and cardiovascular disease* (pp. 195–221). New York: Plenum Press.

Coombs, R. H. (1991). Marital status and personal well-being: A literature review. *Family Relations, 40*, 97–102.

Coyne, J. C., & DeLongis, A. (1986). Going beyond social support: The role of social relationship in adaptation. *Journal of Consulting and Clinical Psychology, 54*, 454–460.

Coyne, J. C., Kessler, R. C., Tal, M., Turnbull, J., Wortman, C. B., & Greden, J. F. (1987). Living with a depressed person. *Journal of Consulting and Clinical Psychology, 55*, 347–352.

Coyne, J. C., Wortman, C. B., & Lehman, D. R. (1988). The other side of support: Emotional overinvolvement and miscarried helping. In B. H. Gottlieb (Ed.), *Marshaling social support: Formats, processes, and effects* (pp. 305–330). Newbury Park, CA: Sage Publications.

Crawshaw, J. E. (1974). Community rehabilitation after myocardial infarction. *Heart and Lung, 3*, 258–266.

Croog, S. H., Levine, S., & Lurie, Z. (1968). The heart patient and the recovery process: A review of the directions of research on social and psychological factors. *Social Science and Medicine, 2*, 111–164.

Davidson, D. M., Houston, N., & DeBusk, R. (1978, September). *Prognostic value of exercise testing early after myocardial infarction.* Paper presented at the Eighth World Congress of Cardiology, Tokyo.

DeBusk, R. F., Houston Miller, N., Superko, H. R., Dennis, C. A., Thomas, R. J., Lew, H. T., Berger, W. E., Heller, R. S., Rompf, J., Gee, D., Kraemer, H. C., Bandura, A., Ghandour, G., Clark, M., Shah, R. V., Fisher, L., & Taylor, C.B. (1994). Case-management system for coronary risk factor modification after acute myocardial infarction. *Annals of Internal Medicine, 120*, 721–729.

Doerr, B. C., & Jones, J. W. (1979). Effect of family preparation on the state anxiety level of the CCU patient. *Nursing Research, 28*, 315–316.

Doherty, W. J., Schrott, H. G., Metcalf, L., & Iasiello-Vailas, L. (1983). Effect of spouse support and health beliefs on medication adherence. *Journal of Family Practice, 17*, 837–841.

Ell, K., & Dunkel-Schetter, C. (1994). Social support and adjustment to myocardial infarction, angioplasty, and coronary artery bypass surgery. In S.A. Shumaker & S. M. Czajkowski (Eds.), *Social support and cardiovascular disease* (pp. 301–332). New York: Plenum Press.

Ell, K. O, & Haywood, L.J. (1984). Social support and recovery from myocardial infarction: A panel study. *Journal of Social Service Research, 4*, 1–9.

Eriksen, W. (1994). The role of social support in the pathogenesis of coronary heart disease. A literature review. *Family Practice, 11*, 201–209.

Ewart, C. K., Taylor, C. B., Kraemer, H. C., & Agras, W. S. (1991). High blood pressure and marital discord: Not being nasty matters more than being nice. *Health Psychology, 10*, 155–163.

Falger, P. R. J. (1983). Behavioral factors, life changes and the development of vital exhaustion and depression in myocardial infarction patients. *International Journal of Behavior Development, 6*, 405–425.

Finlayson, A., & McEwen, J. (1977). *Coronary heart disease and patterns of living.* New York: Prodist.

Fiske, V., Coyne, J. C., & Smith, D. A. (1991). Couples coping with myocardial infarction: An empirical reconsideration of the role of overprotectiveness. *Journal of Family Psychology, 5*, 4–20.

Folks, D. G., Blake, D. J., Freeman, A. M., Sokol, R. S., & Baker, D. M. (1988). Persistent depression in coronary bypass patients reporting sexual maladjustment. *Psychosomatics, 29*, 387–391.

Fontana, A. F., Kerns, R. D., Rosenberg, R. L., & Colonese, K. L. (1989). Support, stress, and recovery from coronary heart disease: A longitudinal causal model. *Health Psychology, 8*, 175–193.

Galan, K. M., Deligonul, U., Kern, M. J., Chaitman, B. R., & Vandormael, M. G. (1988). Increased frequency of restenosis in patients continuing to smoke cigarettes after acute percutaneous transluminal angioplasty. *American Journal of Cardiology, 6*, 260–263.

Garrity, T. F., & Klein, R. F. (1975). Emotional response and clinical severity as early determinants of six-month mortality after myocardial infarction. *Heart and Lung, 4*, 730–737.

Gillis, C. L. (1984). Reducing family stress during and after coronary artery bypass surgery. *Nursing Clinics of North America, 19*, 103–111.

Goldstein, M. G., & Niaura, R. (1992). Psychological factors affecting physical condition: Part 1. Coronary artery disease and sudden death. *Psychosomatics, 33*, 134–145.

Hackett, T. P., & Cassem, N. H. (1969). Factors contributing to delay in responding to signs and symptoms of acute myocardial infarction. *American Journal of Cardiology, 24*, 651–658.

Hanson, B. S., Isacsson, S., & Janzon, L. (1990). Social support and quitting smoking for good: Is there an association? Results from the population study: "Men born in 1914," Malmo, Sweden. *Addictive Behavior, 15*, 221–233.

Hanson, B. S., Isacsson, S., Janzon, L., & Lindell, S. (1989). Social network and social support influence mortality in elderly men. *American Journal of Epidemiology, 130*, 100–111.

Haynes, S. G., Feinlieb, M., Levine, S., Scotch, N., & Kannel, W. B. (1978). The relationship of psychosocial factors to coronary heart disease in the Framingham study: II. Prevalence of coronary heart disease. *American Journal of Epidemiology, 107*, 384–402.

Hayward, C. (1995). Psychiatric illness and cardiovascular disease risk. *Epidemiology Review, 17*, 129–138.

Helgeson, V. S. (1991). The effects of masculinity and social support on recovery from myocardial infarction. *Psychosomatic Medicine, 53*, 621–633.

Hellerstein, H., & Friedman, E. H. (1969). Sexual activity and the post coronary patient. *Medical Aspects of Human Sexuality, 3*, 70–96.

Horwitz, R. I., Viscoli, C. M., Berkman, L., Donaldson, R. M., Horwitz, S. M., Murray, C. J., Ransohoff, D. F., & Sindelar, J. (1990). Treatment adherence and risk of death after myocardial infarction. *Lancet, 336,* 542–545.

House, J. S., Landis, K. R., & Umberson, D. (1988). Social relationships and health. *Science, 241,* 540–545.

House, J. S., Robbins, C., & Metzner, H. L. (1982). The association of social relationships and activities with mortality: Prospective evidence from the Tecumseh Community Health Study. *American Journal of Epidemiology, 116,* 123–140.

Hunink, M. G., Goldman, L., Tosteson, A. N., Mittleman, M. A., Goldman, P. A., Williams, L. W., Tsevat, J., & Weinstein, M. C. (1997). The recent decline in mortality from coronary heart disease, 1980–1990. The effect of secular trends in risk factors and treatment. *Journal of the American Medical Association, 277,* 535–542.

Jenkins, C. D., Stanton, B., Savageau, J. A., Ockene, B. S., Denlinger, P., & Klein, M. D. (1983). Coronary artery bypass surgery: Physical, psychological, social and economic outcomes six months later. *Journal of the American Medical Association, 250,* 782–788.

Kamarck, T. W., Manuck, S., & Jennings, J. R. (1990). Social support reduces cardiovascular reactivity to psychological challenge: A laboratory model. *Psychomatic Medicine, 52,* 42–58.

Kannel, W. B., Sorlie, P., Castelli, W. P., & McGee, D. (1980). Blood pressure and survival after myocardial infarction: The Framingham study. *American Journal of Cardiology, 45,* 326–330.

Kuhn, F. E., & Rackley, C. E. (1993). Coronary artery disease in women: Risk factors, evaluation, treatment, and prevention [Review]. *Archives of Internal Medicine, 153,* 2626–2636.

Kulik, J. A., & Mahler, H. I. M. (1989). Social support and recovery from surgery. *Health Psychology, 8,* 221–238.

Kulik, J. A., & Mahler, H. I. M. (1993). Emotional support as a moderator of adjustment and compliance after coronary artery bypass surgery: A longitudinal study. *Journal of Behavioral Medicine, 16,* 45–63.

Langeluddecke, P., Fulcher, G., Baird, D., Hughes, C., & Tennant, C. (1989). A prospective evaluation of the psychosocial effects of coronary artery bypass surgery. *Journal of Psychosomatic Research, 33,* 37–45.

Lerner, D. J., & Kannel, W. B. (1986). Patterns of coronary heart disease morbidity and mortality in the sexes: A 26-year follow-up of the Framingham population. *American Heart Journal, 111,* 383–390.

Levenson, R. W., & Gottman, J. M. (1983). Marital interaction: Physiological linkage and affective exchange. *Journal of Personality and Social Psychology, 3,* 587–597.

Levenson, R. W., & Gottman, J. M. (1985). Physiological and affective predictors of change in relationship satisfaction. *Journal of Personality and Social Psychology, 49,* 85–94.

Margolin, G., & Wampold, B. (1981). Sequential analysis of conflict and accord in distressed and nondistressed marital partners. *Journal of Consulting and Clinical Psychology, 49*, 554–567.

Mayou, R., Foster, A., & Williamson, B. (1978). The psychological and social effects of myocardial infarcts on wives. *British Medical Journal, 1*, 699–701.

Medalie, J. H., & Goldbourt, U. (1976). Angina pectoris among 10,000 men. *American Journal of Medicine, 60*, 910–921.

Mermelstein, R., Lichtenstien, E., & McIntyre, K. (1983). Partner support and relapse in smoking-cessation programs. *Journal of Consulting and Clinical Psychology, 51*, 465–466.

Michela, J. L. (1987). Interpersonal and individual impacts of a husband's heart attack. In A. Baum & J. Singer (Eds.), *Handbook of psychology and health: Vol. 5. Stress and coping* (pp. 255–300). Hillsdale, NJ: Erlbaum.

Miller, N. H., & Taylor, C. B. (1995). *Lifestyle management in patients with coronary heart disease.* Champaign, IL: Human Kinetics.

Morgan, M. (1980). Marital status, health, illness and service use. *Social Science and Medicine, 14A*, 633–643.

Mumford, E., Schlesinger, H. J., & Glass, G. V. (1982). The effects of psychological intervention on recovery from surgery and heart attacks: An analysis of the literature. *American Journal of Public Health, 72*, 141–151.

Murabito, J. M., Evans, J. C., Larson, M. G., & Levy, D. (1993). Prognosis after the onset of coronary heart disease: An investigation of differences in outcome between the sexes according to initial coronary disease presentation. *Circulation, 88*, 2548–2555.

Notarius, C. I., & Markman, H. J. (1989). Coding marital interaction: A sampling and discussion of current issues. *Behavioral Assessment, 11*, 1–11.

Orth-Gomer, K., Rosengren, A., & Wilhelmsen, L. (1993). Lack of social support and incidence of coronary heart disease in middle-aged Swedish men. *Psychosomatic Medicine, 55*, 37–43.

Papadopoulos, C., Beaumont, C., Shelley, S. I., & Larrimore, P. (1983). Myocardial infarction and sexual activity of the female patient. *Archives of Internal Medicine, 143*, 1528–1530.

Papadopoulos, C., Larrimore, P., Cardin, S., & Shelley, S. I. (1980). Sexual concern and needs of the postcoronary patient's wife. *Archives of Internal Medicine, 140*, 38–41.

Pickering, T. (1996). Why study blood pressure reactivity to stress? [Editorial; comment]. *American Journal of Hypertension, 9*, 941–942.

Pratt, L. A., Ford, D. E., Crum, R. M., Armenian, H. K., Gallo, J. J., & Eaton, W. W. (1996). Depression, psychotropic medication, and risk of myocardial infarction. Prospective data from the Baltimore ECA follow-up. *Circulation, 94*, 3123–3129.

Rankin-Esquer, L. A., Baucom, D. H., Epstein, N., & Burnett, C. K. (1997, November). Do depressed spouses show the same significant relationships among important marital variables as normative community spouses? Paper presented at the 31st Annual Convention of the Association for the Advancement of Behavior Therapy, Miami, FL.

Rankin-Esquer, L. A., Houston Miller, N., Myers, D., & Taylor, C. B. (1997). Marital status and outcome in patients with coronary heart disease. *Journal of Clinical Psychology in Medical Settings, 4*, 417–435.

Reed, D., McGee, D., Yano, K., & Feinleib, M. (1983). Social networks and coronary heart disease among Japanese men in Hawaii. *American Journal of Epidemiology, 117*, 384–397.

Rhodewalt, F., & Smith, T. W. (1990). Current issues in Type A behavior, coronary proneness, and coronary heart disease. In C. R. Snyder & D. R. Forsyth (Eds.), *Handbook of social and clinical psychology* (pp. 197–220). New York: Pergamon Press.

Roviaro, S., Holmes, D. S., & Holmsten, D. H. (1984). Influence of a cardiac rehabilitation program on the cardiovascular, psychological and social functioning of cardiac patients. *Journal of Behavioral Medicine, 7*, 61–81.

Ruberman, W., Weinblatt, E., Goldberg, J. D., & Chaudhary, B. S. (1984). Psychosocial influences on mortality after myocardial infarction. *New England Journal of Medicine, 311*, 552–559.

Rudy, E. B. (1980). Patients' and spouses' causal explanations of a myocardial infarction. *Nursing Research, 29*, 352–356.

Schleifer, S. J., Marcari-Hinson, M. M., Coyle, D. A., Slater, W. R., Kahn, M., Gorlin, R., & Zucker, H. D. (1989). The nature and course of depression following myocardial infarction. *Archives of Internal Medicine, 149*, 1785–1789.

Seeman, T., Berkman, L. F., Kohout, F., Lacroix, A., Glynn, R., & Blazer, D. (1993). Intercommunity variations in the association between social ties and mortality in the elderly: A comparative analysis of three communities. *Annals of Epidemiology, 3*, 448–450.

Shumaker, S. A., & Hill, D. R. (1991). Gender differences in social support and physical health. *Health Psychology, 10*, 102–111.

Skelton, M., & Dominian, J. (1973). Psychological stress in wives of patients with myocardial infarction. *British Medical Journal, 2*, 101–103.

Sokolow, M., & McIlroy, M. B. (1987). *Clinical cardiology* (4th ed.). Los Altos, CA: Lange Medical Publications.

Speedling, E. F. (1982). *Heart attack: The family response at home and in the hospital.* New York: Tavistock.

Stern, M. J., & Pascale, L. (1979). Psychosocial adaptation post-myocardial infarction: The spouse's dilemma. *Journal of Psychosomatic Research, 23*, 83–87.

Surgeon General. (1979, March). Highlights of the 1979 Surgeon General's report on smoking and health. *Journal of Medical Association of Georgia 68*(3), 185–189.

Taylor, C. B., DeBusk, R. F., Davidson, D. M., Houston, N., & Burnett, K. (1981). Optimal methods for identifying depression following hospitalization for myocardial infarction. *Journal of Chronic Diseases, 34*, 1–7.

Thom, T. J. (1987). Cardiovascular disease mortality among United States women. In E. D. Earker, B. Packard, N. K. Wenger, T. B. Clarkson, & H. A. Tyroler (Eds.), *Coronary heart disease in women* (pp. 33–41). New York: Haymarket Doyma.

Thompson, D. R., & Cordle, C. J. (1988). Support of wives of myocardial infarction patients. *Journal of Advanced Nursing, 13*, 223–228.

Trelawny-Ross, C., & Russell, O. (1987). Social and psychological responses to myocardial infarction: Multiple determinants of outcome at six months. *Journal of Psychosomatic Research, 31*, 125–130.

Verbrugge, L. (1979). Marital status and health. *Journal of Marriage and the Family, 41*, 267–285.

Waltz, M. (1986). Marital context and post-infarction quality of life: Is it social support or something more? *Social Science and Medicine, 22*, 791–805.

Weizman, R., Eldar, M., Hod, H., Eshkol, A., Rabinowitz, B, Tyano, S., & Neufeld, H. N. (1991). Effects of uncomplicated acute myocardial infarction on biochemical parameters of stress and sexual function. *Psychosomatics, 32*, 275–279.

Wells, K. B., Stewart, A., Hays, R. D., Burnam, M. A., Rogers, W., Daniel, M., Berry, S., Greenfield, S., & Ware, J. (1989). The functioning and well-being of depressed patients. *Journal of the American Medical Association, 262*, 914–919.

Westman, M., Eden, D., & Shirom, A. (1985). Job stress, cigarette smoking and cessation: The conditioning effects of peer support. *Social Science and Medicine, 20*, 637–644.

Wiklund, I., Oden, A., Sanne, H., Ulvenstam, G., Wilhelmsson, C., & Wilhelmsen, L. (1988). Prognostic importance of somatic and psychosocial variables after a first myocardial infarction. *American Journal of Epidemiology, 128*, 786–795.

Wilhelmsson, C., Vedin, J. A., Elmfeldt, D., Tibblin, G., & Wilhelmsson, L. (1975). Smoking and myocardial infarction. *Lancet 1*, 415–420.

Williams, R. B., Barefoot, J. C., Califf, R. M., Haney, T., Saunders, W., Pryor, D. Hlatky, M. Siegler, I., & Mark, D. (1992). Prognostic importance of social and economic resources among medically treated patients with angiographically documented coronary artery disease. *Journal of the American Medical Association, 267*, 520–524.

Williams, R. B., Haney, T. L., Lee, K. K. Kong, Y., Blumenthal, J. A., Whalen, R. E. (1980). Type A behavior, hostility and coronary atherosclerosis. *Psychosomatic Medicine, 42*, 539–549.

Winefield, H. R. (1982). Male social support and recovery after myocardial infarction. *Australian Journal of Psychology, 34*, 45–52.

Wingard, D. L., & Cohn, B. A. (1987). Disease mortality among women in Alameda County, 1965 to 1973. In E. D. Eaker, B. Packard, N. K. Wenger, T. B. Clarkson, & H. A. Tyroler (Eds.), *Coronary heart disease in women* (pp. 99–105). New York: Haymarket Doyma.

Wishnie, H. A., Hackett, T. P., & Cassem, N. H. (1971). Psychological hazards of convalescence following myocardial infarction. *Journal of the American Medical Association, 215,* 1292–1296.

World Health Organization. (1989). *World health statistics annual.* Geneva, Switzerland: Author.

3

COUPLES COPING WITH RESPIRATORY DISORDERS

KAREN B. SCHMALING AND NILOOFAR AFARI

Breathing is essential to life; therefore, alterations in breathing are threatening to one's well-being. This chapter focuses on respiratory diseases, their associations with couple factors, and the role of partner-involved treatments. The chapter begins by reviewing basic information on the etiology, mechanisms, epidemiology, and prognosis for the most common respiratory diseases: asthma, upper respiratory infections (URIs), chronic obstructive pulmonary disease (COPD), obstructive sleep apnea (OSA), lung cancer, cystic fibrosis (CF), and tuberculosis (TB). It then reviews the association between respiratory illnesses and intimate relationship satisfaction and goes on to discuss assessment and treatment and how they relate to couples.

OVERVIEW OF RESPIRATORY ILLNESSES

Asthma

Asthma is a common illness that affects 14 million persons in the United States (Centers for Disease Control, 1996a), or about 5% of the population. Asthma mortality rates increased steadily from 1979 to 1987, an average of 6.3% per year for young adults age 15–34 (Weiss & Wagener, 1990). It is a costly disease: In the United States, adult asthma care totaled $1.2 billion in direct costs (1990 dollars), not including medications, and $1.3 billion in indirect costs, including lost employment and premature death (Weiss, Gergen, & Hodgson, 1992).

Asthma is characterized by reversible airway obstruction: The airways narrow because of smooth muscle contraction, airway inflammation, and bronchial hyperresponsiveness (National Heart, Lung, and Blood Institute [NHLBI], 1997). Symptoms include wheezing, coughing, dyspnea, and chest tightness (McFadden & Gilbert, 1992). Its course is variable, with periods of remission and exacerbation, but it is not progressive. Asthma exacerbations may develop slowly or more quickly in response to triggers such as exercise, strong emotions, laughter, cold air, temperature changes, allergens, cat dander, or strong smells. There is a significant but complex genetic component to asthma; some genetic predisposition is probably necessary to develop asthma, but not all persons who are genetically predisposed will develop asthma (Mrazek & Klinnert, 1991; Mrazek, Klinnert, Mrazek, & Macey, 1991).

Upper Respiratory Infection

Upper respiratory tract infections (URIs or the common cold) are caused by one of over 200 viruses and are highly communicable. Because of the number of viruses involved, people do not develop immunity to colds, as they may do with other viral diseases; adults experience 2–5 colds per year, totaling nearly 66 million annual cases of the common cold in the United States (Adams & Marano, 1995).

Chronic Obstructive Pulmonary Disease

Chronic obstructive pulmonary disease (COPD) was the fourth leading cause of death in the United States in 1996 (Centers for Disease Control, 1997). COPD is a general term that includes the conditions of chronic bronchitis and emphysema. Chronic bronchitis involves excessive mucus production for several consecutive years; infections and dyspnea are common. Emphysema involves both distension and destruction of certain lung structures, leading to loss of lung elasticity necessary for breathing. COPD may be differentiated from asthma by several factors: Asthma is intermittent, reversible, aggravated by extrinsic triggers such as allergens, and has a relatively acute onset; COPD is chronic, progressive, unresponsive to allergens, and has an insidious onset. However, both COPD and asthma involve shortness of breath, coughing, wheezing, increased secretions, and obstruction in the small airways.

COPD is more common among males. Although onset is insidious, symptoms generally present at ages 40–50 years. The primary risk factor is a history of cigarette smoking, at least 20 pack years, but often 40–60 pack years (pack years = number of packs per day × the number of years smoking). Recurrent bronchial infections and a certain congenital abnormality (i.e., alpha-one antitrypsin deficiency) also may lead to COPD.

Obstructive Sleep Apnea

The collapse or closure of the upper airway during sleep characterizes obstructive sleep apnea (OSA). Sleep arousal generally stops the apneic event; a diagnosis of OSA typically requires at least five apneic events per night. Repeatedly interrupted sleep likely contributes to the daytime sleepiness common among patients with OSA (Guilleminault, 1987), and loud snoring is a hallmark of OSA. Guilleminault noted that the snores of patients with OSA have been reported to be around 65 decibels, above the Occupational Safety and Health Administration's criterion for a safe noise level in the workplace. Thus, the snoring of patients with OSA can contribute to hearing loss and sleep disruptions for patients and their sleeping partners.

The onset of OSA is usually in the 40–60 years age range, with the condition being eight times more common among men than women (Nasser & Rees, 1992). Obesity is another important risk factor for OSA. OSA and COPD often co-occur.

Lung Cancer

Lung cancer is the leading fatal cancer (Wingo, Ries, Rosenberg, Miller, & Edwards, 1998). Malignant neoplasms (cancers) were the second most common cause of death in the United States in 1996 (Centers for Disease Control, 1997). Lung cancers are much more common among men than women (5:1). It is the most common form of cancer for men and has surpassed breast cancer in prevalence among women (Rozenberg, Liebens, Kroll, & Vandromme, 1996). The primary reason for this increase is the rapid growth in cigarette smoking in developing countries (Du et al., 1996; Lazcano-Ponce, Tovar-Guzman, Meneses-Gonzalez, Rascon-Pancheco, & Hernandez-Avila, 1997). Risk factors for lung cancer include smoking; environmental pollutants and industrial exposure; and socioeconomic factors such as urban residence, less education, and lower socioeconomic status (Horne & Picard, 1979). Because only about 20% of smokers develop lung cancer, genetic factors also may play a role (Bartsch & Hietanen, 1996; Groeger et al., 1997). The symptoms associated with lung cancer depend on the site and the stage of the disease; prognosis depends on similar factors, as well as the type of the malignancy.

Cystic Fibrosis

Cystic fibrosis (CF) is an autosomal recessive genetic illness that is characterized by digestive and respiratory problems. Common symptoms are increased production of mucus, sweat, and saliva that obstruct air passages and passageways that carry pancreatic enzymes into the small intestines. CF is a progressive disease that often leads to bronchial inelasticity, chronic infection, and lung scarring; most CF patients die of chronic lung disease. It is the most common life-threatening hereditary disease among White children (Centers for Disease Control, 1997): Between 20,000 and 25,000 persons had CF in the United States in 1995 (Cystic Fibrosis Foundation, 1996). The incidence of CF among live births is about 1 in 3,400 for White and 1 in 12,200 for nonwhite (Kosorok, Wei, & Farrell, 1996).

The illness is always fatal. Although the longevity for CF patients has been increasing in recent years and many patients survive into adulthood, the median life span is still only 29 years (Rosenstein & Zeitlin, 1995). With increased longevity, a sizable portion of individuals with CF establish committed relationships (20% from Levine & Stern, 1982; 31% from Gillen, Lallas, Brown, Yelin, & Blanc, 1995).

Tuberculosis

Tuberculosis (TB), an infection caused by *mycobacterium tuberculosis*, may be widely disseminated throughout the body but primarily affects the lungs. Common symptoms include fatigue, loss of weight and appetite, night sweat and fever, and a persistent cough with bloodstained sputum. The pathogenesis of TB involves localized areas of lung tissue destroyed by the infection. Scarlike fibrous tissue forms to repair the damage, which in turn decreases lung elasticity and impairs breathing. Massive hemorrhages may occur as the disease advances and destroys the lung tissue; death is common if the disease is untreated. Aerosolized droplets that are expelled when talking, coughing, or sneezing spread TB.

TB is generally recognized in adulthood. Nearly 23,000 cases of TB were identified in the United States in 1995, the lowest rate of TB reported in the United States since surveillance began in 1953. However, 36% of all cases occurred among foreign-born persons (Centers for Disease Control, 1996b), and the proportion of cases among foreign-born persons has increased in the past decade. TB is found especially among those infected with HIV, because individuals with weak immune systems are particularly susceptible to TB infection (Schneider & Rosen, 1996). Men account for about two thirds of the cases.

ASSOCIATION OF ILLNESS AND COUPLE FACTORS

Our review of the association between respiratory illnesses and intimate relationship factors is organized around three factors: couple status (e.g., single vs. married), relationship satisfaction, and couple interaction (e.g., Burman & Margolin, 1992). These factors or levels of inquiry are related to one another. Couples characterized by positive interactions with one another (e.g., positive affect, more agreements, less criticisms) are likely to have greater relationship satisfaction (greater self-evaluations of relationship quality). Couple status may change from partnered to separated if couple interactions and relationship satisfaction decline. However, the association of specific relationship behaviors and respiratory illness has been studied only among couples in which one person has asthma.

Asthma

Couple Status

Asthma occurs among people who are single and in couples in similar proportions (Lindegard, 1989). Marriage and subsequent adjustment to life as a couple may be associated with the identification of asthma among susceptible persons. The first 3 years of marriage (or a new member in the family) have been associated with insidious-onset asthma (Teiramaa, 1981). There is evidence that asthma can be triggered by stress (Lehrer, 1998): The stress of a newly committed relationship and concomitant life adjustments may be associated with the first detection of asthma among persons predisposed to its development.

Relationship Satisfaction

There has been limited research concerning the extent to which asthma affects and is affected by relationship satisfaction. In a study of 46 couples in which 1 partner had mild-to-moderate asthma, 27% of the variability in patients' relationship satisfaction was predicted by asthma severity and use of asthma medications (Schmaling, Afari, Barnhart, & Buchwald, 1997). Bronchial reactivity but not airflow limitation was associated with relationship satisfaction, so having more severe but better controlled asthma was associated with more relationship satisfaction. Better medication adherence may lead to better asthma control, despite worse illness severity. Better care of one's asthma may be associated with more relationship satisfaction.

Schmaling, McKnight and Afari (2000) examined the associations of psychosocial variables to pulmonary function over an average of 4 months. Thirty-two participants provided daily ratings of mood and stress (e.g., intimate relationship stress) and measured pulmonary function. Within-subjects autoregression analyses revealed that psychosocial variables were significantly related to pulmonary function among 16 (50%) participants. In particular, intimate relationship stress was a significant predictor of pulmonary function among 4 of 32 participants. Among 1 participant, greater relationship stress was associated with better pulmonary function; among the remaining 3 participants, less relationship stress was associated with better pulmonary function. The inconsistent and sometimes counterintuitive results of these studies suggest that further work is needed to examine other covariates that may illuminate the association between relationship stress and pulmonary function.

Couple Interaction

Two studies have demonstrated that interacting with one's intimate partner in the laboratory can have significant effects on pulmonary function. Schmaling et al. (1996) reviewed six case studies of couples in which one person had severe asthma. Couples discussed relationship-related topics; the person with asthma also completed measures of pulmonary function before and after the interaction tasks. These couple interactions, which lasted about 20 minutes, led to improvements in pulmonary function for 2 patients of about 1 standard deviation in magnitude and decrements in pulmonary function (ranging from about $1/2$ to nearly 2 standard deviations) for the remainder. These case studies suggest that among some patients with asthma, interacting with one's partner is associated with significant changes in pulmonary function.

Similar interaction tasks were used to examine which task-related moods and behavior were associated with change in pulmonary function among 50 couples in which one person had mild-to-moderate asthma (Schmaling, Afari, Hops, Barnhart, & Buchwald, 2000). As in the Schmaling et al. (1996) study, the participants with asthma measured their pulmonary function before and after the interaction tasks with their partners. Change in pulmonary function was significantly related to anxiety: Bronchoconstriction was associated with more anxiety. More stable (less variable) pulmonary function was associated with more active coping and problem-solving behavior.

Summary

The stress of a new marriage may be associated with the first recognition of asthma with an insidious onset. Studies of the association between asthma-related factors and relationship satisfaction suggest that persons with satisfied relationships take better care of their asthma. The assessment of relationship stress and pulmonary function over time, without experimental intervention, has yielded inconsistent results. Acutely anxiety-provoking relationship situations occurring in the laboratory produced decreased pulmonary function. On the other hand, active problem solving during stressful situations appeared to reduce pulmonary sensitivity to the stress. Further work to directly measure the physiological processes (e.g., sympathetic vs. parasympathetic activation) that mediate the associations between stress (acute and chronic), mood, and asthma is needed.

Upper Respiratory Infection

Couple Status

Although no studies have examined specifically the association between relationship status and URIs, several studies have looked at psychosocial factors that may affect susceptibility to the common cold. In a series of ingenious studies, Cohen, Doyle, Skoner, Rabin, and Gwaltney (1997) and Cohen, Tyrrell, and Smith (1991, 1993) studied groups of healthy participants who were given nasal drops containing one of five respiratory viruses; additional control participants were given saline nasal drops. The participants were then quarantined and monitored for the development of infection and symptoms. Results from the 1997 study indicated that those participants with more kinds of social ties, including partners, were less susceptible to common colds. In fact, there was a dose–response relationship between greater diversity in social network and reduced susceptibility to colds. Introversion was associated with greater susceptibility to colds. Smoking, poor sleep quality, alcohol abstinence, low dietary intake of vitamin C, and elevated catecholamine levels (a measure of stress) mediated the relationship between social ties and susceptibility to colds.

Another study compared participants' self-reported cold symptoms with ratings by a physician who was unaware of participants' ratings (Macintyre & Pritchard, 1989). Male participants perceived their cold symptoms as significantly more severe than did female participants. Although not statistically different, single participants tended to overrate the severity of their colds in comparison with participants in relationships.

Relationship Satisfaction

Recent stressful life events, including family-related events, are related to cold onset (Evans & Edgerton, 1991; Stone, Porter, & Neale, 1993). In a prospective study of 79 couples (Stone et al., 1993), desirable and undesirable events in the 5 days before the onset of a URI were predictive of URI symptoms. Family events such as arguments with the partner accounted for the largest proportion of both desirable and undesirable events.

Summary

Being single, having small social networks, and stressful relationship events can be risk factors for developing URIs in persons exposed to URI-causing viruses.

Chronic Obstructive Pulmonary Disease

Couple Status

Smoking tobacco is an important risk factor in the development of COPD or lung cancer. Being single has been linked to high smoking rates (Manfredi, Lacey, Warnecke, & Buis, 1992). Frost, Tollestrup, and Starzyk (1994) found that smoking during the last 15 years of life was associated with divorced status as well as death from lung cancer or COPD. Thus, being a smoker and single may be associated with a high risk for COPD.

Relationship Satisfaction

Among a sample of 82 patients with mild-to-moderate COPD, women tended to report less satisfaction with their relationship than did age- and sex-matched control groups; male COPD patients' relationship satisfaction did not differ from that of control patients (Isoaho, Keistinen, Laippala, and Kivela, 1995). Unger, Jacobs, & Cannon (1996) studied 100 couples with mixed respiratory diagnoses in which COPD prevailed. Global relationship satisfaction was in the satisfied range for this sample. Support from family was associated with better relationship satisfaction of the patients (of both genders) and also for female partners but not for male partners. Support from friends was associated with better relationship satisfaction among male patients in shorter but not longer relationships. This study suggests that larger, supportive social networks help sustain the relationship satisfaction of couples in which one person has COPD; limitations included self-reported medical diagnoses and the lack of objective measures of disease severity, which may have affected the variables of interest.

Other studies have examined the satisfaction level of the partners of patients with COPD. Forty-six female partners of male COPD patients reported that they had more stress and less life satisfaction, had taken on more tasks, and had less sexual activity than did 30 women with healthy partners (Sexton & Munro, 1985). Fifty-four percent of the couples reported that they no longer engaged in any sexual activity. Hanson (1982) studied a group of 128 participants, predominantly 40–70-year-old partnered men, with asthma, emphysema, or a combination (asthma, emphysema, and chronic bronchitis). Participants were asked about the importance and effects of lung disease on various aspects of life. Whereas 91% of participants reported that lung disease was very important to their life in general, 74% reported that it was important to the sexual aspects of their relationship, and

89% believed it to be important for the emotional aspects of their relationship. The authors attributed this difference to the participants' age, reflecting decreased importance of sexual functioning and increased importance of emotional aspects of the relationship. Several studies have noted impotence and decreased sexual activity among men with COPD, a potential source of relationship dissatisfaction among couples.

Lane and Hobfoll (1992) studied the effects of COPD-related symptoms on patient and supporter anger. Specific emotional reactions to illness reflect somewhat different aspects of a relationship than global relationship satisfaction, yet they are often related. Seventy-eight patients with COPD and their supporters were assessed at two points in time, 3 months apart. More COPD symptoms at Time 1 significantly predicted more anger at Time 2, over and above Time 1 anger. In turn, patient anger and irritability were associated with increased supporter anger. Angry reactions to COPD may lead to continually eroding emotional health for both patients and partners over time, which may ultimately contribute to withdrawal of support. Note that 68% of the supporters were partners. The data for the patient–partner dyads were not presented separately from the data of other sorts of supporter relationships (friend, parent, sibling), so the results are not entirely representative of relationships with intimate partners.

Summary

Being single has been associated with high smoking rates in general and specifically with smoking in the last 15 years of life (associated with COPD). Women with COPD report less relationship satisfaction than do healthy women. Female partners of male COPD patients report greater stress and less relationship satisfaction than do women with healthy partners. COPD appears to diminish sexual functioning in men. Anger and irritability about COPD can negatively affect the patient and partner. For all patients, support from family and others can help maintain better relationship satisfaction.

Obstructive Sleep Apnea

Couple Status

Loud snoring is a frequent clinical feature of OSA. In a study of over 5,000 participants 65 years of age and older, 33% of the men and 17% of the women reported loud snoring; OSA was confirmed in 13% of men and 4% of women (Enright et al., 1996). In this study, both loud snoring and OSA were associated with relationship status among men but not among women. Men who had partners reported more loud snoring and were more likely to have OSA than single men.

Relationship Satisfaction

OSA has been called a "disease of listeners": Bed partners report displeasure with snoring, the primary clinical feature of OSA (Bonekat & Krumpe, 1990). Patient and partner reports of snoring and other symptoms of OSA concur modestly with interesting gender differences: For men, partners (women) reported significantly more snoring than did patients, whereas for women, partners (men) reported much less snoring than did patients (Wiggins, Schmidt-Nowara, Coultas, & Samet, 1990).

Cartwright and Knight (1987) characterized relationship and family responsibilities as "an added burden" (p. 244) for patients with OSA. They assessed patient and partner relationship satisfaction and measures of social adjustment and emotional distress among 10 couples. These latter measures were compared with those of 10 divorced patients with OSA. Patients with OSA and their partners were more socially isolated and depressed than were divorced patients with OSA. The Marital Satisfaction Inventory (MSI; Snyder, 1979; Snyder, Lachar, & Wills, 1988) profiles, completed by the partners only, indicated more global distress and conflicts related to child rearing compared with normative values. OSA has been repeatedly linked to erectile difficulties among male patients (Guilleminault, 1987). Couple and family responsibilities may exacerbate rather than buffer the impact of OSA.

Summary

Men in relationships seem more likely to have loud snoring and OSA than single men, possibly because of greater symptom reports by a partner. In addition, women (patients or partners) seem more likely to report snoring than men. Partners of OSA patients report greater global relationship distress than those living with healthy persons. Patients must contend with their OSA as well as the challenges of partner dissatisfaction and problems with sexual functioning.

Lung Cancer

Couple Status

Most studies assessing the risk for the development of subsequent lung cancer suggest that smokers not in relationships are at greater risk for the development of lung cancer than smokers in relationships (Burnley, 1992; Chiazze, Watkins, & Fryar, 1992; Frost et al., 1994).

Having an intimate partner seems to be critical for survival and quality of life while living with lung cancer (Ganz, Lee, & Siau, 1991). During the terminal phase of the illness, effective support from partners can enhance the patients' psychological adjustment (Goldberg & Wool, 1985).

Relationship Satisfaction

Many patients with lung cancer and their partners adapt well without professional psychosocial involvement (Goldberg & Wool, 1985). Social network seems to be a more critical factor than health or physical status in the psychosocial adjustment of the partner (Goldberg, Wool, Glicksman, & Tull, 1984). Given that smoking is associated with lung cancer, the bulk of the literature in this area has focused on the relationship between family and relationship factors and smoking cessation (see chapter 11, by Palmer, Baucom, and McBride, in this volume).

Summary

The majority of reseach suggests that single smokers are at greater risk for developing lung cancer than smokers with partners. In addition, being in a relationship is associated with improved survival from lung cancer and better psychological adjustment during the terminal phase of the illness. Little research exists on the association between relationship satisfaction and lung cancer variables. The existing literature suggests that patients and partners adapt well to the relationship consequences of the illness.

Cystic Fibrosis

Couple Status

Few CF patients are in relationships, given their relatively short life expectancy. Because more men survive into adulthood (Rosenfeld, Davis, FitzSimmons, Pepe, & Ramsey, 1997), more men with CF are in relationships than women with CF. Patients in relationships are generally older at the age of CF diagnosis and have better pulmonary functioning (Coffman, Levine, Althof, & Stern, 1984).

Relationship Satisfaction

Most of the literature on relationship satisfaction and CF focuses on parental couple satisfaction when a child in the family has CF (see chapter 12, Gaither, Bingen, and Hopkins, in this volume). The literature regarding the relationships of adults with CF has focused on the sexual adjustment of CF patients in relationships. Generally, there is no association between sexual functioning and illness severity; sexual problems, if any, are related to lack of desire (Coffman et al., 1984; Levine & Stern, 1982) and are most common among women patients. Among 48 single adult patients with CF and 55 age-similar single healthy persons, female patients reported significantly lower levels of desire than healthy women; however, CF and healthy male participants were similar in terms of sexual milestones and activity (Coffman et al., 1984).

In a study of CF patients and caregivers, including parents and partners, 45% of partners reported experiencing moderate or high caregiver burden (Patton et al., 1997). This same group of researchers studied the partners of 26 adult patients with CF and found that the partners showed comparable or greater levels of psychological distress than did patients: Fatigue was the most frequent problem among the partners (Patton et al., 1998).

Summary

Patients with CF in relationships seem to have better pulmonary function than single patients. Among partnered patients, those who report sexual problems tend to be women; decreased sexual desire is the most commonly noted problem. There is significant caregiver burden on partners of CF patients, which may be affected by relationship factors. Fatigue is the most frequent partner complaint; perhaps partner fatigue may affect the patient's sexual desire? This hypothetical association and other possible associations between relationship variables and CF variables await future research efforts.

Tuberculosis

The diagnosis and treatment of TB in one partner has been found to lead to divorce or broken engagements; this phenomenon occurs more frequently among women with TB than men (Liefooghe, Michiels, Habib, Moran, & DeMuynck, 1995). To date, there have been no studies of the relationship satisfaction of couples in which one person has TB.

Summary of Illnesses

This review of respiratory illnesses and intimate relationship factors indicates a marked lack of research. Only among couples with asthma have the effects of the couple interaction been examined in terms of pulmonary function. People in relationships are less likely to have asthma, lung cancer, or CF than are single people. However, OSA has been found to be more common among men with partners than among single men, but this could be confounded with the increased likelihood of men's bed partners bringing the symptoms to medical attention. Data regarding the associations between respiratory illnesses and relationship satisfaction were more commonly found in the literature. In general, global relationship distress is associated with illness. However, only a few studies have examined the direction of these effects, and most studies rely on retrospective reports of relationship events vis-à-vis respiratory illnesses. These studies indicate that premorbid relationship events (e.g., the adjustment to becoming a committed couple) may prompt illness among persons with intermittent respiratory conditions (e.g., URIs or asthma). Conversely, it appears that living with chronic and severe respiratory problems (e.g., CF, OSA, or COPD) may lead to decreased relationship satisfaction for both patient and partner. In particular, sexual dysfunction or lack of sexual desire was noted to be associated with these conditions. The effects of the burden of the illness on the healthy partner have received scant attention and are worthy of future research, as are more studies using prospective designs.

ASSESSMENT

Medical

Pulmonary Function Tests

Airflow can be assessed easily through spirometry or pulmonary function testing. In their simplest form, these tests consist of a maximum effort of exhaling as hard and as fast as possible, after a full inspiration. Three important parameters are derived from these tests. Forced expiratory volume in the first second of the exhalation (FEV_1) is expressed as the volume of liters of air expelled in this time period. This parameter is decreased in COPD, symptomatic asthma, and CF. The vital capacity (FVC) is the total, maximum volume of air exhaled after a maximal inspiration. The ratio of FEV_1/FVC indicates airflow limitation, to the extent it is decreased.

Lung volume varies as a function of age, gender, and height. It increases until the mid-30s and then decreases with age, increases with height, and is nearly one third greater in men than in women of the same height and age.

Chest Radiographs

Chest radiographs (X rays) are important in the diagnosis of several of the conditions described in this chapter. For example, patients with TB, CF, COPD, or lung cancer have abnormal chest radiographs; however, most asthma patients have normal studies (O'Connor & Weiss, 1994). Scarring and inflammation of the lung tissue in TB, CF, and COPD and the presence of malignant masses in the lung are easily detected.

Laboratory Tests

TB is diagnosed through cultured samples of the patient's sputum; the determination of which combination of medications a specific strain of the organism is and is not resistant to determines subsequent medical treatment. In the case of asthma, the assessment of serum IgE concentration can be used as a measure of allergic sensitization leading to asthma and the efficacy of allergen avoidance interventions (O'Connor & Weiss, 1994).

Other Medical Tests

Arterial blood gas measurements such as concentration of oxygen (PO_2) and carbon dioxide (PCO_2) correlate modestly with pulmonary function during acute asthma exacerbations. Elevations of PCO_2 are generally seen in the presence of ventilatory impairment and predict the need for artificial ventilation (O'Connor & Weiss, 1994). Arterial blood gas measurements also are used in assessing the severity of COPD.

Behavioral–Psychological

Assessment of Airflow

The peak flow meter is a portable device (approximately 8 in. in length and a few ounces in weight) often used to monitor airflow in patients with asthma. Peak flow meters are available from medical supply companies and cost about $10; no physician prescription is needed. The peak flow maneuver is similar to the forced expiratory maneuver that produces FEV_1; peak flow correlates highly with FEV_1 (cf. Connolly & Chan, 1987). Typically, patients are told to do three peak expiratory maneuvers and record the highest number. A behavioral-monitoring program may involve recording peak flows on a regular basis (e.g., before medications, on awakening, and before bedtime) and as needed, to verify the need for reliever (or rescue) medication (see below). A chart of normal peak flow values by gender, age, and height is typically enclosed with a new peak flow meter to be used as a guideline for below-normal values. However, for patients with more severe asthma, it may be preferable to establish a baseline of their "personal best," on which they base the decision to take extra medication, rather than population norms.

Assessment of Medication Adherence

Patients with respiratory problems may be prescribed multiple kinds of inhaled or oral medications (see the review below). In particular, inhaled medications delivered by a metered dose inhaler (MDI) are subject to poor behavioral technique. The position of the MDI vis-à-vis the mouth, head and neck position, timing of the inhalation through the actuation (releasing) of the medication, length of breath holding, and time elapsed between doses all affect medication delivery, absorption and, consequently, effectiveness. Poor technique may lead to undertreatment and poor control of illness. Behavioral scientists can observe their patients' usual technique and offer feedback. An exemplary publication from the NHLBI's National Asthma

Education Program (1991) outlines the steps involved in the correct use of MDIs and includes pictures of appropriate positioning. Dry powder inhalers may take less coordination than MDIs. Other devices may ease the use of regular MDIs. A spacer or holding chamber is attached to a regular MDI, the medication is actuated into it, and the patient inhales, so no coordination of actuation and inhalation is needed. Interpersonal issues, such as embarrassment about taking medications in front of others or not wanting to worry the partner, may be important factors in nonadherence and should be assessed.

Questionnaires

There have been no questionnaires developed that address the special concerns of couples with respiratory difficulties or relationship issues among persons with respiratory difficulties. Several questionnaires specific to asthma have useful scales to assess relevant interpersonal issues for some patients. Also, questionnaires that assess relationship satisfaction are well suited for use among persons with respiratory difficulties.

The Dyadic Adjustment Scale (DAS; Spanier, 1976) and the MSI (Snyder, 1979; Snyder et al., 1988) are two of the most commonly used self-report relationship questionnaires. The DAS is a 32-item instrument designed to assess the quality of the relationship, as perceived by the couple. The total score can be used as a global measure of satisfaction in an intimate relationship. The instrument also assesses four aspects of the relationship: dyadic satisfaction, dyadic cohesion, dyadic consensus, and affectional expression. The DAS can be used to assess commitment and willingness to work on the relationship. The MSI is a multidimensional self-report measure of couple interaction with one validity scale, one global affective scale, and nine additional scales that focus on specific areas of couple interaction. There are normative data from nondistressed, distressed, and divorcing couples' profiles on the MSI; furthermore, two partners' evaluation of the relationship can be compared. Both the DAS and MSI can elucidate specific relationship factors or activities, such as household tasks and matters of recreation, affected by one partner's respiratory problems.

The Knowledge, Attitude, and Self-Efficacy Asthma Questionnaire (Wigal et al., 1993) is a 60-item self-report questionnaire that was developed to assess asthma patients' attitudes, knowledge, and confidence in their ability to manage the illness. Whereas the Knowledge subscale may be an indicator of lack of understanding about what to do to prevent or manage asthma, the Attitude and Self-Efficacy subscale scores can be affected by the patients' partners' stance with respect to the illness. Items such as "My family can help me get the upper hand on my asthma" and "I feel OK about asking for help during asthma attacks when I need to" can be used to explore relationship factors that may be affecting the patients' attitude and self-efficacy concerning asthma management.

Respiratory illnesses affect quality of life, which in turn can affect intimate relationships, as well as the patients' use of medications and medical services. The Asthma Quality of Life Questionnaire (Marks, Dunn, & Woolcock, 1992) is a 20-item questionnaire with Breathlessness, Mood Disturbance, Social Disruption, and Concerns for Health subscales. The Social Disruption items include statements such as "Asthma has interfered with my social life" and "I've been restricted in the sports, hobbies, or other activities I can engage in because of my asthma," limitations that can significantly affect the patients' as well as the couples' lifestyle.

Negative affect (Priel, Heimer, Rabinowitz, & Hendler, 1994), anxiety (Kinsman, Dirks, & Jones, 1982), and depression (Janson, Bjornsson, Hetta, & Boman, 1994), all of which can be instigated by relationship difficulties, have been shown to affect perceptions of symptom severity in asthma. Perceptions of severity may in turn affect management of these symptoms and medical utilization. Thus, the use of psychological distress measures can be beneficial in a comprehensive assessment of patients with respiratory difficulties. The Brief Symptom Inventory (BSI; Derogatis, 1993) is a 53-item self-report symptom inventory designed to assess the psychological distress status of psychiatric and medical patients. The BSI is the shorter form of the Symptom Checklist-90 (Derogatis & Cleary, 1977). The primary symptom dimensions measured by the BSI are Somatization, Obsessive–Compulsive, Interpersonal Sensitivity, Depression, Anxiety, Hostility, Phobic Anxiety, Paranoid Ideation, and Psychoticism. This instrument has been used widely in the assessment of psychological distress related to physiological stress and illness (cf. Derogatis, 1993). Patients' as well as partners' psychological distress, as measured by the BSI, can affect patients' perceptions of health functioning and medical utilization (Afari & Schmaling, in press).

The Medical Outcomes Study (MOS; Tarlov et al., 1989) was a 2-year observational study designed to understand how specific aspects of the health care system affect the outcome of medical care. As part of this study, a Short-Form Health Survey (SF–36; Ware & Sherbourne, 1992) was developed to measure heath status and well-being in over 9,000 adults. Since then, the SF–36 has been used extensively in research and clinical practice. The SF–36 assesses eight domains related to health problems: Physical Functioning, Role-Physical, Bodily Pain, Social Functioning, Mental Health, Role-Emotional, Vitality, and General Health. In the MOS, people with chronic lung problems had significantly lower scores on all scales of the SF–36 than the patients with no chronic conditions (Stewart et al., 1989). In addition, better quality of life, as measured by the SF–36 scales, has been associated with better pulmonary functioning in asthma patients (Bousquet et al., 1994). As with previously discussed measures, the social functioning items can be used to explore relationship issues with respect to patient's health functioning.

TREATMENT

Medical

Medical treatment varies widely with illness. A comprehensive review of possible treatment regimens indicated for each respiratory illness is beyond the scope of this chapter, so we offer instead a brief overview of the treatments most commonly used for each illness and the potential interpersonal ramifications associated with each approach.

Medication

Asthma may be classified into several levels of severity; matching medications with severity level or step is consistent with practice guidelines (NHLBI, 1997). Asthma medications may be separated into *controller* and *reliever* (or rescue) medications. Examples of the former are corticosteroids taken long term in inhaled (e.g., flunisolide) or oral (e.g., prednisone) forms that are used to decrease inflammation. Examples of reliever medications are inhaled, short-acting beta$_2$ agonists (e.g., albuterol) that relieve acute bronchospasm by relaxing the smooth muscles. Mild asthma, characterized by mild intermittent symptoms, may be treated effectively with as needed use of reliever medications. Severe persistent asthma usually requires regular use of controller and reliever medications. The medication regimen for patients with COPD also varies with severity and may include the controller and reliever medications described above, as well as oxygen therapy (see below) among patients with significant airflow limitations. TB requires a multidrug regimen after in vitro drug susceptibility testing identifies the drug combination most effective to treat an individual patient's organism (Centers for Disease Control, 1993). Because a major cause of drug resistance (e.g., in the treatment of TB) and treatment failure is nonadherence with prescribed treatment, the direct observation of medication ingestion may be indicated to ensure adequate treatment and decrease public health risk.

Patterns of medication use and adherence have been associated with relationship status and satisfaction. In a 2-year study of adherence with an inhaled medication regimen (ipratropium bromide or placebo) among nearly 4,000 participants with COPD, satisfactory or better adherence was found among 48% of the sample. The most consistent predictor of adherence was relationship status; patients in relationships were about 1.5 times more likely to adhere than single patients (Rand, Nides, Cowles, Wise, & Connett, 1995). Asthma patients with high life stress and little social support were found to require nearly three times the daily dose of prednisone as those with similarly high life stress but abundant social support, after controlling for illness severity (De Araujo, Van Arsdel, Holmes, & Dudley, 1973).

Long-Term Oxygen Therapy

Oxygen therapy improves survival (Nocturnal Oxygen Therapy Trial Group, 1980), neurocognitive functioning (Krop, Block, & Cohen, 1973), and functional status among patients with COPD. Oxygen therapy is often experienced as cumbersome and limiting by the patient; it requires the use of portable oxygen canisters and nasal cannulas. Wearing the cannulas is an adjustment, as is the vigilance required to ensure that adequate oxygen is available in the portable canisters.

Lung Transplant

Lung transplant is an invasive, intensive treatment for patients with end-stage lung diseases who have been unresponsive to medical treatment (Patterson, 1997). The lung conditions that are potentially appropriate for transplantation include obstructive diseases (e.g., COPD) and suppurative diseases (e.g., CF; Smith, 1997).

Lung transplants are performed at about 70 centers in the United States (Smith, 1997). There are more potential lung recipients than available organs. For example, between 1988 and 1992, the number of registrants waiting for a lung increased 1,277%, and during 1991, the median wait for an organ was 291 days (Edwards, Breen, Guo, Ellison, & Daily, 1992). Twelve percent to 30% (Edwards et al., 1992; Smith, 1997) of potential lung transplant recipients die while waiting for an organ. The waiting process is emotionally challenging for the partners of the patients; longer waits for a heart transplant were associated with greater negative impact and stress on the patients' partners (Collins, White, & Jalowiec, 1996), attributable to the partners shouldering more family responsibilities during the waiting period.

Transplantation is considered appropriate when the patient's functional status is low, life expectancy is limited to 1 or 2 years, and the condition has been unresponsive to medical treatment. Transplant candidates are evaluated carefully before they are placed on a waiting list for an organ. Standard pretransplant evaluation guidelines include medical and psychosocial issues (L. W. Miller et al., 1995; Smith, 1997). The social support network of the patient is a crucial component of the evaluation (Craven, Bright, & Dear, 1990). Programs generally require that patients have someone who can accompany and assist them until they have recovered from the procedure (Craven et al., 1990). A survey of 84 physicians from 52 transplant programs revealed that 81% felt that "no social support system" should be an absolute or potential contraindication for a heart transplant (L. W. Miller et al., 1995). For comparison purposes, over 90% felt that current alcohol or tobacco abuse or Axis II psychiatric disorders were absolute or potential contraindications.

Chacko, Harper, Kunik, and Young (1996) found that among 31 lung or heart–lung transplant patients, 52% had partners, and 68% and 23% met criteria for an Axis I or Axis II diagnosis, respectively. Lung transplant patients with an Axis I disorder were more likely to have impaired home functioning and sexual problems than patients without an Axis I disorder. Relationship satisfaction was most impaired among lung transplant patients with both Axis I and Axis II disorders and least impaired among those without such disorders. In summary, the presence of psychiatric disorders is related to dissatisfied intimate relationships and poor functioning in the home environment among lung transplant patients.

Lung transplants are not a panacea. Comparisons of the 2-year survival rates among patients with COPD and CF who did versus who did not receive a transplant indicate a 13% advantage in the transplanted sample (59% vs. 72% survival rate for COPD; 50% vs. 63% for CF). However, after a lung transplant, recipients' quality of life improves dramatically. Nearly 3 years after transplant, functional status was within the normal range among 59 lung recipients (Littlefield et al., 1996). A caveat to these encouraging results should be noted: 69% of these 59 transplant recipients were in relationships. The recipients also were asked to estimate the improvement in their quality of life after transplantation in eight areas. Whereas the participants rated their overall quality of life as 98% improved, the lowest relative areas of improvement were noted for sex life and intimate relationship (both 47% improved). Relatively less improvement in intimate relationships may be due to the emotional, instrumental, and financial drain imposed by the transplantation procedure and its preparation and recovery periods. Partners may assume the transplant will fix the patient's problems (Craven et al., 1990); negative feelings may occur when recovery is not quick, dramatic, or complete.

Treatment for OSA

The most common treatments for OSA are surgery and continuous positive airway pressure (CPAP; Guilleminault, 1987). The surgical procedure of uvulopalatopharyngoplasty involves the removal of redundant tissue that may contribute to airway blockage. CPAP involves wearing a mask, in which air pressure is delivered to keep the upper airway from collapsing, while sleeping. The CPAP apparatus may be experienced as uncomfortable or unbearable (among patients with claustrophobia), leading to poor treatment adherence.

Trials of CPAP for the treatment of OSA have been found to effectively reverse the chronic hypoxemia associated with OSA, resulting in less neurocognitive difficulties. CPAP also relieved impaired nocturnal penile tumescence among 5 of 15 men with OSA (Karacan & Karatas, 1995). OSA may contribute to erectile dysfunction through lowering testosterone. Seven patients with OSA and consequent decreased sexual interest and serum testosterone who underwent uvulopalatopharyngoplasty were found to have less apnea, renewed sexual interest, normal sexual functioning, and increased serum testosterone 3 months after the procedure (Santamaria, Prior, & Fleetham, 1988).

Treatment for CF

A recent summary of CF treatment included the following components: enzyme replacement to correct pancreatic insufficiency; correction of nutritional and vitamin deficiencies; clearance of lower airway pulmonary obstructions; antibiotic treatment for pulmonary infections; and medications for antinflammatory, bronchodilating, and secretion thinning-and-clearing effects (Ramsey, 1996). Thus, treatment for CF is complex and time-consuming. Bilateral lung transplantation may be indicated (Patterson, 1997).

Couples Therapy

To date, we know of no trials of couples therapy for any respiratory illness or its associated difficulties or sequelae, although it has been suggested repeatedly that such interventions would be useful. For example, couple involvement in the treatment of asthma may decrease stressful dysfunctional interactions that may trigger asthma symptoms and increase the likelihood of partner support of optimal medical decision making and intervention during symptom exacerbations (Lehrer, Sargunaraj, & Hochron, 1992). Indeed, couples therapy has been termed the "treatment of choice" for patients in relationships coping poorly with COPD (Post & Collins, 1981–1982). Poor coping may be the consequence of the patient's failure to adjust expectations to be consistent with decreasing functional capacities. This failure leads to chronic frustration, anger, blaming, and emotional arousal. Post and Collins have stated that effective coping with COPD involves limiting emotional arousal in addition to modifying expectations to be consistent with functional capacity. Lane and Hobfoll's (1992) research, reviewed above, which found that patient anger seemed to escalate over time and led to increased partner anger, lends further support to the potential usefulness of limiting emotional arousal. Thus, strategies that reduce patient emotional arousal may lead to increased stability of partner availability.

Enhancing partner's knowledge of and participation in the patient's treatment also may be useful. For example, Cartwright and Knight (1987) have suggested that the partners of patients with OSA should be educated about the disorder and its treatment and directly involved in some aspects of treatment, such as weight loss. Partners often administer some aspects of treatment to patients with OSA, for example, to perform the chest clapping maneuver, to loosen secretions and enhance the patient's ability to clear the secretions, or to help oxygen-dependent patients fill their portable oxygen tanks. However, we know of no studies that have examined the effects of these sorts of partner involvement in the treatments on relationship satisfaction or examples of intervention efforts aimed at maximizing partner and patient adjustment to these processes.

Smoking cessation is the most important behavior change a person can undertake to reduce health risks, such as the development of COPD or lung cancer. Treatment outcome research on partner-involved smoking cessation is reviewed in chapter 11.

Taken together, couple interventions related to respiratory illnesses may be *partner assisted* or *disorder specific* (Baucom, Shoham, Mueser, Daiuto, & Stickle, 1998). Examples of partner-assisted treatments might include psychoeducation about the nature of the illness and its treatments and systematic training of the partner to be involved in specific aspects of treatment (e.g., how the partner can support or assist in the patient's adherence to his or her medication regimen, CPAP for OSA, weight loss, smoking cessation, exercise, or rehabilitation). Examples of disorder-specific treatments might include the inclusion of the partner in communication, problem-solving, and emotion-regulation training, to minimize stress and arousal arising from the relationship and enhance the patient's ability to modulate her or his reactions to stresses that do occur. Disorder-specific treatments may exert direct effects on the illness. For example, improving effective communication may enhance emotion modulation, thereby balancing autonomic tone and decreasing emotionally provoked bronchoconstriction among patients with asthma. Given the apparent association between relationship and illness factors, couples treatment should be emphasized in future research efforts.

Interventions designed to change target behaviors such as communication and problem-solving skills have long been the mainstays of couples therapy (Stuart, 1980). Although change-based interventions for couples are associated with improvements in many domains (see review by Baucom et al., 1998), recent work has focused on enhancing acceptance. Acceptance complements and provides another means to bring about change. Acceptance as a desired therapeutic outcome has been studied in the context of both chronic illnesses and couples therapy. Much of the literature on acceptance of illness has focused on chronic pain (Kabat-Zinn, 1984; Kabat-Zinn, Lipworth, & Burney, 1985; McCracken, 1998). In a study of 160 adults (McCracken, 1998), greater acceptance of chronic pain was associated with reports of lower pain intensity, less psychological distress, less physical and psychosocial disability, higher level of activity, and better work status. Acceptance of pain also predicted better patient functioning independent of perceived pain intensity. Kabat-Zinn (1984; Kabat-Zinn et al., 1985) has demonstrated large and significant reductions in pain perception and affective correlates of pain when patients with chronic pain practiced mindfulness meditation, a psychological stance of nonevaluative observation. These changes were present up to 1.5 years after treatment completion. Acceptance of chronic pain or illness also has been associated with greater perceived self-control (Lenhart & Ashby, 1996) and active and problem-solving coping strategies (Schuessler, 1992).

The utility of acceptance as a treatment strategy for respiratory diseases has not been studied widely. In a qualitative study of 6 adolescents with asthma, Kintner (1997) described several stages of coming to terms with having asthma: initial awareness, acknowledgment, gaining knowledge, resigned acceptance, reasoning, drawing conclusions, and acceptance. Acceptance was defined in terms of taking control over the illness and its imposed limitations, vigilance regarding the need for treatment, and openness to learning about the illness. Distinction is made between acceptance and resigned acceptance; the latter involves giving up or not having control. Another qualitative study of 30 adult asthma patients (Adams, Pill, & Jones, 1997) revealed that acceptance of the label or diagnosis of asthma was related to compliant use of controller medication.

The use of acceptance in couples therapy is most evident in Jacobson and Christensen's integrative couple therapy (ICT; Jacobson & Christensen, 1996). In ICT, emotional acceptance strategies are used in combination with more traditional behavior-change strategies, such as behavioral exchange and communication training. Emotional acceptance is defined as a shift in the interpersonal context of the relationship so that the complainant experiences a change in emotional response to a conflict in addition to or instead of a change in the problematic behavior (Koerner, Jacobson, & Christensen, 1994). Interventions like this alter the meaning of the problem behavior (coming home late no longer means rejection of the partner), increase empathy through reframing, objectify the problem into an "it" to bring the couple together against a common obstacle, increase tolerance for partners' negative behavior, and increase self-care (Koerner et al., 1994). Research is forthcoming on the efficacy of this approach.

Among couples with chronic illness, acceptance may be critical to overcoming the effects of chronic illness on relationships (McCurry & Schmidt, 1994). The definition of acceptance can include consent or agreement, unconditional positive regard, and surrender, all of which can be applied individually or within a couple or family system. McCurry and Schmidt have suggested that acceptance can help partners of people with chronic illness who view themselves as failures or inadequate or feel embarrassed, irritated, disappointed, or fearful of the effects of the illness.

We now present an example of the potential integration of partner-assisted and disorder-specific strategies, using both acceptance and change interventions, in the treatment of a couple in which one partner had asthma.

Case Example

Leslie, a 30-year-old freelance architect, had moderate asthma since childhood. At the time of the interview, Leslie's asthma was relatively well controlled through the regular use of beta agonists and inhaled steroids. Leslie's partner, Juan, a 32-year-old engineer, had no medical illnesses and was not taking any medications. Leslie and Juan had known each other for 3 years. They had been living together since their move to Seattle in the previous year, instigated by Juan's job, although Leslie was happy to have moved to the West Coast. She was interested in attending medical school and was pursuing opportunities in Seattle.

Leslie and Juan were assessed regarding their relationship functioning and its relation to Leslie's asthma. On a measure of relationship satisfaction (DAS), both Juan and Leslie received scores in the lower end of the satisfied range, with Leslie reporting less satisfaction than Juan (total DAS scores were 98 and 106, respectively). Both indicated that they occasionally to frequently disagreed on matters of recreation and leisure, time spent together, demonstration of affection, and household tasks. When asked to discuss a relationship issue, Leslie wanted to talk about the problem of not spending enough time together: "I don't feel like I get enough time or that I'm a priority. . . . When you're not working, something needs to happen to make me feel important." Leslie's biggest complaint was that Juan spent a lot of time commuting or at work. They were asked to try to solve this problem together. Their proposed solutions were rather general, included spending more time together when Juan did not have work deadlines and talking and interacting more when Juan was at home and not working. Compared with the group of 50 couples in the Schmaling et al. (2000) study, Leslie and Juan's problem-solving skills were below average. Leslie had activities that she liked and wanted Juan to participate in, but he seemed uninterested or too busy. In turn, Leslie seemed to interpret his nonparticipation as a rejection of her and felt hopeless:

> *Leslie:* I like being able to walk on the beach. I do that stuff by myself but would like it more with you.
> *Juan:* I don't have time for that stuff.
> *Leslie:* If you liked it, you'd find time for it. . . . It's [Juan's work] always going to be this busy.

Leslie's pulmonary function reduced 8% over the 15 minutes that they discussed this issue of spending time together. Thus, her emotional arousal and their poor problem-solving skills may have contributed directly to decrements in her pulmonary function.

Assessing the effects of asthma on the relationship revealed that both Leslie and Juan were frustrated by the limitations of their activities due to asthma. Leslie described asthma as "a thorn in my side . . . something to always think about." She also was frustrated by Juan's seeming not to take her illness seriously and not offering to dust and vacuum, tasks that could precipitate an asthma exacerbation. Juan was concerned about Leslie's use of asthma medications; he said, "You use the inhaler too much." In actuality, Leslie used her inhalers as prescribed. But the severity of her asthma was such that over a 4-month-long monitoring period, almost two thirds of her highest morning peak flows were more than 2 standard deviations below her expected value for someone her age and height. Thus, her asthma was not as well controlled as it could have been, and more medication use may have been appropriate. Juan's perception that she was using her inhalers too much was inaccurate. Toward the end of a discussion about her asthma, the following exchange occurred:

> *Leslie:* Maybe I use asthma as an excuse to get attention from you.
> *Juan:* So the upshot of this is you want me to clean the house more.
> *Leslie:* That would be nice.

Although Juan and Leslie did not receive treatment, this information is instructive and could be the basis for a comprehensive approach to enhancing her asthma management, their interactions, and general relationship satisfaction. In terms of partner-assisted interventions, both Leslie and Juan would benefit from further education about the pathophysiology and treatment of asthma and what could be done to minimize her symptoms, such as environmental control and medication use. A conjoint visit to Leslie's physician may have been helpful, especially if they could review her daily monitoring, which indicated that her asthma was not well controlled. The physician would likely have suggested changes in her drug treatment regimen, at which time Juan could ask questions about drugs to treat asthma, hopefully leading to more realistic and informed expectations on his part. Problem-solving training would have helped them identify more specific solutions and work out implementation plans for problems such as decreasing Leslie's exposure to house dust. Other potential solutions, beyond Juan taking over (when he was already stating he had "no time" to do and which might have further decreased their available time together) would have been identified, such as hiring cleaning help or swapping chores with neighbors.

One of the interesting features of their interaction is that Leslie desires more emotional intimacy and connection; however, she does not communicate clearly what "being a priority" to Juan might look like, and Juan interacts with her on an instrumental level. The goal of disorder-specific intervention would be to enhance Leslie's emotion regulation and acceptance skills, thereby enhancing autonomic tone and decreasing the risk of emotional "pathogens" to her asthma. Standard change techniques of communication and problem-solving training also have their role in this regard. Increasing Leslie's ability for emotionally accurate communication, for example, stating what she hopes for from Juan, would increase the likelihood that he would respond in beneficial ways for both of them. Problem-solving sessions also could focus on spending time together and how to develop shared activities interesting and enjoyable to both of them and unlikely to trigger Leslie's asthma. Emotion regulation and acceptance interventions might include enhancing Juan's empathy for Leslie's sense of loss related to her asthma and Leslie's empathy for Juan's demanding job situation, her repertoire of pleasant activities that do not require Juan's presence, and her emotion mindfulness and balancing skills (e.g., Linehan, 1993).

Leslie was contacted approximately 4 months after the above information was obtained. She reported that she had been accepted into a premedicine program on the East Coast and was moving there. Juan would stay in Seattle, with the future of their relationship unknown.

INTEGRATIVE MODEL

On the basis of the literature reviewed in this chapter, Figure 3.1 depicts a model that includes premorbid (predisposing, risk, and precipitating), physiological, and interpersonal factors and their potential interaction among persons with respiratory disorders. This general model may be applicable to the range of respiratory disorders, although data are lacking to support the hypothesized connections for many of the disorders. The model also implies potential points of couple-involved intervention: All of the risk

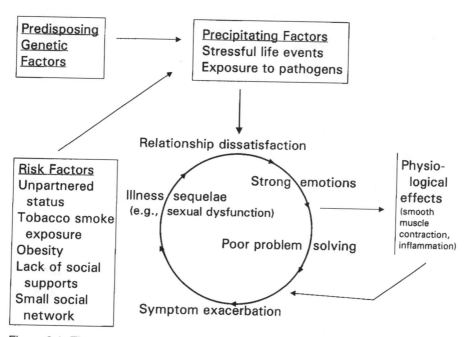

Figure 3.1. The potential role of relationship factors in respiratory illnesses.

factors and elements of the interpersonal circle are potentially modifiable variables.

As noted previously, some respiratory illnesses are associated with genetic predisposition (e.g., asthma, CF, and sometimes COPD and lung cancer), so relationships are formed long after the putative risk. However, some illnesses may be amenable to couples treatment aimed at changing the risk behavior, such as smoking cessation to decrease COPD and lung cancer and weight loss to treat OSA. Small or dissatisfying social support systems seem to be a common risk factor for respiratory illnesses. Among couples, partners could help expand the couple's support system, thereby enhancing the patient's support system. Other respiratory illnesses are associated with exposures to viral or bacterial pathogens in the environment (e.g., URIs, TB), and in some cases (i.e., URIs), the data seem to indicate that relationship stress may precipitate illness. Thus, decreasing relationship stress may avert illness.

Intermittent respiratory conditions in particular (e.g., asthma, and to some extent COPD) may be directly influenced by relationship factors. The autonomic nervous system (ANS) portion of the peripheral nervous system comprises sympathetic and parasympathetic pathways. Although the ANS was at one time believed to be outside of voluntary control, we now know that respiratory behaviors can be conditioned (e.g., D. J. Miller & Kotses, 1995) and that relaxation and some biofeedback treatments have been associated with improved pulmonary function (see Lehrer et al., 1992, for a review). Interacting with one's intimate partner is a potent source of emotional arousal. Strong emotions and passive responses to stress may be associated with bronchoconstriction through autonomic mediation (Lehrer, 1998). Skills-building interventions to improve emotion regulation, relaxation, and use of active problem-solving strategies may enhance autonomic tone, thereby decreasing smooth muscle contraction and inflammation (Lehrer, 1998; Mrazek & Klinnert, 1991). Couples treatment also may decrease the burden of the illness on the partner, benefiting the patient. For example, the partner who modulates responses to stressful relationship events may facilitate more modulated and effective responses by the patient. The efficacy of such interventions for couples coping with respiratory illnesses awaits future systematic study.

CONCLUSIONS AND FUTURE DIRECTIONS

Our review of the association between respiratory illnesses and relationship factors of status, satisfaction, and interaction suggests that being in a relationship can protect some patients from the negative consequences of their illness. Relationship satisfaction and functioning can be adversely affected by the presence of a respiratory condition in one of the partners. In turn, couple interactions and their emotional sequelae can play a role in health functioning of the patient and possibly the non-ill partner as well. The paucity of the literature on these topics provides fertile ground for future research. Specifically, the effects of couples interaction on pulmonary function and other illness-related variables such as functional status can be explored in couples where one partner has lung cancer, COPD, or CF. The potential differential association between relationship factors and illness variables for acute versus chronic respiratory illnesses would be of great interest. Finally, psychotherapeutic approaches to couples with respiratory illnesses have been wholly uninvestigated.

REFERENCES

Adams, P. F., & Marano, M. A. (1995). Current estimates from the National Health Interview Survey, 1994. *Vital and health statistics* (DHHS Publication No. DHS 96-1521).

Adams, S., Pill, R., & Jones, A. (1997). Medication, chronic illness and identity: The perspective of people with asthma. *Social Science and Medicine, 45*, 189–201.

Afari, N., & Schmaling, K. B. (in press). Asthma patients and their partners: Gender differences in the relationship between psychological distress and patient functioning. *Journal of Asthma.*

Bartsch, H., & Hietanen, E. (1996). The role of individual susceptibility in cancer burden related to environmental exposure. *Environmental Health Perspectives, 104*, S569–S577.

Baucom, D. H., Shoham, V., Mueser, K. T., Daiuto, A. D., & Stickle, T. R. (1998). Empirically supported couple and family interventions for marital distress and adult mental health problems. *Journal of Consulting and Clinical Psychology, 66*, 53–88.

Bonekat, H. W., & Krumpe, P. E. (1990). Diagnosis of obstructive sleep apnea. *Clinical Reviews in Allergy, 8*, 197–213.

Bousquet, J., Knani, J., Dhivert, H., Richard, A., Chicoya, A., Ware, J. E., & Michel, F. B. (1994). Quality of life in asthma: 1. Internal consistency and validity of the SF–36 questionnaire. *American Journal of Respiratory and Critical Care Medicine, 149*, 371–375.

Burman, B., & Margolin, G. (1992). Analysis of the association between marital relationships and health problems: An interactional perspective. *Psychological Bulletin, 112*, 39–63.

Burnley, I. H. (1992). Mortality from selected cancers in NSW and Sydney, Australia. *Social Science and Medicine, 35*, 195–208.

Cartwright, R. D., & Knight, S. (1987). Silent partners: The wives of sleep apneic patients. *Sleep, 10*, 244–248.

Centers for Disease Control. (1993). Initial therapy for tuberculosis in the era of multidrug resistance: Recommendations of the Advisory Council for the Elimination of Tuberculosis. *Morbidity and Mortality Weekly Reports, 42*, 1–8.

Centers for Disease Control. (1996a). Asthma surveillance programs in public health departments—United States. *Morbidity and Mortality Weekly Reports, 45*, 802–804.

Centers for Disease Control. (1996b). Tuberculosis morbidity—United States, 1995. *Morbidity and Mortality Weekly Reports, 45*, 365–370.

Centers for Disease Control. (1997). Mortality patterns—Preliminary data, United States, 1996. *Morbidity and Mortality Weekly Reports, 46*, 941–944.

Chacko, R. C., Harper, R. G., Kunik, M., & Young, J. (1996). Relationship of psychiatric morbidity and psychosocial factors in organ transplant candidates. *Psychosomatics, 37*, 100–107.

Chiazze, L., Jr., Watkins, D. K., & Fryar, C. (1992). A case-control study of malignant and nonmalignant respiratory disease among employees of a fiberglass manufacturing facility. *British Journal of Industrial Medicine, 49*, 326–331.

Coffman, C. B., Levine, S. B., Althof, S. E., & Stern, R. C. (1984). Sexual adaptation among single young adults with cystic fibrosis. *Chest, 86*, 408–412.

Cohen, S., Doyle, W. J., Skoner, D. P., Rabin, B. S., & Gwaltney, J. M., Jr. (1997). Social ties and susceptibility to the common cold. *Journal of the American Medical Association, 277*, 1940–1944.

Cohen, S., Tyrrell, D. A., & Smith, A. P. (1991). Psychological stress and susceptibility to the common cold. *New England Journal of Medicine, 325*, 606–612.

Cohen, S., Tyrrell, D. A., & Smith, A. P. (1993). Negative life events, perceived stress, negative affect, and susceptibility to the common cold. *Journal of Personality and Social Psychology, 64*, 131–140.

Collins, E. G., White, W. C., & Jalowiec, A. (1996). Impact of the heart transplant waiting process on spouses. *Journal of Heart and Lung Transplantation, 15*, 623–630.

Connolly, C. K., & Chan, N. S. (1987). Relationship between different measures of respiratory function in asthma. *Respiration, 52*, 22–33.

Craven, J. L., Bright, J., & Dear, C. L. (1990). Psychiatric, psychosocial, and rehabilitative aspects of lung transplantation. *Clinics in Chest Medicine, 11*, 247–257.

Cystic Fibrosis Foundation. (1996, August). *Patient registry 1995 annual report data.* Bethesda, MD: Author.

De Araujo, G., Van Arsdel, P. P., Holmes, T. H., & Dudley, D. L. (1973). Life change, coping ability and chronic instrinsic asthma. *Journal of Psychosomatic Research, 17*, 359–363.

Derogatis, L. R. (1993). *Brief Symptom Inventory: Administration, scoring and procedures manual* (3rd. ed.). Minneapolis: National Computer Systems.

Derogatis, L. R., & Cleary, R. A. (1977). Confirmation of the dimensional structure of the SCL–90–R: A study in construct validation. *Journal of Clinical Psychology, 33*, 981–989.

Du, Y. X., Cha, Q., Chen, X. W., Chen, Y. Z., Huang, L. F., Feng, Z. Z., Wu, X. F., & Wu, J. M. (1996). An epidemiological study of risk factors for lung cancer in Guangzhou, China. *Lung Cancer, 14,* S9–S37.

Edwards, E. B., Breen, T. J., Guo, T., Ellison, M. D., & Daily, O. P. (1992). The UNOS OPTN waiting list: 1988 through November 30, 1992. *Clinical Transplants,* 61–75.

Enright, P. L., Newman, A. B., Wahl, P. W., Manolio, T. A., Haponik, E. F., & Boyle, P. J. R. (1996). Prevalence and correlates of snoring and observed apneas in 5,201 older adults. *Sleep, 19,* 531–538.

Evans, P., & Edgerton, N. (1991). Life events and mood as predictors of the common cold. *British Journal of Medical Psychology, 64,* 35–44.

Frost, F., Tollestrup, K., & Starzyk, P. (1994). History of smoking from the Washington State death certificate. *American Journal of Preventive Medicine, 10,* 335–339.

Ganz, P. A., Lee, J. J., & Siau, J. (1991). Quality of life assessment: An independent prognostic variable for survival in lung cancer. *Cancer, 67,* 3131–3135.

Gillen, M., Lallas, D., Brown, C., Yelin, E., & Blanc, P. (1995). Work disability in adults with cystic fibrosis. *American Journal of Respiratory and Critical Care Medicine, 152,* 153–156.

Goldberg, R. J., & Wool, M. S. (1985). Psychotherapy for the spouses of lung cancer patients: Assessment of an intervention. *Psychotherapy and Psychosomatics, 43,* 141–150.

Goldberg, R. J., Wool, M. S., Glicksman, A. S., & Tull, R. M. (1984). *Relationship of social environment and patients' physical status to depression in lung cancer patients and spouses.* Unpublished manuscript, Brown University, Providence, RI.

Groeger, A. M., Esposito, V., Mueller, M. R., Caputi, M., Kaiser, H. E., & Giordano, A. (1997). Advances in the understanding of lung cancer. *Anticancer Research, 17,* 2519–2522.

Guilleminault, C. (1987). Obstructive sleep apnea syndrome: A review. *Psychiatric Clinics of North America, 10,* 607–621.

Hanson, E. I. (1982). Effects of chronic lung disease on life in general and on sexuality: Perceptions of adult patients. *Heart and Lung, 11,* 435–441.

Horne, R. L., & Picard, R. S. (1979). Psychosocial risk factors for lung cancer. *Psychosomatic Medicine, 41,* 503–514.

Isoaho, R., Keistinen, T., Laippala, P., & Kivela, S. L. (1995). Chronic obstructive pulmonary disease and symptoms related to depression in elderly persons. *Psychological Reports, 76,* 287–297.

Jacobson, N. S., & Christensen, A. (1996). *Integrative couple therapy: Promoting acceptance and change.* New York: Norton.

Janson, C., Bjornsson, E., Hetta, J., & Boman, G. (1994). Anxiety and depression in relation to respiratory symptoms and asthma. *American Journal of Respiratory and Critical Care Medicine, 149,* 930–934.

Kabat-Zinn, J. (1984). An outpatient program in behavioral medicine for chronic pain patients based on the practice of mindfulness meditation: Theoretical considerations and preliminary results. *ReVision, 7*, 71–72.

Kabat-Zinn, J., Lipworth, L., & Burney, R. (1985). The clinical use of mindfulness meditation for the self-regulation of chronic pain. *Journal of Behavioral Medicine, 8*, 163–190.

Karacan, I., & Karatas, M. (1995). Erectile dysfunction in sleep apnea and response to CPAP. *Journal of Sex and Marital Therapy, 21*, 239–247.

Kinsman, R. A., Dirks, J. F., & Jones, N. F. (1982). Psychomaintenance of chronic illness. In T. Millon & C. J. Green (Eds.), *Handbook of clinical health psychology* (pp. 435–466). New York: Plenum Press.

Kintner, E. (1997). Adolescent process of coming to accept asthma: A phenomenological study. *Journal of Asthma, 34*, 547–561.

Koerner, K., Jacobson, N. S., & Christensen, A. (1994). Emotional acceptance in integrative behavioral couple therapy. In S. C. Hayes, N. S. Jacobson, V. M. Follette, & M. J. Dougher (Eds.), *Acceptance and change: Content and context in psychotherapy* (pp. 109–118). Reno, NV: Context Press.

Kosorok, M. R., Wei, W. H., & Farrell, P. M. (1996). The incidence of cystic fibrosis. *Statistics in Medicine, 15*, 449–462.

Krop, H. D., Block, A. J., & Cohen, E. (1973). Neuropsychological effects of continuous oxygen therapy in chronic obstructive pulmonary disease. *Chest, 64*, 317–322.

Lane, C., & Hobfoll, S. E. (1992). How loss affects anger and alienates potential supporters. *Journal of Consulting and Clinical Psychology, 60*, 935–942.

Lazcano-Ponce, E. C., Tovar-Guzman, V., Meneses-Gonzalez, F., Rascon-Pancheco, R. A., & Hernandez-Avila, M. (1997). Trends of lung cancer mortality in Mexico. *Archives of Medical Research, 28*, 565–570.

Lehrer, P. M. (1998). Emotionally triggered asthma: A review of research literature and some hypotheses for self-regulation therapies. *Applied Psychophysiology and Biofeedback, 23*, 13–41.

Lehrer, P. M., Sargunaraj, D., & Hochron, S. (1992). Psychological approaches to the treatment of asthma. *Journal of Consulting and Clinical Psychology, 60*, 639–643.

Lenhart, R. S., & Ashby, J. (1996). Cognitive coping strategies and coping modes in relation to chronic pain disability. *Journal of Applied Rehabilitation Counseling, 27*, 15–18.

Levine, S. B., & Stern, R. C. (1982). Sexual function in cystic fibrosis: Relationship to overall health status and pulmonary disease severity in 30 married patients. *Chest, 81*, 422–428.

Liefooghe, R., Michiels, N., Habib, S., Moran, M. B., & DeMuynck, A. (1995). Perception and social consequences of tuberculosis: A focus group study of tuberculosis patients in Sialkot, Pakistan. *Social Science and Medicine, 41*, 1685–1692.

Lindegard, B. (1989). Marital state, psoriasis, urticaria, and asthma. *Dermatologica, 179*, 55–56.

Linehan, M. M. (1993). *Skills training manual for treating borderline personality disorder.* New York: Guilford Press.

Littlefield, C., Abbey, S., Fiducia, D., Cardella, C., Greig, P., Levy, G., Maurer, J., & Winton, T. (1996). Quality of life following transplantation of the heart, liver, and lungs. *General Hospital Psychiatry, 18*, 36S–47S.

Macintyre, S., & Pritchard, C. (1989). Comparisons between the self-assessed and observer-assessed presence and severity of colds. *Social Science and Medicine, 29*, 1243–1248.

Manfredi, C., Lacey, L., Warnecke, R., & Buis, M. (1992). Smoking-related behavior, beliefs, and social environment of young Black women in subsidized public housing in Chicago. *American Journal of Public Health, 82*, 267–272.

Marks, G. B., Dunn, S. M., & Woolcock, A. J. (1992). A scale for the measurement of quality of life in adults with asthma. *Journal of Clinical Epidemiology, 45*, 461–472.

McCracken, L. M. (1998). Learning to live with the pain: Acceptance of pain predicts adjustment in persons with chronic pain. *Pain, 74*, 21–27.

McCurry, S. M., & Schmidt, A. (1994). Acceptance, serenity, and resignation in elderly caregivers. In S. C. Hayes, N. S. Jacobson, V. M. Follette, & M. J. Dougher (Eds.), *Acceptance and change: Content and context in psychotherapy* (pp. 237–251). Reno, NV: Context Press.

McFadden, E. R., & Gilbert, I. A. (1992). Asthma. *New England Journal of Medicine, 327*, 1928–1937.

Miller, D. J., & Kotses, H. (1995). Classical conditioning of total respiratory resistance in humans. *Psychosomatic Medicine, 57*, 148–153.

Miller, L. W., Kubo, S. H., Young, J. B., Stevenson, L. W., Loh, E., & Costanzo, M. R. (1995). Report of the Consensus Conference on Candidate Selection for Heart Transplantation. *Journal of Heart and Lung Transplantation, 14*, 562–571.

Mrazek, D. A., & Klinnert, M. (1991). Asthma: Psychoneuroimmunologic considerations. In R. Ader, D. L. Felten, & N. Cohen (Eds.), *Psychoneuroimmunology* (2nd. ed., pp. 1013–1035). San Deigo, CA: Academic Press.

Mrazek, D. A., Klinnert, M. D., Mrazek, P., & Macey, T. (1991). Early asthma onset: Consideration of parenting issues. *Journal of the American Academy of Child and Adolescent Psychiatry, 30*, 277–282.

Nasser, S., & Rees, P. J. (1992). Sleep apnoea: Causes, consequences and treatment. *British Journal of Clinical Practice, 46*, 39–43.

National Heart, Lung, and Blood Institute. (1991). National Asthma Education Program: Expert panel report. *Journal of Allergy and Clinical Immunology, 88*, 425–534.

National Heart, Lung, and Blood Institute. (1997, July). *National Asthma Education and Prevention Program Expert Panel Report 2: Guidelines for the diagnosis and management of asthma* (NIH Publication No. 97–4051). Bethesda, MD: Author.

Nocturnal Oxygen Therapy Trial Group. (1980). Continuous or nocturnal oxygen therapy in hypoxemic chronic obstructive lung disease: A clinical trial. *Annals of Internal Medicine, 93,* 391–398.

O'Connor, G. T., & Weiss, S. T. (1994). Clinical and symptom measures. *American Journal of Respiratory and Critical Care Medicine, 149,* S21–S28.

Patterson, G. A. (1997). Indications: Unilateral, bilateral, heart–lung, and lobar transplant procedures. *Clinics in Chest Medicine, 18,* 225–230.

Patton, S. R., Landel, J. L., Holsclaw, D., Kaplan, M., Nguyen, J., Klein, D., & Lomas, P. (1998). The hidden patients: The psychological health of partners of adults with cystic fibrosis. *Annals of Behavioral Medicine, 20* [Abstract], S114.

Patton, S., Landel, J., Holsclaw, D., Kaplan, M., Nguyen, J., Lomas, P., & Klein, D. (1997, November). *Caregivers of adults with cystic fibrosis: Burden and its relationship to distress.* Paper presented at the 25th Annual Convention of the Association for the Advancement of Behavior Therapy, Miami Beach, FL.

Post, L., & Collins, C. (1981–1982). The poorly coping COPD patient: A psychotherapeutic perspective. *International Journal of Psychiatry in Medicine, 11,* 173–182.

Priel, B., Heimer, D., Rabinowitz, B., & Hendler, N. (1994). Perceptions of asthma severity: The role of negative affectivity. *Journal of Asthma, 31,* 479–484.

Ramsey, B. W. (1996). Management of pulmonary disease in patients with cystic fibrosis. *New England Journal of Medicine, 335,* 179–188.

Rand, C. S., Nides, M., Cowles, M. K., Wise, R. A., & Connett, J. (1995). Long-term metered-dose inhaler adherence in a clinical trial. *American Journal of Respiratory and Critical Care Medicine, 152,* 580–588.

Rosenfeld, M., Davis, R., FitzSimmons, S., Pepe, M., & Ramsey, B. (1997). Gender gap in cystic fibrosis mortality. *American Journal of Epidemiology, 145,* 794–803.

Rosenstein, B. J., & Zeitlin, P. L. (1995). Prognosis in cystic fibrosis. *Current Opinion in Pulmonary Medicine, 1,* 444–449.

Rozenberg, S., Liebens, F., Kroll, M., & Vandromme, J. (1996). Principal cancers among women: Breast, lung and colorectal. *International Journal of Fertility and Menopausal Studies, 41,* 166–171.

Santamaria, J. D., Prior, J. C., & Fleetham, J. A. (1988). Reversible reproductive dysfunction in men with obstructive sleep apnoea. *Clinical Endocrinology, 28,* 461–470.

Schmaling, K. B., Afari, N., Barnhart, S., & Buchwald, D. S. (1997). The association of disease severity, functional status and medical utilization with relationship satisfaction among asthma patients and their partners. *Journal of Clinical Psychology in Medical Settings, 4,* 373–382.

Schmaling, K. B., Afari, N., Hops, H., Barnhart, S. B., & Buchwald, D. B. (2000). *The effects of couple interaction on pulmonary function among patients with asthma.* Manuscript submitted for publication.

Schmaling, K. B., McKnight, P., & Afari, N. (2000). *A prospective study of the association between mood, stress, and pulmonary function.* Manuscript submitted for publication.

Schmaling, K. B., Wamboldt, F., Telford, L., Newman, K. B., Hops, H., & Eddy, J. M. (1996). Interaction of asthmatics and their spouses: A preliminary study of individual differences. *Journal of Clinical Psychology in Medical Settings, 3,* 211–218.

Schneider, R. F., & Rosen, M. J. (1996). Respiratory infections in patients with HIV infection. *Current Opinion in Pulmonary Medicine, 2,* 246–252.

Schuessler, G. (1992). Coping strategies and individual meanings of illness. *Social Science and Medicine, 34,* 427–432.

Sexton, D. L., & Munro, B. H. (1985). Impact of a husband's chronic illness (COPD) on the spouse's life. *Research in Nursing and Health, 8,* 83–90.

Smith, C. M. (1997). Patient selection, evaluation, and preoperative management for lung transplant candidates. *Clinics in Chest Medicine, 18,* 183–197.

Snyder, D. K. (1979). Multidimensional assessment of marital satisfaction. *Journal of Marriage and the Family, 41,* 813–823.

Snyder, D. K., Lachar, D., & Wills, R. M. (1988). Computer-based interpretation of the Marital Satisfaction Inventory: Use in treatment planning. *Journal of Marital and Family Therapy, 14,* 397–409.

Spanier, G. B. (1976). Measuring dyadic adjustment: New scales for assessing the quality of marriage and similar dyads. *Journal of Marriage and the Family, 38,* 15–28.

Stewart, A. L., Greenfield, S., Hays, R. D., Wells, K., Rogers, W. H., Berry, S. D., McGlynn, E. A., & Ware, J. E. (1989). Functional status and well-being of patients with chronic conditions: Results from the Medical Outcomes Study. *Journal of the American Medical Association, 262,* 907–913.

Stone, A. A., Porter, L. S., & Neale, J. M. (1993). Daily events and mood prior to the onset of respiratory illness episodes: A non-replication of the 3–5 day "desirability dip." *British Journal of Medical Psychology, 66,* 383–393.

Stuart, R. B. (1980). *Helping couples change: A social learning approach to marital therapy.* New York: Guilford Press.

Tarlov, A. R., Ware, J. E., Greenfield, S., Nelson, E. C., Perrin, E., & Zubkoff, M. (1989). The Medical Outcomes Study: An application of methods for monitoring the results of medical care. *Journal of the American Medical Association, 262,* 925–930.

Teiramaa, E. (1981). Psychosocial factors, personality and acute-insidious asthma. *Journal of Psychosomatic Research, 25,* 43–49.

Unger, D. G., Jacobs, S. B., & Cannon, C. (1996). Social support and marital satisfaction among couples coping with chronic obstructive airway disease. *Journal of Social and Personal Relationships, 13,* 123–142.

Ware, J. E., & Sherbourne, C. D. (1992). The MOS 36-item Short-Form Health Survey (SF–36). *Medical Care, 30,* 473–483.

Weiss, K. B., Gergen, P. J., & Hodgson, T. A. (1992). An economic evaluation of asthma in the United States. *New England Journal of Medicine, 326,* 862–866.

Weiss, K. B., & Wagener, D. K. (1990). Changing patterns of asthma mortality: Identifying target populations at high risk. *Journal of the American Medical Association, 264,* 1683–1687.

Wigal, J. K., Stout, C., Brandon, M., Winder, J. A., McConnaughy, K., Creer, T. L., & Kotses, H. (1993). The Knowledge, Attitude, and Self-Efficacy Asthma Questionnaire. *Chest, 104,* 1144–1148.

Wiggins, C. L., Schmidt-Nowara, W. W., Coultas, D. B., Samet, J. M. (1990). Comparison of self- and spouse reports of snoring and other symptoms associated with sleep apnea syndrome. *Sleep, 13,* 245–252.

Wingo, P. A., Ries, L. A. G., Rosenberg, H. M., Miller, D. S., & Edwards, B. K. (1998). Cancer incidence and mortality, 1973–1995: A report card for the U.S. *Cancer, 82,* 1197–1207.

4

RHEUMATIC ILLNESS AND RELATIONSHIPS: COPING AS A JOINT VENTURE

SHARON DANOFF-BURG AND TRACEY A. REVENSON

The rheumatic diseases constitute more than 100 illnesses and conditions, affecting nearly 40 million people in the United States. By 2020, it is expected that nearly 60 million Americans will have some form of rheumatic disorder (Helmick, Lawrence, Pollard, Lloyd, & Heyse, 1995). The most frequently diagnosed rheumatic illnesses include osteoarthritis (OA), fibromyalgia, rheumatoid arthritis (RA), and gout. In the public consciousness, arthritis may evoke an image of annoying aches and pains experienced primarily by older people, an image reinforced by advertisements for nonprescription pain relievers. In reality, although each disease has distinguishing features, the rheumatic diseases share the characteristics of severe, unpredictable pain episodes and joint involvement, all which erode patients' quality of life.

The writing of this chapter was supported in part by an Arthritis Foundation postdoctoral fellowship awarded to Sharon Danoff-Burg and a grant from the Professional-Staff Congress, City University of New York, awarded to Tracey A. Revenson.

This chapter focuses primarily on RA, which has received the most attention from researchers interested in psychosocial aspects of rheumatic illness. After describing the illness, its treatment, and its impact on the person and on the healthy partner, we turn to the importance of relationships for people with rheumatic disease, with attention to how close interpersonal relationships can affect health and well-being in positive and negative ways. Next, psychosocial interventions for rheumatic disease are reviewed, with a focus on treatments that include partners and other family members; questions will be raised regarding the appropriate level of intervention. We conclude by offering recommendations for future research using an illness-in-context framework.

BACKGROUND

Description of the Illness

RA is a chronic, systemic disease of unknown etiology, thought to be an autoimmune disorder. Its cardinal manifestation of joint inflammation results in severe and often unremitting pain, degenerative joint destruction, and concomitant physical disability. Common symptoms include joint pain, swelling, and tenderness, as well as morning stiffness and fatigue. In the majority of cases there is a steady progression toward increasing disability over the life span. What is important for mental health professionals to know is that the course of RA is unpredictable and highly variable, with symptoms that flare and remit. Thus, a person with RA is likely to experience unpredictable transitions from periods of relative comfort to periods of severe pain and is thus living with a chronic (if non-life-threatening) condition.

RA affects 1%–2% of the U.S. adult population. The distribution of RA spans the globe and affects people of all ethnic groups. As with other illnesses, individuals with fewer economic and social resources are likely to have more disease-related problems. Despite stereotypes of arthritis as an older person's disease (based on images of OA, which involves bone degeneration caused by lifelong "wear and tear"), the average age of onset of RA is between 25 and 50 years, although the incidence and prevalence of the disease increase with age. The impact of RA and the other rheumatic diseases on society is difficult to measure. As Callahan, Rao, and Boutaugh (1996) noted, "the impact of arthritis is often underestimated because of difficulties in quantifying many of its consequences and because of its high prevalence among older persons and women" (p. 401). However, the annual cost of the musculoskeletal conditions in the United States is estimated to be $72.3 billion in direct costs of medical care and $77.1 billion in indirect costs such as lost wages (Yelin & Callahan, 1995). The total cost of RA alone is estimated to account for 0.3% of the gross domestic product (Yelin, 1996).

The Gender Variable

One cannot discuss rheumatic illness without considering gender. In fact, the editor of the journal *Arthritis Care and Research* has called for arthritis to receive recognition as a significant women's health issue (Callahan, 1996). Simply put, "being a woman is the primary risk factor for the rheumatic diseases" (Hannan, 1996, p. 424), and RA is no exception. RA affects 2.5 times as many women as men. Arthritis in all of its forms is the most common self-reported chronic condition affecting women (Centers for Disease Control and Prevention, 1995). The biologic reasons for these gender differences are not understood at present.

Recent data suggest that women and men with RA experience different patterns of symptoms (Seachrist, 1996): Men are more likely to develop joint erosion and fibrosis of the lungs, whereas women are more likely to have surgery for small joints in the hands and feet and to experience dry eyes and mouth. Katz and Criswell (1996) have found that women evaluate their RA symptoms as more severe than do men and that this is due to more severe disease among women rather than overreporting of symptoms or overrating of symptom severity.

Evidence also exists that RA is more disabling for women than for men, even after controlling for age (Allaire, 1996). Functional disability is likely to affect men and women differently due to societal gender roles regarding division of labor inside and outside of the home (Reisine & Fifield, 1992); this topic is explored in more depth later in the chapter.

Treatment

Currently, RA cannot be cured or reversed. Treatment focuses on slowing disease progression (i.e., decreasing pain, inflammation, and joint damage) while increasing physical function and quality of life. Traditionally, a pyramid approach to treatment was advocated, beginning with nonsteroidal anti-inflammatory drugs (e.g., aspirin, ibuprofen, naproxen) and rest. If patients did not respond, then corticosteroids were added. The third line of defense was to add a disease-modifying antirheumatic drug (DMARD) such as methotrexate or sulphasalazine. In recent years, however, rheumatologists have moved to a more aggressive treatment strategy in which the pyramid is turned upside down: DMARDs are used early in treatment to prevent or reduce irreversible joint destruction (Kellick, Martins-Richards, & Chow, 1998). In addition to pharmacotherapy, patient education regarding pain management and coping skills, physical therapy, and occupational therapy are central components of a multimodal treatment plan. Individuals with severe and permanent joint destruction often benefit from surgical intervention such as joint replacement.

As with other chronic illnesses, the effectiveness of medical treatment is related to the degree to which patients adhere to prescribed regimens.

Factors that affect adherence include open communication between patients and health care providers, self-efficacy beliefs regarding ability to manage pain and carry out the treatment plan, characteristics of the home environment, and demands of the medical regimen (Agras, 1989; Bradley, 1989; Newman, Fitzpatrick, Revenson, Skevington, & Williams, 1996). Complex regimens are more difficult to follow, as are those that change frequently. These issues are particularly relevant to the management of RA in that for many patients a number of treatments will be tried before an effective one is found, and treatment plans change as disease progression occurs and current treatment becomes less effective.

What are termed *alternative* or *complementary* therapies by the medical profession are sought and used by many people with rheumatic disease. One study found that 84% of individuals with arthritis or musculoskeletal disorders had used an unconventional remedy within the past 6 months (Cronan, Kaplan, Posner, Blumberg, & Kozin, 1989). Some of these practices are accepted treatment strategies within behavioral medicine (e.g., relaxation techniques, exercise, prayer) and find no opposition among rheumatologists. Others, however, present cause for concern. For example, some products derived from plant sources (e.g., Comphrey, Kombucha tea) are purported to help arthritis but have the potential to cause great harm (Manley, 1997). For these reasons, patients should be encouraged to seek their physicians' guidance before trying unconventional remedies and not to forgo conventional medicine, which can actually reduce or halt joint destruction, in lieu of alternative treatment.

Impact on the Patient

Lifestyle Changes

Frequent pain episodes and increasing physical disability precipitate major changes in lifestyle for many people with RA as well as for their family members. Most directly, individuals with RA report restrictions in social, recreational, and leisure activities. These changes in activity level may occur not only because of physical limitations such as difficulties with mobility and severe pain but also because of experienced or feared stigmatization and rejection. In an ongoing study of coping with RA conducted by us, one participant explained, "Due to the longevity of the illness and at times the severity, several friends drifted away, unable to cope with my fatigues and inability to participate in activities." Another person, diagnosed in her 20s, commented, "Friends dropped me like a hot potato." Concerns about being rejected or stigmatized also can lead people with RA to pull away from intimacy with others. One woman in our study described how at times she chooses to withhold honesty in hope of preserving her relationships: "When people ask 'How are you?' I say 'Fine' even when I feel awful because I don't want to alienate people."

Activities previously taken for granted may become difficult, requiring the person to find new ways to perform tasks or to redefine roles at home and at work. Increased dependence on others may be a source of stress. In the words of one woman with RA in the above study, "I was raised to depend on no one except God and myself. . . . Reaching out to others for assistance is not something I can do with any kind of ease or grace."

RA has a profound effect on employment status, with many people unable to maintain their job as the disability worsens. Approximately half the persons with RA who are working at the time of disease onset become work disabled (Callahan et al., 1996). Loss of income may further affect the ability to engage in activities or recruit assistance. In addition, restrictions in the ability to perform daily activities associated with caring for children and other family members have been shown to hamper the self-worth and perceived competence of many women with RA. In a landmark study of female homemakers with RA (landmark because it reconceptualized the issue of illness interference from a gendered perspective), Reisine, Goodenow, and Grady (1987) found that the illness interfered not only with instrumental tasks such as cooking and cleaning but also with nurturant aspects of the homemaker role, such as making arrangements and maintaining family ties. Moreover, nurturant limitations had a greater impact on women's satisfaction with their functioning than did instrumental limitations.

Depression

During the 1940s and 1950s, studies suggested an "arthritic personality" that predisposed particular individuals to RA (see K. O. Anderson, Bradley, Young, McDaniel, & Wise, 1985). The patient with this personality type was characterized as depressed, restricted in capacity for emotional expression, dependent, perfectionistic, and interested in outdoor sports. In the 1970s, serious methodological flaws of these studies were noted, and the explanation that qualities such as depressed mood are consequences rather than causes of the disease has come to be accepted.

McCracken (1991) has noted that "there is now accumulating evidence that RA can impact nearly every segment of the patient's behavior including affective, cognitive, and social aspects" (p. 57). Despite this multitude of potential stressors, most individuals with RA do not experience clinical depression. However, they are more likely to experience depression than people without serious chronic illnesses and are about as likely to experience depression as people with other types of serious chronic illness (DeVellis, 1993). There is some evidence that the prevalence of depression may be lower among people with RA than with other rheumatic diseases such as systemic lupus erythematosus (SLE; Liang et al., 1984) and fibromyalgia (Walker et al., 1997), although these studies have methodological weaknesses (e.g., small samples). Recently reported estimates of the prevalence of depression among patients with RA range from 15% to 34%, with most studies reporting figures closer to the low end of this range (Creed & Ash, 1992; Creed, Murphy, & Jayson, 1990; DeVellis, 1993; Frank, Chaney, Clay, & Kay, 1991; Katz & Yelin, 1993). However, these figures are based primarily on self-report scales measuring depressive symptoms rather than on diagnostic interviews or instruments administered by clinicians and therefore may be somewhat unreliable in capturing the true prevalence of depressive disorders in this population.

Risk factors for depression among persons with RA include high daily stress, low perceived ability to cope with pain, and high degree of physical disability (Wright et al., 1996). In addition, among patients with RA, women, younger adults, and people with fewer economic and social resources have been found to have greater depressive symptoms (Newman, Fitzpatrick, Lamb, & Shipley, 1989; Wright et al., 1998).

Impact on the Partner

Caring for and providing support to an intimate partner who is ill can be deeply rewarding, but it also can be very stressful. Partners in this position may find themselves experiencing conflicting roles: They are the primary source of support for the person with rheumatic illness, yet they are also in need of support for themselves. In fact, "healthy" partners may be facing their own serious medical problems, particularly as they grow older.

Common stressors experienced by partners of individuals with rheumatic disease include helplessness in response to seeing their partner in pain, frustration with the partner's physical limitations and changes in mood, reduction in shared pleasurable activities, and fear and uncertainty regarding the future (Revenson & Majerovitz, 1990; see also Foxall, Kollasch, & McDermott, 1989). People may feel reluctant to burden their ill partners with their own needs. For example, Revenson and Majerovitz (1990) found that some wives of men with RA reported having lessened their own requests for support so as not to increase their husbands' distress. At the same time, patients may fear burdening their partners. For example, a study of 74 women with SLE found that over 80% reported hiding symptoms and feelings about their illness from their partner (Druley, Stephens, & Coyne, 1997).

Despite multiple illness-related stressors, the spouses in the Revenson and Majerovitz (1990) study reported levels of depression, stress, and marital adjustment comparable to normative samples of adults. Stress was buffered by having strong support from a close network of family and friends, particularly at times when the arthritis symptoms were severe or the disease more advanced. Thus, living with a person who has RA creates a set of new and identifiable stressors for partners but does not lead automatically to extreme levels of distress.

Impact on the Relationship

Sexuality

The aforementioned study (Revenson & Majerovitz, 1990) found that sex was a concern for many partners of individuals with RA. We continue to hear these concerns in our current research and popular media sources. A woman in our study of coping with RA remarked bluntly, "My spouse is afraid to touch me at bedtime for fear of hurting me." The cover story of the May–June 1998 issue of *Arthritis Today* magazine, read by thousands of patients with arthritis, was titled "Sexual Healing" and was written in response to readers' questions about sex and arthritis symptoms (e.g., pain, fatigue, joint limitations), body image, and fear of losing one's partner.

However, a number of studies underscore the fact that although rheumatic disease can interfere with sexual functioning, the overall sexual satisfaction and needs of couples with and without rheumatic illness may not be dramatically different. Majerovitz and Revenson (1994) found that couples coping with rheumatic illness did not experience significantly more sexual dissatisfaction than did a matched sample of couples in which neither partner had a chronic illness. In another study, individuals without chronic illness reported similar levels of interest in sexual counseling as did people with RA, and for both the patient and the comparison sample, sexual dissatisfaction was not related to interest in learning to enhance sexual functioning (Blake, Maisiak, Alarcon, Holley, & Brown, 1987). It appears that the strongest predictor of sexual satisfaction among couples with rheumatic illness is severity of the disease (Curry, Levine, Jones, & Kurit, 1993; Majerovitz & Revenson, 1994). For example, in the Majerovitz and Revenson study, greater physical disability was related to lower sexual satisfaction among both members of the couple, and spouses also reported lower sexual satisfaction when their partners reported more arthritis pain.

Shifting Responsibilities

As Pearlin and Turner (1987) have written, "Disruptive events acquire much of their stressful character not by their own direct impact but by disrupting and dislocating the more *structured* elements of people's lives" (p. 148, italics added). Illness often requires long-established patterns of family activities to be rearranged and the partner to take on additional responsibilities, particularly as disability increases (Revenson & Lanza, 1994). For some people, these new responsibilities may be particularly challenging when they are not in accordance with traditional gender roles. For example, a husband may begin to do more cleaning and child care as his wife's level of disability increases, or a wife who has not worked outside of the home may seek employment when her husband is unable to continue his job because of arthritis.

Here is how one man in our recent research described the effects of his disability on the family:

> My wife is forced to go to work, which causes other problems around the house, i.e., cleaning, washing, errands, etc. My wife never had to go to work before. . . . We never have time for ourselves. My wife is always stressed and tries to alleviate my stress. She never has time to sit with my 6-year-old to study. My kids are used to her being home and taking them places. I can't.

In accordance with national trends, women with rheumatic disease continue to shoulder more of the household burdens than their male partners. Revenson and Lanza (1994) found that although married women with RA did a somewhat smaller proportion of household labor than did wives of men with RA or wives in a healthy comparison sample, they were still carrying out approximately 75% of all the household responsibilities handled by the couple (i.e., household labor not done by paid or family help). Moreover, women were responsible for more of the daily maintenance tasks such as cooking, cleaning, and child care, and when ill women's household burden was decreased, it was more often relegated to paid help than to the husband.

These findings replicate those of national studies of healthy couples (Hochschild, 1989) but have different implications for couples coping with rheumatic illness. An inequitable distribution of household labor can become extremely problematic when pain, joint swelling, and symptom flares are neither predictable, controllable, nor time limited. Thus, division of household labor needs to be flexible for couples in which one partner has RA. The findings also may explain why husbands and wives often disagree on what constitutes helpful support (Melamed & Brenner, 1989).

The influence of gender socialization cannot be underestimated here. Women are likely to feel a responsibility to keep the family and home intact, but for couples with rheumatic illness, this may occur at great personal and emotional cost. Whether in the role of patient or caregiver, women often assume a disproportionate share of the responsibility for maintaining the family's organization and functioning. Whereas these responsibilities may be logical extensions of women's traditional roles, they also may create added strains on the marriage.

ASSOCIATION OF ILLNESS AND COUPLE FACTORS

Importance of Interpersonal Relationships

In numerous studies of patients with RA, social support provided by family and friends has been associated with lower depression (Brown, Wallston, & Nicassio, 1989; Fitzpatrick, Newman, Archer, & Shipley, 1989; Goodenow, Reisine, & Grady, 1990; Penninx et al., 1997; Revenson,

Schiaffino, Majerovitz, & Gibofsky, 1991) and with enhanced self-esteem (Druley & Townsend, 1998; Fitzpatrick, Newman, Lamb, & Shipley, 1988), psychological adjustment (Affleck, Pfeiffer, Tennen, & Fifield, 1988), and life satisfaction (Smith, Dobbins, & Wallston, 1991). The mediating processes underlying these associations have received less attention.

For example, many of the studies linking support to well-being are cross-sectional, leaving open the possibility that the presence of depression drives people away from intimacy and affects relationship quality (Coyne, 1976). Depressed individuals may not solicit support or accept it when offered, in effect dismantling their support resources for the long term and maintaining their depressed mood. It is not clear whether depressed persons actually receive less support; they may perceive themselves as receiving less support, possibly because the support received was not the type desired or was offered at the wrong time (Revenson, 1990). Alternately, depressed persons may refuse offers of support in an attempt to maintain a sense of autonomy and not let the illness control their life.

A single close relationship with an intimate partner can prevent social isolation (Lowenthal & Haven, 1968). To date, most of the research on close, intimate relationships has focused on heterosexual, married persons. People who are married tend to have larger social networks and more extended family ties (Sherbourne & Hays, 1990), suggesting a greater reservoir of available support. A number of epidemiological studies demonstrate that a greater number of ties and greater (perceived) support are related to better physical and mental health and lowered mortality (House, Landis, & Umberson, 1988). In keeping with the broader literature on health advantages associated with marriage (Burman & Margolin, 1992; Ross, Mirowsky, & Goldstein, 1990), there is evidence that individuals with rheumatic illness who have a partner fare better: Women and men with RA who are married have been shown to exhibit a lower rate of functional disability progression over time than people with RA who are unmarried (Ward & Leigh, 1993).

Of course, such positive effects do not come attached to the marriage license; marital quality must be considered in addition to marital status (Burman & Margolin, 1992). Indeed, happily married women with RA experience greater physical and psychological well-being than unhappily married or unmarried women with RA (Roth-Roemer & Kurpius, 1996). Legal marriage is neither a necessary nor sufficient condition for the emergence of emotional and health benefits. Rather, it appears that a unique form of social support operates in successful couples' relationships. As Revenson (1994) explained about married couples with chronic illness,

> Spouses are on the front lines of providing support to their ill partner. Spouses provide love and affection, especially the assurance that the patient is loved despite any adverse changes that illness has wrought on the physical body, personality, or quality of the marriage. They provide

tangible assistance with day-to-day responsibilities and special needs created by treatment. They validate the patient's emotions or coping choices, and help their partners reappraise the meaning of the illness. They share the existential and practical concerns about how the illness may affect the marriage and family in the future. They provide continuity and security in a life disrupted in many ways. (p. 122)

The Downside of Relationships

Clinicians know well that it is important to consider not only the positive aspects of intimate relationships but also the problematic ones that may erode mental health. Revenson et al. (1991) has likened social support to a double-edged sword, because the support offered can be perceived by the recipient as either helpful or unhelpful and consequently can be either protective or detrimental to one's health and well-being.

A number of studies have shown the impact of negative support on well-being among people with RA. For example, in one study, people with RA were asked directly what others said or did that added further strain to their coping efforts (Affleck et al., 1988); the most frequently reported behaviors were minimization of the severity of the pain or illness, pessimistic comments, and expressed pity or solicitousness. Another study made clear that almost any type of support can be perceived by the recipient as helpful or unhelpful (Lanza, Cameron, & Revenson, 1995).

Not surprisingly, people with RA report both supportive and nonsupportive interactions with the same individuals (Revenson et al., 1991), but the negative elements of those relationships are more predictive of depression than are the positive elements. Negative interactions may reflect unvoiced expectations that, when not met, take on greater meaning and lead to the discounting of positive aspects of the relationship. In fact, negative interpersonal interactions may be better conceptualized as stressors than as indicators of lack of support, in that they potentiate the effects of other stressors (Coyne & DeLongis, 1986). Nonetheless, for people with RA, it appears that having a relationship characterized by high levels of both positive and problematic (i.e., unhelpful or upsetting) support is better than having little or no positive support (Revenson et al., 1991).

In an early study of interpersonal processes among couples with RA, Manne and Zautra (1989) found that wives with RA whose husbands made critical comments were more psychologically distressed. Although that finding makes common sense, the investigators illuminated the mediating process: Women whose husbands made critical comments were more likely to engage in the coping strategy of wishful thinking than the strategies of cognitive restructuring or information seeking, which were used more often by wives who perceived their husbands as supportive. Moreover, the content of the husbands' critical remarks suggested that their disapproval was fueled by limitations and disruptions in activities imposed by the illness.

The Manne and Zautra (1989) study focused on obviously negative comments, interpersonal interactions never intended to be supportive. But even in the healthiest relationships, well-intended support efforts can backfire. How and when does this occur? Support involves an interpersonal transaction between a provider and a recipient and is located at a particular point in time and life context (Revenson, 1990). For instance, at times, the ill person may not want the help or comfort that is offered; she or he may feel that the partner is being too controlling or too protective or that the partner is offering support for the wrong reasons. As one woman with RA said of her husband and best friend, "Although they encourage me to fight the pain, they sometimes help too much. I think they do it because *they* don't like to see the pain" (Revenson et al., 1991, p. 812).

Couples may simply disagree about which actions are helpful, as illustrated by a study of 35 couples with arthritis who had been married for a long time (Melamed & Brenner, 1989). Asked to indicate which spousal behaviors were not supportive, couples reached agreement on only a few actions: expressing irritation, expressing anger, and ignoring the ill spouse. The high degree of disagreement as to which behaviors were supportive suggests that most behaviors are helpful at some times but not at others and that the perception of support is subtle.

It has been proposed that people with RA are especially sensitive to interpersonal conflict. A study by Zautra, Burleson, Matt, Roth, and Burrows (1994) found that interpersonal conflict accounted for more than twice the variance in depression for women with RA compared with those with OA. In addition, study participants with RA who reported high levels of depressive symptoms or felt that their coping was ineffective showed higher levels of stimulatory hormones (prolactin, cortisol, and estradiol), which in turn were associated with greater disease activity. Zautra et al. speculated that people with RA may be more reactive to interpersonal stressors because they live with the prospect of severe disability and future dependence on others to carry out activities of daily living. Additional evidence of increased sensitivity to interpersonal conflict is provided by Druley and Townsend (1998). Comparing married persons with and without arthritis, these researchers found that self-esteem was more strongly related to negative marital interactions among individuals with arthritis, even though there was no difference between the two groups in the amount of negative marital interactions experienced.

Support needs change over the course of the illness in response to changing treatment regimens, self-image, disability, pain, and symptoms. What may be useful one day may be (or may be perceived as) inappropriate the next. For people to benefit, the type of support offered must fit with the type desired. This is not a simple equation, because finding the right match requires not only successful communication and understanding between partners but also a sense of timing. In a study comparing helpful and unhelpful support (Lanza et al., 1995), tangible assistance, such as help with chores and errands, was reported as the most helpful type of support around the time of diagnosis, when patients were confronting lifestyle adjustments and adaptation to treatment regimens. Informational support was the least helpful during this time, particularly when it came from family members (who were perceived to be uninformed). For patients with long-term rheumatic disease, the majority of helpful support episodes involved tangible or emotional support, most likely because the disability was more severe. Emotional support, particularly from spouses, was identified as helpful throughout the course of the illness. Unhelpful transactions occurred when expected support was not received, such as when partners minimized patients' pain. In one woman's words, "[My husband] couldn't accept that [the arthritis] was debilitating. . . . He was denying it and saying it was nothing, and for a long time, made light of it" (Lanza et al., 1995, p. 454). Partners' definitions of what is helpful or unhelpful need to be communicated clearly and may be an important topic on which to focus psychological intervention.

Coping at the Level of the Couple

There have been numerous studies of how individual-level coping by people with RA affects their emotional well-being (see Newman & Revenson, 1993; Zautra & Manne, 1992). But coping does not occur in a social void, and one partner's coping affects the other's. Although coping is usually conceptualized as conscious thoughts and behaviors that are directed toward ameliorating, solving, or managing stressful situations and the emotions they elicit (Aldwin, 1994), coping efforts can be defined narrowly or broadly. For example, how a couple deals with the division of household labor can be considered coping, although it has never appeared on a standardized checklist of coping strategies.

There are few studies of coping with illness at the level of the couple. A recent theoretical approach involves the notion of *relationship-focused coping*, or strategies used to deal directly with problems in the relationship, as opposed to coping with the changeable stressors of the illness and one's emotional distress (see, e.g., Coyne & Fiske, 1992; O'Brien & DeLongis, 1997). A second approach is to examine the congruence or "fit" of partners' coping efforts (Revenson, 1995). Just as helpful social support depends on a match between what the provider gives and what the recipient needs, the effectiveness of couples' coping may depend on how well partners' coping strategies fit together. Congruence may be defined as either similarity or complementarity, depending on the stressful situation being confronted.

A study of married couples in which one partner had rheumatic illness (Revenson, 1995) examined three dimensions of congruence from couples' coping profiles (determined by cluster analysis): the predominant strategy or strategies used by the members of the couple, the intensity of each partner's coping efforts, and the degree to which partners' strategies were similar or dissimilar. Similarity in husbands' and wives' coping strategies or in the intensity of their efforts did not predict the best adjustment outcomes; instead, complementarity was related to better adjustment. This is not surprising. As Eckenrode (1991) has written,

> In close relationships, we may also see a certain degree of synchrony or orchestration that takes place as each person seeks to cope with a common stressor or when one individual attempts to support the other in coping with stressors he or she is individually facing. (p. 5)

Furthermore, the study showed that couples' coping styles emerge within specific illness contexts, for example, the degree of distress experienced by the partner and spouse, the occurrence of concurrent life stressors, and the duration of the illness also appear to shape coping.

The cross-sectional nature of this study poses a number of intriguing questions about the evolution of couples' coping patterns over time. Can we really consider illness a common stressor? Does one partner's choice of coping strategy change how the other person copes? Do partners knowingly coordinate coping efforts, whether capitalizing on similarities or differences, to get all of the coping tasks done? Do partners' coping efforts become more congruent over time as ineffective strategies or those that impede the other partner's coping are discarded and successful ones are adopted or recycled?

ASSESSMENT AND INTERVENTION

Assessment

Schmaling and Sher (1997) have written that "no assessment instruments exist that are meant for couples where one person is ill that are generally applicable to a variety of illnesses" (p. 337). They have suggested that clinicians use assessment procedures that have been validated on distressed or nondistressed couples, such as assessment of relationship satisfaction. In addition, we suggest that clinicians assess discrepancy in partners' representations of the illness and its meaning for their own lives and for the relationship. Discrepancy in perceptions of how each member of the couple gives and receives support and how each partner copes (including the efficacy of coping efforts) also should be explored. These differing beliefs and behaviors may then serve as a foundation for treatment planning and guide therapeutic goals.

Depression is the most commonly studied psychosocial variable in arthritis research and one for which illness-specific assessment issues have been raised. As with other physical illnesses, the assessment of depression in persons with RA can be difficult. First, symptoms of the illness (e.g., fatigue) may overlap with symptoms of depression, and the diagnosis of one might mask the other. Second, some medications used to treat RA, such as corticosteroids, can induce depressive symptoms, further complicating the clinical picture. Depression can worsen the pain and disability associated with rheumatic disease, leading patients and physicians alike to interpret difficulties caused by depression as a worsening of the rheumatic disease process; this in turn can lead to unnecessary changes in the medical regimen while the depression is left untreated. Depression also has been shown to result in poorer adherence to medical treatment and misutilization of health care services (DeVellis, 1993).

The problem of assessment arises in research as well as clinical practice. Most research studies rely on self-report scales of depressive symptoms such as the Center for Epidemiologic Studies Depression Scale (CES–D; Radloff, 1977), which were not meant to diagnose mood disorders with clinical validity. Yet many researchers continue to use cutoff scores obtained from one sample in a diagnostic fashion. A major assessment issue is the problem of *criterion contamination*, or the extent to which scales confound symptoms of depression with symptoms of rheumatic disease (DeVellis, 1993). A secondary analysis of data from three studies revealed that the CES–D overestimated the prevalence and severity of depressive symptoms among persons with RA, but the magnitude of this bias was modest (Blalock, DeVellis, Brown, & Wallston, 1989). Moreover, the investigators found that removing items representing the somatic symptoms that might be part of both depression and RA did not affect the CES–D's reliability, validity, or correlation with other variables.

Before concluding this section, we wish to note that developing or using standardized assessment tools may emphasize the focus on pathology (vs. adaptation) inherent in the medical model. Assessment instruments should include the evaluation of strengths and competencies as well as problems or difficulties.

Intervention

One of the great appeals of the constructs of coping and social support is that they are amenable to change through psychosocial intervention. The majority of psychological, supportive, and educational interventions for people with rheumatic disease are aimed at individual-level change and have focused on increasing self-efficacy beliefs, managing pain, and expanding the patient's repertoire of coping skills (Lanza & Revenson, 1993). But as all the chapters in this volume make clear, illness is experienced within the context of interpersonal relationships. Thus, it may be helpful not only to include partners in treatment but also to focus on the day-today and long-term effects of living with a serious physical illness on the relationship itself.

In the following sections we discuss clinical implications derived from existing research. We review the few controlled studies of psychosocial interventions for arthritis that have involved partners or other family members and then suggest new directions that interventions can take. Although the lion's share of literature has focused on group (patient education) interventions, many of the findings and techniques are applicable to the treatment of individual couples.

Involving Partners in Treatment

There are many potential advantages to including partners in psychosocial treatment for rheumatic illness. Couples who come to treatment together may have higher rates of attendance and may report greater enjoyment of the treatment process. Groups composed of patients and their partners allow couples to learn from each other and may bring individual couples closer together by providing a safe place for them to discuss difficult topics, explore conflicts, and express feelings. Couples may share their frustrations about the uncertainty of living with RA and their fears and hopes for the future, they may learn to clarify and communicate which types of support are helpful in which situations for which partners, and they may identify and then build on complementary coping efforts.

One risk of a group intervention that does not include both members of the couple is that difficulties or maladaptive patterns within the relationship will not be recognized and improved but instead will be perpetuated or intensified (Gonzalez, Steinglass, & Reiss, 1989). Yet for some couples it may be more helpful to attend separate therapy or support groups, which allow members to ventilate thoughts and feelings without fear of upsetting their partner.

Social relationships outside of those maintained by the couple appear to be particularly important. Involvement in partner support groups is one way that partners may establish relationships with others experiencing similar circumstances. This may be especially helpful for men, for whom the intimate partner is often the primary or even sole social tie and for whom seeking help may be particularly difficult. Although the existence of a strong support network may be most critical later in the disease course, when disability is greatest (Revenson & Majerovitz, 1991), partners should be encouraged to develop such networks early, so that they are in place when needed most. The partner with rheumatic illness also should be encouraged to develop, maintain, and strengthen relationships with close friends and relatives, so that these supports are available during flare-ups as well as during periods of relative stasis.

Partners in the role of caregiver should be helped to understand that garnering support for themselves will improve their ability to help their partner cope and in turn will benefit the relationship. Consider the example of a woman who felt guilty participating in activities that were not directly related to caring for her ill husband. Coyne (1995) suggested that a clinician could help her by using the metaphor of an oxygen mask during an airplane emergency: "In the event of decompression, please adjust your own mask before trying to be of assistance to anyone else. That way, you will be much more effective" (p. 118).

Controlled Studies Involving Partners

Do partners enhance individual-level treatment? A few studies using multimodal techniques provide some evidence.

Cognitive–behavioral treatment. Many psychological interventions for RA involve cognitive–behavioral therapy (CBT). CBT for arthritis patients involves education about the illness and training in pain management skills such as relaxation techniques, goal setting and activity pacing, and cognitive restructuring. Controlled-outcome studies have documented the effectiveness of CBT for decreasing self-reported pain associated with RA (e.g., Appelbaum, Blanchard, Hickling, & Alfonso, 1988; Bradley et al., 1987; O'Leary, Shoor, Lorig, & Holman, 1988; Parker et al., 1988). However, results have varied and often have been disappointing with regard to maintenance of treatment gains at follow-up.

The participation of family members rarely has been examined in studies attempting to isolate the active ingredients of treatment. A notable exception is an investigation of whether a family support component would improve a 6-week CBT intervention for RA (Radojevic, Nicassio, & Weisman, 1992). The CBT with family support intervention was superior to the other groups (CBT without family support, education with family support, no-treatment control) with regard to severity and number of swollen joints, although no differences in self-reported pain or distress emerged. At a 2-month follow-up, however, there was no difference between the two CBT groups. This finding was due to maintenance of treatment gains among those who received the CBT plus family support intervention, coupled with improvement in the CBT-only group.

A study by Keefe et al. (1996) resulted in similar findings. Patients with OA of the knees were randomly assigned to one of three groups: a cognitive–behavioral pain-coping-skills-training (CST) group, a CST group with spouse assistance, or an arthritis education group with spousal support. Results indicated that the CST group with spousal assistance, compared with the education group with spousal support, showed decreased pain, mood disturbance, and pain behavior, as well as increased self-efficacy and use of pain-coping strategies. The spouse-assisted CST group showed greater improvements than the CST group without spouse assistance, but these differences were not statistically significant.

Although these studies do not provide unequivocal evidence for including a family support component in treatment, involvement of family members may be critical for particular patients, for example, those for whom family interactions interfere with adaptive behaviors. And as has been shown in other domains, family programs with a cognitive–behavioral orientation may be more helpful than family programs with a supportive–educational format (Mazzuca, 1982).

Arthritis self-management program. The most widely disseminated psychosocial intervention for people with arthritis is the Arthritis Self-Management Program, a structured group intervention typically led by trained laypersons with arthritis. The program combines education about arthritis with cognitive–behavioral techniques. Benefits of the program appear to be relatively long-lasting and include increased knowledge and self-care behaviors (e.g., exercise, relaxation) and decreased pain (Lorig & Holman, 1989; Lorig, Lubeck, Kraines, Seleznick, & Holman, 1985). Attendance of family members is encouraged but optional. We could not find any studies examining whether patients attending with family members achieve better results.

Facilitating Support in Couples

Practitioners can work toward a number of goals with couples to enhance support: (a) teaching patients and their intimate partners how to develop and maintain close interpersonal communication, (b) teaching patients how to recognize and accept the help and emotional encouragement provided by their partner, (c) improving partners' skills for determining patients' support needs and for offering help, and (d) facilitating positive appraisals of support. These four goals are not mutually exclusive, nor are they incompatible with other illness-related goals. For example, interventions that help patients or other family members positively evaluate the meaning of the illness in their life simultaneously may affect support transactions. The key is to conceptualize support as dyadic transactions with each partner as both a provider and recipient of support.

In designing interventions to strengthen family support for individuals faced with rheumatic disease, clinicians should avoid making two potentially erroneous assumptions: first, that there is a support deficit and, second, that the referred patient should be the locus of the intervention. The practitioner should not assume that the patient is experiencing a shortage of naturally occurring support. Some people seek support groups or psychotherapy as an additional source of support, not as compensation for lack of support from their family. Nor can a professional support intervention compensate for predominantly negative interactions with family members, which may indicate deeper and potentially longer lasting problems (Coyne & DeLongis, 1986). Low levels of partner support may actually be an indication of broader discord within the relationship. In such cases, it is this discord, not the lack of support, that may lead to psychological problems and should be the focus of treatment.

Recognizing that close relationships can be liabilities as well as assets, and that rheumatic disease affects the mental health of family members as well as patients, we raise several questions to help guide practitioners dealing with family support issues. Given the limited research evidence available, we prefer to raise questions for consideration rather than to issue firm guidelines for practice.

What kinds of partner support should be encouraged? There is no single or simple answer to this question. Different types of support are more or less helpful depending on the fit between the type of support provided and that needed, the stage of the illness, and the patient's mental state. Who is providing support may be as important as what support in considering an optimal match. In many cases, misfit occurs because the needs of the support provider and those of the support recipient are incongruent, often because support needs have not been communicated adequately. It is important to promote open communication between partners, including feedback but not criticism, when the help that is offered is not the help that is desired.

Who should be targeted for intervention? The majority of support interventions, as with most health education efforts, are directed toward the patient (Lanza & Revenson, 1993). However, as evident from the research presented in this chapter, couple or family relationships should also be the loci of interventions. Intimate partners in particular bear a large proportion of the stresses and burdens engendered by the illness, because they are often the primary or sole provider of social support in the other partner's life. In the study of spouses of people with RA described earlier (Revenson & Majerovitz, 1991), the stress-buffering role of network support was particularly strong for couples in which the patient had more severe arthritis. Translating this finding into an intervention strategy, partners of individuals with chronic illness should be encouraged in the early stages of the illness to build support networks outside the relationship, both within their existing social milieu and through more formal groups of others facing similar stresses.

Interventions involving both members of the couple could focus on how the illness affects the relationship (rather than either individual). Many partners worry about burdening an ill partner with their own worries and hesitate to ask the ill partner for support. Current research suggests that one of the by-products of including partners in psychosocial interventions is the voicing of those silent thoughts and feelings.

At what point in the illness might intervention help most? Disease duration and stage are important aspects of the illness context, because they reflect specific treatment regimens and coping tasks. As discussed earlier, different types and amounts of support may be more helpful at different points in the illness. The rate at which the disease progresses and the frequency with which treatment demands change are other factors to consider. A less rapid disease process probably allows a gradual and smoother adaptation, as anticipatory coping efforts may be made. A disease course marked with frequent transitions from health to illness, sometimes without warning, may prove a harder road to follow. The words of one woman with RA in our recent research illustrate this challenge:

> Before being diagnosed, family members would yell at me for walking slow and not being able to do things around the house. They thought I was lazy. Now they understand that there are times when I am more able to do work around the house and there are times that the fatigue and pain overcome me. (Danoff-Burg & Revenson, 1999)

The stress-buffering hypothesis (Cohen & Wills, 1985) suggests that support is most beneficial during periods when illness-related stress is high. Thus, interventions that help patients and their family members cope with flare-ups or surgery may be most effective.

The fact that rheumatic diseases are chronic, long-term illnesses can affect support providers' ability to provide long-term support effectively. As social support needs change, caregivers must learn when to give and when to withhold help, because providing too much support or providing it at the wrong time may erode the patient's autonomy and self-worth. Support attempts may fail because individuals tire of being the supporter or act in ways that demean the recipient (Coyne, Wortman, & Lehman, 1988; Manne & Zautra, 1989).

Is any support better than no support? Most support interventions assume that if support is good, more support is even better. Increased attention must be devoted to the unintended negative consequences of support interventions. Just as medication may cause adverse side effects, so can social support. For example, research into self-help groups suggests that for particular patients, social comparisons with others who are better or worse off may impede adjustment (Affleck, Tennen, Pfeiffer, Fifield, & Rowe, 1987; Hinrichsen, Revenson, & Shinn, 1985). Although similar others who are coping well with their illness may serve as strong role models, patients who are not coping well, particularly those at advanced stages of the illness, may provide frightening fantasies of what lies ahead. In one intervention study (Shearn & Fireman, 1985), a few participants mentioned fears of meeting more disabled people in the support group.

Just as support groups are not always perceived as helpful, well-intended support efforts from family members are not necessarily perceived as such by the patient. Although some research suggests that support from family members may increase patients' adherence to treatment (e.g., Chaney & Peterson, 1989), other studies suggest that recipients may view such support as a form of social control, which recipients then fight against (Rook, 1990).

Practitioners should help family members learn to encourage patients' coping efforts, provide emotional support, and offer help that does not undermine the patient's self-esteem.

Although this chapter has focused on couples' support, note that partners may not be able to meet all of each other's needs, perhaps because of the illness-related stresses they share or perhaps because of prior life experiences. Older patients may have few friends or family members to whom they can turn. In such cases, adjunct support provided by informal helping networks (e.g., neighbors, support groups) or professional helping networks (e.g., psychologists, social workers, visiting nurses) may be required. It is important to consider interventions directed toward marshaling the support of one or more key members of the existing network, as well as interventions designed to create new networks (Daltroy & Liang, 1988; Gottlieb, 1988).

What about emotional support from health care providers? Coyne and Fiske (1992) have reminded us not to leave the medical professional out of the equation. Interactions with health care providers can have profound influence on patients' adaptation to illness. Some patients may be particularly vulnerable to perceived criticism from support providers, including medical professionals. It is also possible for interactions with health care providers to affect the couple's relationship. For example, conflict may arise if partners leave a medical visit with contradictory interpretations of the instructions or information provided. When this occurs, couples may respond by struggling on their own instead of requesting clarification from the medical professional (Coyne, 1995).

Relationships with health care providers also can change over time, as patients move from crisis phases to more stable, long-term phases of medical care (Newman et al., 1996). For example, an initial diagnosis may require informational support from all sources, but particularly from the physician, as the patient makes a decision regarding which course of treatment to pursue. Soon after, emotional and problem-focused support from the partner may be critical in learning to adhere to a treatment regimen that must be woven into daily life, and emotional support from health care providers also may make this adjustment easier. For these reasons, it is important that medical and behavioral medicine training programs emphasize the importance of the patient's interpersonal environment, including relationships with medical professionals, as a major determinant of treatment outcome (Parker et al., 1993).

FUTURE DIRECTIONS

We believe that couples' coping with illness can be best studied within an illness-in-context perspective, which emphasizes that health and psychosocial adaptation to illness are functions not only of person characteristics but also of the broader interpersonal, social, political, and cultural contexts (Revenson, 1994). The contextual approach has been applied to analyses of the relation between personality and disease (Revenson, 1990), the role of sociodemographic factors on psychophysiological responses such as heart rate and blood pressure (N. B. Anderson & McNeilly, 1991), and the effects of HIV on women (Ickovics, Thayaparan, & Ethier, in press). A contextual approach serves as deep structure for developing research questions, a framework that exposes the interconnections among the many factors that influence couples' coping.

The sociocultural context includes variables such as age, gender, socioeconomic status, and educational level. These demographic markers may be proxy variables denoting health-promoting or health-damaging psychological processes, or they may serve as moderators of the relationship between illness stress and adaptation. The *interpersonal* context represents the full spectrum of an individual's social relations, including relations not only between the couple but also with their families, friends, and health care professionals. The *situational* context alludes to the specific stresses that an illness presents (e.g., pain or disability) as well as other co-occurring major and minor stresses. The *temporal* context refers to the timing of illness within couples' relationships, the effect of psychosocial variables on health at different stages of the disease and treatment, and the influence of disease stage or severity on interpersonal relationships and psychological well-being.

Three aspects of a contextual perspective are worth noting with regard to designing research on couples' coping with illness. First, these contexts are not mutually exclusive; individuals exist within a number of interdependent systems or contexts. As an example, an investigator might find that partner support (the interpersonal context) may bolster self-esteem and competence, but only for women (the sociocultural context) and only in the early stages of illness (the temporal context) when the couple is adapting to a new treatment regimen that requires vigilance (the situational context). As this example illustrates, contextual domains overlap.

Second, a contextual approach addresses the reciprocal relationships between individuals and the social systems with which they interact. For couples, the coping process involves transactions not only between the two partners but also between the couple and other family members, the couple and friends, and the couple and health care professionals. The psychosocial effects of illness extend in a ripple effect from one partner to the other, throughout the entire social system and back again. One must look not merely at the passive reaction of one partner to the other's coping behavior but also at how each partner directly or covertly influences the other person's cognitions, emotions, and actions. For example, it is not enough to know that a partner was attempting to be supportive; it is also critical to assess whether that support was perceived as helpful by the recipient.

Third, variables beyond the level of the individual are critical to understanding a contextual perspective. Admittedly, it is difficult to untangle the effects of the illness on each partner from the effects of illness on the relationship. Each coping task that patients confront has a counterpart in family functioning. For instance, medical uncertainty about prognosis and disease progression is mirrored in uncertainty about future functioning of the family or social unit (e.g., how the unit will restructure itself if the patient becomes severely disabled).

We can begin to construct a blueprint for studying couples' coping with RA that revolves around these different aspects of context. Let us take the interpersonal context first, examining the dyadic interaction of the partners. The starting point for this interaction is arbitrary; either partner may initiate a situation to which the other responds, or a particular illness-related stressor may require partners to coordinate coping efforts. Appraising the degree to which a feature of the illness is stressful, each partner tries a variety of coping strategies to minimize distress and maintain family functioning. The other partner's reaction to this coping creates, over time, a set of conditions to which the first partner responds. The second partner then tries to act or react in a way that will minimize her or his partner's distress but may instead exacerbate it. Thus, couples' adaptation to illness can be described as a reciprocal process whereby the patient's distress affects the partner's coping and support provisions, which in turn affects the patient's distress and coping, which in turn affects the partner, and so on.

Although family members' responses to illness are important determinants of adaptation, the family's coping repertoire may be constrained by the medical context. Pain, disability, and appraisals of uncertainty may be stronger determinants of family coping than either individual attributes or family interactional styles. Even the most adaptive families may not be able to cope successfully with constant pain and severe disability. For example, the disruption of daily life by medical treatment, its side effects, and the uncertainty it presages about future health may create a highly stressful context. The provision of increased support may be appreciated during critical times, such as during a flare-up, but at other times may be interpreted as unnecessary, unhelpful, or threatening to self-esteem.

The temporal context also shapes coping processes. Different coping tasks present themselves at different stages of illness (Newman & Revenson, 1993). For example, on being informed that one partner has RA, couples are faced with the immediate coping tasks of making critical decisions (e.g., where to receive care or how to handle medical costs), taking care of daily responsibilities at home and work, informing the family, setting aside—at least temporarily—other demands, and acknowledging the threat that the diagnosis places on the identity of the patient and the couple. At different times in the illness, medication regimens change, which results in disease improvements or additional side effects; at the same time, social relationships need to be maintained, and family responsibilities may change once again. The rate at which the disease progresses and the frequency with which treatment demands change may influence coping, and what may be effective coping at one time may not be at another.

CONCLUSION

In a 1992 editorial in *Arthritis Care and Research*, Bradley expressed concern that psychologists who conduct arthritis research generally do not make their work accessible to other health professionals. He challenged behavioral scientists to demonstrate that their research is relevant to clinical practice.

Clearly, the current research on psychological aspects of rheumatic disease only taps the surface and remains anchored in a traditional treatment perspective, focused on pathology and individual-level outcomes. At this time, we know little about what constitutes effective coping for couples with rheumatic illness. Moreover, what may be effective coping at one time in the illness or at a particular developmental stage in a couple's life may not be at another. In this regard, important clinical questions remain, such as how illness stage and duration affect support needs and how family members can best be involved in treatment. It is time to braid together the knowledge we have on individual adjustment, the natural progression of the disease, and couples' interactions, to begin developing interventions that focus on strength and resilience.

REFERENCES

Affleck, G., Pfeiffer, C., Tennen, H., & Fifield, J. (1988). Social support and psychosocial adjustment to rheumatoid arthritis. *Arthritis Care and Research, 1,* 71–77.

Affleck, G., Tennen, H., Pfeiffer, C., Fifield, J., & Rowe, J. (1987). Downward comparison and coping with serious medical problems. *American Journal of Orthopsychiatry, 57,* 570–578.

Agras, W. S. (1989). Understanding compliance with the medical regimen: The scope of the problem and a theoretical perspective. *Arthritis Care and Research, 2*(Suppl. 3), S2–S7.

Aldwin, C. M. (1994). *Stress, coping, and development.* New York: Guilford Press.

Allaire, S. H. (1996). Gender and disability associated with arthritis: Differences and issues. *Arthritis Care and Research, 9,* 435–440.

Anderson, K. O., Bradley, L. A., Young, L. D., McDaniel, L. K., & Wise, C. M. (1985). Rheumatoid arthritis: Review of psychological factors related to etiology, effects, and treatment. *Psychological Bulletin, 98,* 358–387.

Anderson, N. B., & McNeilly, M. (1991). Age, gender and ethnicity as variables in psychophysiological assessment: Sociodemographics in context. *Psychological Assessment, 3,* 376–384.

Appelbaum, K. A., Blanchard, E. B., Hickling, E. J., & Alfonso, M. (1988). Cognitive–behavioral treatment of a veteran population with moderate to severe rheumatoid arthritis. *Behavior Therapy, 19,* 489–502.

Blake, D. J., Maisiak, R., Alarcon, G. S., Holley, H. L., & Brown, S. (1987). Sexual quality-of-life of patients with arthritis compared to arthritis-free controls. *Journal of Rheumatology, 14,* 570–576.

Blalock, S. J., DeVellis, R. F., Brown, G. K., & Wallston, K. A. (1989). Validity of the Center for Epidemiological Studies Depression scale in arthritis populations. *Arthritis and Rheumatism, 32,* 991–997.

Bradley, L. A. (1989). Adherence with treatment regimens among adult rheumatoid arthritis patients: Current status and future directions. *Arthritis Care and Research, 2*(Suppl. 3), S33–S39.

Bradley, L. A. (1992). Challenges facing psychologists in arthritis research. *Arthritis Care and Research, 5,* 1–2.

Bradley, L. A., Young, L. D., Anderson, K. O., Turner, A. R., Agudelo, C. A., McDaniel, L. K., Pisko, E. J., Semble, E. L., & Morgan, T. M. (1987). Effects of psychological therapy on pain behavior of rheumatoid arthritis patients: Treatment outcome and 6-month follow-up. *Arthritis and Rheumatism, 30,* 1105–1114.

Brown, G. K., Wallston, K. A., & Nicassio, P. M. (1989). Social support and depression in rheumatoid arthritis: A one-year prospective study. *Journal of Applied Social Psychology, 19,* 1164–1181.

Burman, B., & Margolin, G. (1992). Analysis of the association between marital relationships and health problems: An interactional perspective. *Psychological Bulletin, 112,* 39–63.

Callahan, L. F. (1996). Arthritis as a women's health issue. *Arthritis Care and Research, 9,* 159–161.

Callahan, L. F., Rao, J., & Boutaugh, M. (1996). Arthritis and women's health: Prevalence, impact, and prevention. *American Journal of Preventive Medicine, 12,* 401–409.

Centers for Disease Control and Prevention. (1995). Prevalence and impact of arthritis among women—United States, 1989–1991. *Morbidity and Mortality Weekly Report, 44,* 329–334.

Chaney, J. M., & Peterson, L. (1989). Family variables and disease management in juvenile rheumatoid arthritis. *Journal of Pediatric Psychology, 14,* 389–403.

Cohen, S., & Wills, T. A. (1985). Stress, support and the buffering hypothesis. *Psychological Bulletin, 98,* 310–357.

Coyne, J. C. (1976). Depression and the response of others. *Journal of Abnormal Psychology, 85,* 186–193.

Coyne, J. C. (1995). Intervention in close relationships to improve coping with illness. In R. F. Lyons, M. J. L. Sullivan, & P. G. Ritvo (Eds.). *Relationships in chronic illness and disability* (pp. 96–122). Thousand Oaks, CA: Sage.

Coyne, J. C., & DeLongis, A. (1986). Going beyond social support: The role of social relationships in adaptation. *Journal of Consulting and Clinical Psychology, 54,* 454–460.

Coyne, J. C., & Fiske, V. (1992). Couples coping with chronic and catastrophic illness. In T. J. Akamatsu, M. A. P. Stephens, S. E. Hobfoll, & J. Crowther (Eds.), *Family health psychology* (pp. 129–149). Washington, DC: Hemisphere.

Coyne, J. C., Wortman, C. B., & Lehman, D. R. (1988). The other side of support: Emotional overinvolvement and miscarried helping. In B. H. Gottlieb (Ed.), *Marshaling social support* (pp. 305–330). Newbury Park, CA: Sage.

Creed, F., & Ash, G. (1992). Depression in rheumatoid arthritis: Aetiology and treatment. *International Review of Psychiatry, 4,* 23–34.

Creed, F., Murphy, S., & Jayson, M. V. (1990). Measurement of psychiatric disorder in rheumatoid arthritis. *Journal of Psychosomatic Research, 34,* 79–87.

Cronan, T. A., Kaplan, R. M., Posner, L., Blumberg, E., & Kozin, F. (1989). Prevalence of the use of unconventional remedies for arthritis in a metropolitan community. *Arthritis and Rheumatism, 32,* 1604–1607.

Curry, S. L., Levine, S. B., Jones, P. K., & Kurit, D. M. (1993). Medical and psychosocial predictors of sexual outcome among women with systemic lupus erythematosus. *Arthritis Care and Research, 6,* 23–30.

Daltroy, L. H., & Liang, M. H. (1988). Patient education in the rheumatic diseases: A research agenda. *Arthritis Care and Research, 1,* 161–169.

Danoff-Burg, S., & Revenson, T. A. (1999). [Data collected at City University of New York Graduate Center]. Unpublished research findings.

DeVellis, B. M. (1993). Depression in rheumatologic diseases. *Balliere's Clinical Rheumatology, 7,* 241–257.

Druley, J. A., Stephens, M. A. P., & Coyne, J. C. (1997). Emotional and physical intimacy in coping with lupus: Women's dilemmas of disclosure and approach. *Health Psychology, 16,* 506–514.

Druley, J. A., & Townsend, A. L. (1998). Self-esteem as a mediator between spousal support and depressive symptoms: A comparison of healthy individuals and individuals coping with arthritis. *Health Psychology, 17,* 255–261.

Eckenrode, J. (1991). *The social context of coping.* New York: Plenum.

Fitzpatrick, R., Newman, S., Archer, R., & Shipley, M. (1989). Social support, disability, and depression: A longitudinal study of rheumatoid arthritis. *Social Science and Medicine, 33,* 605–611.

Fitzpatrick, R., Newman, S., Lamb, R., & Shipley, M. (1988). Social relationships and psychological well-being in rheumatoid arthritis. *Social Science and Medicine, 27,* 399–403.

Foxall, M. J., Kollasch, C., & McDermott, S. (1989). Family stress and coping in rheumatoid arthritis. *Arthritis Care and Research, 2,* 114–121.

Frank, R. G., Chaney, J. M., Clay, D. L., & Kay, D. R. (1991). Depression in rheumatoid arthritis: A re-evaluation. *Rehabilitation Psychology, 36,* 219–230.

Gonzalez, S., Steinglass, P., & Reiss, D. (1989). Putting the illness in its place: Discussion groups for families with chronic medical illnesses. *Family Process, 28,* 69–87.

Goodenow, C., Reisine, S. T., & Grady, K. E. (1990). Quality of social support and associated social and psychological functioning in women with rheumatoid arthritis. *Health Psychology, 9,* 266–284.

Gottlieb, B. H. (Ed.). (1988). *Marshaling social support.* Newbury Park, CA: Sage.

Hannan, M. T. (1996). Epidemiologic perspectives on women and arthritis: An overview. *Arthritis Care and Research, 9,* 424–434.

Helmick, C. G., Lawrence, R. C., Pollard, R. A., Lloyd, E., & Heyse, S. P. (1995). Arthritis and other rheumatic conditions: Who is affected now, and who will be affected later? *Arthritis Care and Research, 8,* 203–211.

Hinrichsen, G. A., Revenson, T. A., & Shinn, M. (1985). Does self-help help? An empirical investigation of scoliosis peer support groups. *Journal of Social Issues, 41,* 65–87.

Hochschild, A. (1989). *The second shift.* New York: Avon.

House, J. S., Landis, K. R., & Umberson, D. (1988). Social relationships and health. *Science, 241,* 540–545.

Ickovics, J. R., Thayaparan, B., & Ethier, K. A. (in press). Women and AIDS: A contextual analysis. In A. Baum, T. A. Revenson, & J. E. Singer (Eds.). *Handbook of health psychology.* Hillsdale, NJ: Erlbaum.

Katz, P. P., & Criswell, L. A. (1996). Differences in symptom reports between men and women with rheumatoid arthritis. *Arthritis Care and Research, 9,* 441–448.

Katz, P. P., & Yelin, E. H. (1993). Prevalence and correlates of depressive symptoms among persons with rheumatoid arthritis. *Journal of Rheumatology, 20,* 790–796.

Keefe, F. J., Caldwell, D. S., Baucom, D., Salley, A., Robinson, E., Timmons, K., Beaupre, P., Weisberg, J., & Helms, M. (1996). Spouse-assisted coping skills training in the management of osteoarthritic knee pain. *Arthritis Care and Research, 9,* 279–291.

Kellick, K. A., Martins-Richards, J., & Chow, C. (1998). Management of arthritis. *Lippincott's Primary Care Practice, 2,* 66–80.

Lanza, A. F., Cameron, A. E., & Revenson, T. A. (1995). Perceptions of helpful and unhelpful support among married individuals with rheumatic diseases. *Psychology and Health, 10,* 449–462.

Lanza, A. F., & Revenson, T. A. (1993). Social support interventions for rheumatoid arthritis patients: The cart before the horse? *Health Education Quarterly, 20,* 97–117.

Liang, M. H., Rogers, M., Larson, M., Eaton, H. M., Murawski, B. J., Taylor, J. E., Swafford, J., & Schur, P. H. (1984). The psychosocial impact of systemic lupus erythematosus and rheumatoid arthritis. *Arthritis and Rheumatism, 27,* 13–19.

Lorig, K., & Holman, H. R. (1989). Long-term outcomes of an arthritis self-management study: Effects of reinforcement efforts. *Social Science and Medicine, 29*, 221–224.

Lorig, K., Lubeck, D., Kraines, R. G., Seleznick, M., & Holman, H. R. (1985). Outcomes of self-help education for patients with arthritis. *Arthritis and Rheumatism, 28*, 680–685.

Lowenthal, M. F., & Haven, C. (1968). Interaction and adaptation: Intimacy as a critical variable. *American Sociological Review, 33*, 20–30.

Majerovitz, S. D., & Revenson, T. A. (1994). Sexuality and rheumatic disease: The significance of gender. *Arthritis Care and Research, 7*, 29–34.

Manley, H. (1997, November–December). Considering the alternatives? *Arthritis Today*, 18–25.

Manne, S. L., & Zautra, A. J. (1989). Spouse criticism and support: Their association with coping and psychological adjustment among women with rheumatoid arthritis. *Journal of Personality and Social Psychology, 56*, 608–617.

Mazzuca, S. A. (1982). Does patient education in chronic disease have therapeutic value? *Journal of Chronic Diseases, 35*, 521–529.

McCracken, L. M. (1991). Cognitive–behavioral treatment of rheumatoid arthritis: A preliminary review of efficacy and methodology. *Annals of Behavioral Medicine, 13*, 57–65.

Melamed, B. G., & Brenner, G. F. (1989). Social support and chronic medical stress: An interaction-based approach. *Journal of Social and Clinical Psychology, 9*, 104–117.

Newman, S. P., Fitzpatrick, R., Lamb, R., & Shipley, M. (1989). The origins of depressed mood in rheumatoid arthritis. *Journal of Rheumatology, 16*, 740–744.

Newman, S., Fitzpatrick, R., Revenson, T. A., Skevington, S., & Williams, G. (1996). *Understanding rheumatoid arthritis*. London: Routledge.

Newman, S., & Revenson, T. A. (1993). Coping with rheumatoid arthritis. *Balliere's Clinical Rheumatology, 7*, 259–280.

O'Brien, T. B., & DeLongis, A. (1997). Coping with chronic stress: An interpersonal perspective. In B. H. Gottlieb (Ed.). *Coping with chronic stress* (pp. 161–190). New York: Plenum.

O'Leary, A., Shoor, S., Lorig, K., & Holman, H. (1988). A cognitive–behavioral treatment for rheumatoid arthritis. *Health Psychology, 1*, 527–544.

Parker, J. C., Bradley, L. A., DeVellis, R. M., Gerber, L. H., Holman, H. R., Keefe, F. J., Lawrence, T. S., Liang, M. H., Lorig, K. R., Nicassio, P. M., Revenson, T. A., Rogers, M. P., Wallston, K. A., Wilson, M. G., & Wolfe, F. (1993). Biopsychosocial contributions to the management of arthritis disability. *Arthritis and Rheumatism, 36*, 885–889.

Parker, J. C., Frank, R. G., Beck, N. C., Smarr, K. L., Buescher, K. L., Phillips, L. R., Smith, E. I., Anderson, S. K., & Walker, S. E. (1988). Pain management in rheumatoid arthritis patients. *Arthritis and Rheumatism, 31*, 593–601.

Pearlin, L. I., & Turner, H. A. (1987). The family as a context of the stress process. In S. V. Kasl & C. L. Cooper (Eds.), *Stress and health: Issues in research methodology* (pp. 143–165). New York: Wiley.

Penninx, B. W. J. H., Van Tilburg, T., Deeg, D. J. H., Kriegsman, D. M. W., Boeke, A. J. P., & Van Eijk, J. T. M. (1997). Direct and buffer effects of social support and personal coping resources in individuals with arthritis. *Social Science and Medicine, 44,* 393–402.

Radloff, L. S. (1977). The CES–D scale: A self-report depression scale for research in the general population. *Applied Psychological Measurement, 1,* 385–401.

Radojevic, V., Nicassio, P. M., & Weisman, M. H. (1992). Behavioral intervention with and without family support for rheumatoid arthritis. *Behavior Therapy, 23,* 13–30.

Reisine, S. T., & Fifield, J. (1992). Expanding the definition of disability: Implications for planning, policy, and research. *The Milbank Quarterly, 70,* 491–508.

Reisine, S. T., Goodenow, C., & Grady, K. E. (1987). The impact of rheumatoid arthritis on the homemaker. *Social Science and Medicine, 25,* 89–95.

Revenson, T. A. (1990). Social support processes and chronically ill elders: Patient and provider perspectives. In H. Giles, N. Coupland, & J. Wiemann (Eds.). *Communication, health, and the elderly* (pp. 92–113). Manchester, England: University of Manchester Press.

Revenson, T. A. (1994). Social support and marital coping with chronic illness. *Annals of Behavioral Medicine, 16,* 122–130.

Revenson, T. A. (1995, August). *On with the dance: Couples' coping with illness.* Paper presented at the 103rd Annual Convention of the American Psychological Association, New York.

Revenson, T. A., & Lanza, A. F. (1994, August). *Married with illness: Influence of gender on support and coping.* Paper presented at the 102nd Annual Convention of the American Psychological Association, Los Angeles.

Revenson, T. A., & Majerovitz, S. D. (1990). Spouses' support provision to chronically ill patients. *Journal of Social and Personal Relationships, 7,* 575–586.

Revenson, T. A., & Majerovitz, S. D. (1991). The effects of chronic illness on the spouse: Social resources as stress buffers. *Arthritis Care and Research, 4,* 63–72.

Revenson, T. A., Schiaffino, K. M., Majerovitz, S. D., & Gibofsky, A. (1991). Social support as a double-edged sword: The relation of positive and problematic support to depression among rheumatoid arthritis patients. *Social Science and Medicine, 7,* 807–813.

Rook, K. (1990). Social networks as a source of social control in older adults' lives. In H. Giles, N. Coupland, & J. M. Wiemann (Eds.), *Communication, health and the elderly* (pp. 45–63). Manchester, England: Manchester University Press.

Ross, C. E., Mirowsky, J., & Goldstein, K. (1990). The impact of the family on health: The decade in review. *Journal of Marriage and the Family, 52,* 1059–1078.

Roth-Roemer, S., & Kurpius, S. E. R. (1996). Beyond marital status: An examination of marital quality and well-being among women with rheumatoid arthritis. *Women's Health, 2,* 195–205.

Schmaling, K. B., & Sher, T. G. (1997). Physical health and relationships. In W. K. Halford & H. J. Markman (Eds.), *Clinical handbook of marriage and couples* (pp. 323–345). New York: Wiley.

Seachrist, L. (1996, July–August). RA's gender differences. *Arthritis Today*, p. 8.

Shearn, M. A., & Fireman, B. H. (1985). Stress management and mutual support groups in rheumatoid arthritis. *American Journal of Medicine, 78,* 771–775.

Sherbourne, C. D., & Hays, R. D. (1990). Marital status, social support, and health transitions in chronic disease patients. *Journal of Health and Social Behavior, 31,* 328–343.

Smith, C. A., Dobbins, C. J., & Wallston, K. A. (1991). The mediational role of perceived competence in psychological adjustment to rheumatoid arthritis. *Journal of Applied Social Psychology, 21,* 1218–1247.

Walker, E. A., Keegan, D., Gardner, G., Sullivan, M., Katon, W. J., & Bernstein, D. (1997). Psychosocial factors in fibromyalgia compared with rheumatoid arthritis: I. Psychiatric diagnoses and functional disability. *Psychosomatic Medicine, 59,* 565–571.

Ward, M. M., & Leigh, J. P. (1993). Marital status and the progression of functional disability in patients with rheumatoid arthritis. *Arthritis and Rheumatism, 26,* 581–588.

Wright, G. E., Parker, J. C., Smarr, K. L., Johnson, J. C., Hewett, J. E., & Walker, S. E. (1998). Age, depressive symptoms, and rheumatoid arthritis. *Arthritis and Rheumatism, 41,* 298–305.

Wright, G. E., Parker, J. C., Smarr, K. L., Schoenfeld-Smith, K., Buckelew, S. P., Slaughter, J. R., Johnson, J. C., & Hewett, J. E. (1996). Risk factors for depression in rheumatoid arthritis. *Arthritis Care and Research, 9,* 264–272.

Yelin, E. (1996). The costs of rheumatoid arthritis: Absolute, incremental, and marginal estimates. *Journal of Rheumatology, 23,* 47–51.

Yelin, E., & Callahan, L. F. (1995). The economic cost and social and psychological impact or musculoskeletal conditions. *Arthritis and Rheumatism, 38,* 1351–1362.

Zautra, A., J., Burleson, M. H., Matt, K. S., Roth, S., & Burrows, L. (1994). Interpersonal stress, depression, and disease activity in rheumatoid arthritis and osteoarthritis patients. *Health Psychology, 13,* 139–148.

Zautra, A. J., & Manne, S. L. (1992). Coping with rheumatoid arthritis: A review of a decade of research. *Annals of Behavioral Medicine, 14,* 31–39.

5

COUPLES AND COPING WITH CANCER: HELPING EACH OTHER THROUGH THE NIGHT

W. KIM HALFORD, JENNIFER L. SCOTT, AND JILL SMYTHE

I was stunned. The thing was I felt so well; having cancer was like a bolt out of the blue. (Brenda, describing when she first found out she had breast cancer)

***

I had been having trouble urinating for years. Deep down I knew something was wrong, but I couldn't bring myself to go to the doctor. When I did find out it was prostate cancer I just froze with fear. I had no idea that it could be treated, I just assumed that it would be the end of me. I didn't tell Jean [his wife] for a couple of days; I just didn't know how to tell her. (Jim, talking about his struggle to go for treatment for symptoms of prostate cancer)

***

Preparation of this chapter was supported by Queensland Cancer Fund Grant "Psychological and Educational Interventions to Promote Effective Coping With Breast and Gynecological Cancers: A Controlled Trial" to W. Kim Halford, Bruce G. Ward, and Jennifer L. Scott.

My husband and I had a good cry together. That was important because I knew that he was scared. I would have worried about how he was coping if he had avoided showing me how he felt. (Michelle, recalling the first night at home after her husband found out he had prostate cancer)

***

I thought cancer was cancer, you know . . . "the big C," and everybody died from it. I didn't realize there are so many different types of cancer with different treatments and that people could be cured of cancer. Bert [her husband] kept reminding me that most people get better, it kept me going . . . kept me positive. (Andrea, describing how her husband helped her to challenge fearful thoughts after her diagnosis with bowel cancer)

These quotes from some of our patients capture the fear, confusion, and struggle that couples experience when one partner is diagnosed and treated for cancer. From the time when someone first becomes aware of the possibility that he or she may have cancer through the processes of diagnosis, treatment, and recovery (and many patients diagnosed with cancer do recover), most people in committed relationships look to their partner for support. The extent that the partners are able to support each other is crucial in determining the psychological adjustment of both partners and probably improves rates of recovery and survival from cancer (Baum & Posluszny, 1999).

Currently, more than 8 million Americans have had cancer, with two thirds of these people diagnosed 5 or more years ago and many cured of the disease (Landis, Murray, Bolden, & Wingo, 1998). Consequently, health care providers view many types of cancers as chronic illnesses. The primary focus of psychological aspects of care is assisting patients and their loved ones to cope emotionally and physically with diagnosis and treatments and to recover and reclaim their lives. Although a minority of diagnosed cancers are fatal, many patients and their loved ones mistakenly believe that all cancers are terminal conditions that inexorably lead to swift death.

In this chapter, we describe the processes of couple adaptation to diagnosis and treatment of cancer, with a focus on coping with the most common cancers that have good prognoses. We begin with some background information on the nature of cancer and its treatment. Then we describe the common psychological reactions to cancer of patients and their partners, the mediators of those reactions, and the possible impact of psychological adjustment on medical outcomes. We outline psychological intervention that assists couples in which a female partner has been diagnosed with breast or gynecological cancer. The goals of the program, how to assess couples' needs, and the intervention are described. Although our clinical and research work primarily has involved couples where the women have early-stage breast or gynecological cancers, we believe that the intervention can be generalized to other cancers and to couples in which there is a male patient. The chapter concludes with a review of some practical challenges in the delivery of cancer support services and suggests directions for future research.

THE NATURE OF CANCER AND ITS TREATMENT

Cancer is a general term given to more than 200 diseases characterized by disorders of cell growth involving unrestrained, indiscriminate cell production. These cell masses potentially can invade and destroy surrounding tissues and metastasize (spread), via the blood or lymphatic system, to seed the growth of new cancers in other parts of the body. Eventually, many cancer cells lose their biologic function but are still dependent on the body for nutritional supply (Murphy, Lawrence, & Lenhard, 1995). Thus, cancer is essentially "a parasite formed from the patient's own tissues" (Wingate & Wingate, 1988, p. 91).

Epidemiology

If a person survives for 5 years after the initial diagnosis of cancer, his or her probability of death from the cancer is not significantly different from people who have not been diagnosed with cancer; hence, 5-year survivorship is often used as an index of cure (Murphy et al., 1995). The most frequently occurring forms of cancer in the United States have good prognoses. The most commonly diagnosed cancers in men and women are prostate and breast cancers, respectively (Landis et al., 1998). An estimated 184,500 men will be diagnosed with prostate cancer, and 178,700 women will be diagnosed with breast cancer each year, more than twice the number of people who will be diagnosed with the second most common cancer for both men and women, lung cancer. The 5-year survivorship of prostate cancer is 78% and for breast cancer is 79%.

The good prognosis of many cancers does not mean that mortality from cancers is infrequent. Cancers are second only to heart disease as the major cause of death in American men and women (Murphy et al., 1995). Current trends suggest cancers may soon be the leading cause of death, because the percentage of deaths related to heart disease (33.5% of all mortality) has been decreasing over the past three decades, whereas cancer mortality has risen, to account for 23.5% of all deaths (Murphy et al., 1995). The major reason for this increase has been the rise in the incidence of lung cancer. Five-year survivorship from lung cancer is only 12% for men and 15% for women, and approximately 140,000 people are expected to die annually from lung cancer in the United States. If this disease is excluded, cancer death rates over the past 30 years remain constant in males, whereas deaths in females have decreased.

Five-year survival rates for cancers are associated with disease staging and grade, as well as diagnostic sites. The 5-year survival rate for many types of localized cancers is in the order of 92% of cases but drops markedly to rates below 45% for later stage disease. For example, the third most common form of cancer in females is gynecological cancers, with an estimated 80,400 women diagnosed annually. The survival rates for gynecological cancers range from almost 100% for carcinoma of the cervix in situ, which is likely to be discovered at an early stage through routine screening procedures, to 41% for ovarian cancer, which frequently is detected only at an advanced stage.

Treatment

There are three common forms of cancer treatments: *surgery, radiation therapy,* and *medical oncology,* and their use in isolation or in combination is indicated by diagnostic and staging results. Surgery aims to resect, or remove, the mass. Radiation therapy aims to shrink tumor size or eradicate cells through exposure to doses of radioactive substances. Medical oncology involves systemic forms of treatment, such as chemotherapy (administration of cytotoxic drugs to reduce the size of tumors or kill cancerous cells) and the use of agents such as biologic response modifiers. Biologic response modifiers aim to enhance the biological responsiveness of the person to the tumor and disrupt the tumor–host relationship (Murphy et al., 1995).

ADAPTING TO CANCER

A patient diagnosed with cancer faces multiple challenges. First, there is the initial shock of the diagnosis, of being told that a serious and possibly life-threatening disease exists in one's body. For most patients, there is also fear and uncertainty about treatment and prognosis. Surgery usually is required, often followed by chemotherapy, radiotherapy, or some combination of the two. The treatments frequently have significant side effects and are disruptive to normal routines. At the same time, patients and their loved ones struggle with fears about possible death, disability, or disfigurement. Fortunately, for many people, cancer diagnosis and treatment are followed by recovery, but adaptation can be stressful.

Common Psychological Responses in Patients and Partners

Initial Reactions

The diagnosis and treatment of cancer have a significant psychological impact on almost everyone who has this experience (Derogatis et al.,

1983; Mendelsohn, 1990; Pettingale, Burgess, & Greer, 1988). Initial responses of shock, emotional numbness, hostility, and increased levels of depression and anxiety occur in many patients (Andersen, Anderson, & deProsse, 1989a; Derogatis et al., 1983; Fallowfield, Baum, & Maguire, 1986; Gottschalk & Hoigaard-Martin, 1986; Hughes, 1982). Most patients experience concerns relating to the possibility of abandonment or death, impaired functioning, and possible threat to finances through treatment costs and lost earnings (Cordova et al., 1995; Moyer & Salovey, 1996; Psychological Aspects of Breast Cancer Study Group (PABCSG), 1987; Spencer et al., 1999). Other common psychological reactions include concerns about lack of personal control over the treatment and course of the illness (Silberfarb, 1984), uncertainty about the outcome (Silberfarb, 1984), intrusive thoughts and subsequent avoidance responses (Palmer, Tucker, Warren, & Adams, 1993), concern with physical symptoms (PABCSG, 1987), and concern about cancer recurrences (Kemeny, Wellisch, & Schain, 1988).

For some patients, the reactions to cancer diagnosis are so severe that they meet criteria for a diagnosis of an affective or anxiety disorder. For example, 5% to 10% of patients following breast cancer diagnosis meet the criteria for posttraumatic stress disorder (PTSD), which is primarily observed among survivors of severe life-threatening traumas such as combat or assault situations (Cordova et al., 1995). In addition, up to half of patients with cancer may meet criteria for a range of other disorders, including adjustment and major affective disorders such as depression (Derogatis et al., 1983; Fallowfield et al., 1986). People who suffer from these more severe reactions tend to experience greater difficulty in role functioning within their family and workplace, especially while undergoing cancer treatments (Cordova et al., 1995).

Emotional distress and significant adjustment difficulties, such as depression, anxiety, and sexual difficulties, often are present in partners of people diagnosed with cancer (Cassileth, Lusk, Strouse, Miller, Brown, & Cross, 1985; Omne-Ponten, Holmberg, Bergstrom, Sjoden, & Burns, 1993; Ptacek, Pierce, Dodge, & Ptacek, 1997). Partners of patients who have experienced severe negative psychological reactions to cancer diagnosis may be especially vulnerable to adjustment problems (Northouse, Dorris, & Charron-Moore, 1995). The most frequently reported concerns for spouses tend to focus on the disease itself (Gotay, 1984) and on the survival of their partner (Northouse, 1989). There is a high concordance between patient and partner on psychological adjustment (Baider, Koch, Esacson, & Kaplan De-Nour, 1998; Northouse et al., 1995; Northouse, Templin, Mood, & Oberst, 1998). That is, the partners of patients coping poorly also tend to be coping poorly.

Body Image and Sexuality

The diagnosis and treatment of cancers in parts of the body associated with sexuality often lead patients to experience problems with body image or sexual identity. For example, women treated for breast and gynecological cancers commonly report difficulties accepting their appearance and feel they are less attractive or feminine (e.g. Andersen & Jochimsen, 1985; Andersen, Woods, & Copeland, 1997; Schain, d'Angelo, Dunn, Lichter, & Pierce, 1994). After treatment for gynecological cancer, approximately 50% of women report problems in sexual functioning (Andersen, 1993; Andersen et al., 1997), and approximately 30% of women report sexual dysfunction developing in their partner (Andersen, Anderson, & deProsse, 1989b; Morris, Greer, & White, 1977). Most men treated with surgery and radiotherapy for prostate cancer report problems with sexual functioning (Andersen & Lamb, 1995). High rates of relationship and sexual difficulties are common even in patients with early-stage disease.

Sexual problems may occur across all phases of the sexual response cycle, often involving decreases or impairment to sexual interest (Hughson, Cooper, McArdle, & Smith, 1988; Tang, Siu, Lai, & Chung, 1996), sexual drive and satisfaction (Tang et al., 1996), and frequency of intercourse (Andersen & Jochimsen, 1985). Increases in pain during intercourse for women (Andersen, 1996; Andersen et al., 1989b) and difficulty adjusting to changes in intimacy and sexual relations with partners (Andersen, 1993) also are common.

Existential Issues

Confronting a life-threatening illness such as cancer often leads people to reevaluate important life priorities (Halldorsdottir & Hamrin, 1996; Pensiero, 1995). Indeed, some researchers have used the term *existential plight* to describe the predicament faced by patients when their very existence is endangered (Weisman & Worden, 1976). This experience may be transient for some, whereas for others it may elicit a considerable range of emotional changes, including uncertainty, vulnerability, isolation, discomfort, and redefinition (Halldorsdottir & Hamrin, 1996). The process of redefinition involves a reevaluation of roles and goals, as well as changes in priorities, such as the need to be at peace with oneself and to have the presence and support of family, friends, and health professionals (Halldorsdottir & Hamrin, 1996).

Long-Term Adjustment

Despite the considerable acute trauma and disruption experienced by patients as a result of diagnosis and treatment of cancer, the majority of indexes of psychological distress return to premorbid levels with time (Grassi & Rosti, 1996; Hoskins, 1995, 1997). However, there is considerable variability within the course of psychological recovery after cancer diagnosis and treatment. For example, 20% to 25% of women diagnosed with breast or gynecological cancer suffer significant depression or anxiety 6 years after the initial diagnosis (Andersen, 1993; Cordova et al., 1995; Fallowfield et al., 1986; Irvine, Brown, Crooks, Roberts, & Browne, 1991; Vinokur, Threatt, Caplan, & Zimmerman, 1989). A substantial minority of patients with cancer (estimated to be 10%–15%) meet criteria for PTSD up to 10 years after diagnosis (Cordova et al., 1995). People with severe adjustment disorder also are likely to experience decline in their sense of control, adequacy of intimate social support, and access to broader social network relationships (Ell, Nishimoto, Morvay, Mantell, & Hamovitch, 1989).

Some quality-of-life domains remain impaired in spite of the resolution of mood and other psychosocial outcomes (Andersen et al., 1989a). For example, in a substantial proportion of women with breast and gynecological cancers, problems with body image, feelings of femininity, and intimate relationships and sexual functioning persist for many years (Andersen et al., 1989a; Morris et al., 1977; Schover, Fife, & Gershenson, 1989; Wolberg, Romsaas, Tanner, & Malec, 1989).

Factors Mediating Adjustment

Cancer Type and Treatment

Both the stage of cancer and associated prognosis mediate psychological adjustment. People with more advanced stage disease display greater distress, more negative attitudes toward themselves and the future, greater concern with physical symptoms, and more interpersonal difficulties (Cassileth, Lusk, Miller, Brown, & Miller, 1985; Cella & Tross, 1986; PABCSG, 1987). The greater difficulties associated with advanced stage of disease probably are attributable to the need for intensive, invasive, and urgent treatments, which are often distressing (Andersen, 1993; Bremer, Moore, Bourbon, Hess, & Bremer, 1997; Schover et al., 1995). In addition, higher levels of distress almost certainly result from the fact that long-term survival may be unlikely and increased levels of debilitation or pain may be experienced in later stages of the disease (Andersen, 1993). Patient age interacts with stage of disease, so that the most severe distress is evident with advanced cancers in younger patients (Vinokur et al., 1989). In younger patients, the threat of death seems particularly distressing, possibly because of a perception of a large loss of anticipated life expectancy.

Coping Strategies

Patient coping style is predictive of longer term psychological adjustment to cancer (Grassi & Rosti, 1996; Heim, Valach, & Schaffner, 1997). Precise definition of effective coping with cancer has been hindered by researchers using a wide variety of imprecisely defined constructs such as "emotional expression" (Classen, Koopman, Angell, & Spiegel, 1996), "fighting spirit" (Friedman, Nelson, Baer, Lane, & Smith, 1990; Grassi & Rosti,

1996), and "acceptance" (Carver et al., 1993). Each of these styles of coping has been associated with enhanced adjustment to cancer (Dunkel-Schetter, Feinstein, Taylor, & Falke, 1992). The common element to all is *active* coping, as distinct from *avoidant* coping. Behaviors associated with active coping include patients seeking information about their disease, treatment, prognosis, and what they need to do to help themselves. These behaviors are associated with enhanced emotional adjustment (Dunkel-Schetter et al., 1992; Orr, 1986; Stanton & Snider, 1993; Taylor, Lichtman, & Wood, 1984; Timko & Janoff-Bulman, 1985). Further, patients who use multiple coping methods, selected according to the demands of the problem faced, have fewer mood disturbances than other patients (Carver et al., 1993; Gotay, 1984; Grassi & Molinari, 1988; Hilton, 1989).

Most people with cancer use more than one method of coping, and the methods used often change over time (Gotay, 1984; Grassi & Molinari, 1988; Hilton, 1989). Different coping styles may be more effective in facilitating adjustment at particular stages of the treatment process (Epping-Jordan et al., 1999; Glanz & Lerman, 1992; Heim, Augustiny, Schaffner, & Valach, 1993). For example, after diagnosis and before treatment there is often relatively little action patients can take to alter their situation. In this context, emotion-focused coping in which social support is sought may be most helpful (Burgess, Morris, & Pettingale, 1988; Glanz & Lerman, 1992; Lavery & Clarke, 1996; Orr, 1986; Stanton & Snider, 1993). After cancer treatment, more active coping, such as returning to pleasant activities and engaging in health-enhancing behaviors, may promote adjustment (Carver et al., 1993; Dunkel-Schetter et al., 1992; Heim et al., 1997; Orr, 1986).

Cognitions are widely recognized in psychology as crucial in determining coping with stress (Abramson, Seligman, & Teasdale, 1978; Folkman, Lazarus, Dunkel-Schetter, De Longis, & Gruen, 1986; Peterson & Seligman, 1987), and particular types of cognitions are associated with certain types of illness coping (Litt, 1988; O'Leary, Shoor, Lorig, & Holman, 1988; Spiegel, 1995). For example, cognitions of confidence or self-efficacy in one's ability to cope with the potential challenges posed by cancer predict better mood and quality of life (Telch & Telch, 1986).

Social Support and the Couple Relationship

Social support, in particular, partner support for patients in committed relationships, is a major influence on psychological adjustment to cancer. Being married is associated with lower mortality from a wide range of illnesses, and this is also true for cancer (House, Robbins, & Metzner, 1982; Kosenvuo, Kaprio, Kesaniemi, & Sarna, 1980; Ren, 1997). However, an even stronger predictor of health outcomes in illness than marital status is the quality of marital interactions, in particular, the level of support the spouses provide to each other in coping with illness (Burman & Margolin, 1992).

High perceived social support is associated with less depression, anxiety, and general maladjustment to cancer in patients (Bloom & Spiegel, 1984; Grassi & Rosti, 1996; Hoskins, 1995; Northouse, 1988). More specifically, high emotional expressiveness and cohesion in the relationship predict better adjustment (Bloom, 1982; Friedman et al., 1988). In the spouses of patients with cancer, the level of social support provided to the spouse by the patient predicts long-term adjustment to the patient's cancer as well as both partners' marital satisfaction (Ptacek et al., 1997). Thus, mutual social support by partners predicts well-being for both patients and spouses.

Predictors of Sexual Functioning

The extent of body image and sexual difficulties is correlated with the cancer treatment required. For example, relative to women with breast cancer undergoing lumpectomy, women undergoing mastectomy report greater distress about body image (Bartelink, van Dam, & van Dongen, 1985; Glanz & Lerman, 1992; Lee et al., 1992; Schain et al., 1994) and surgical scars (Lee et al., 1992) and feel more ashamed of their breasts (Bartelink et al., 1985; Kemeny et al., 1988; Margolis, Goodman, & Rubin, 1990). Mastectomy patients also report more problems with sex than do lumpectomy patients (e.g., Lee et al., 1992; Noguchi et al., 1993; Schain et al., 1994) and more feelings of being less attractive and sexually desirable (Kemeny et al., 1988; Lasry et al., 1987; Margolis et al., 1990; Steinberg, Juliano, & Wise, 1985). Although it often is assumed that it is the surgical procedures themselves that account for the differential responses of women undergoing lumpectomy versus mastectomy, patients self-select treatment options. It is possible that those patient characteristics that influence treatment decisions also influence appraisals of the choices made, particularly the impact on intimate relationships and sexual adjustment. For example, women's expectations of their attractiveness to their partner may influence their choice of treatment and may predict their long-term psychological adjustment (Stanton et al., 1998).

Patients' cognitions about sexuality after treatment may be particularly important in determining adjustment. For example, cognitions about sexual aspects of oneself such as attractiveness and sexuality (referred to as *sexual self-schema*) are associated with women's sexual adjustment after treatments for gynecological cancers (Andersen et al., 1997). Furthermore, these cognitions account for significant variance in sexual adjustment after controlling for self-reported premorbid intercourse frequency, extent of treatments, and menopausal symptoms (Andersen et al., 1997).

Impact of Psychological Adjustment on Survival

There is some evidence that better psychological adjustment affects cancer-free periods and survival rates. In particular, high social support is associated with lower mortality from cancer (Carlsson & Hamrin, 1994; Christensen, Wiebe, Smith, & Turner, 1994) and longer disease-free periods (Hislop, Waxler, Coldman, Elwood, & Kan, 1987). Research on the effects of coping style on survival has produced mixed results. In some studies, possession of a "fighting spirit" (Greer, Morris, & Pettingale, 1994; Greer, Morris, Pettingale, & Haybittle, 1990) and postoperative optimism (Hislop et al., 1987) were associated with extended recurrence-free survival after cancer. In a methodologically rigorous longitudinal study of young adults with melanoma, persistent avoidance of thoughts about cancer predicted poor disease status 1 year after treatment, after we controlled for initial disease parameters such as staging and extent of disease (Epping-Jordan, Compas, & Howell, 1994). However, other studies with early-stage breast cancer patients (Holland et al., 1986) and melanoma patients (Cassileth, Lusk, Miller, et al., 1985) found no association between coping style and time to relapse.

Andersen, Kiecolt-Glaser, and Glaser (1994) have proposed a biobehavioral model outlining two mechanisms by which psychological responses influence health outcomes in cancer. First, psychological adjustment to cancer may affect health behaviors, such as compliance to medical regimes, exercise (Eskola et al., 1978), drug intake (Jerrells, Marietta, Bone, Weight, & Eckardt, 1988), sleep (Palmblad, Petrini, Wasserman, & Akerstedt, 1979), and nutrition (Chandra, 1983). In turn, these health behaviors may influence health outcomes through their effect on the immune system (Herbert & Cohen, 1993). Second, physiological changes associated with psychological maladjustment may have a direct influence on immune function. For example, both depression and high stress can be immunosuppressive through pathways such as central nervous system activation of the sympathetic nervous system (Felten et al., 1987) or neuroendocrine immune pathways with the release of hormones.

In summary, the evidence of the impact of psychological adjustment on cancer outcomes is intriguing. It is possible that promotion of better social support and coping can enhance disease-free periods and survival rates. Such an effect may be the consequence of either the promotion of health-enhancing behaviors or the psychophysiological changes resulting from stress affecting immune functioning.

COUPLE INTERVENTION AND ADAPTATION TO CANCER

Our couples-based intervention—Cancer Coping for Couples (CanCOPE)—is a six-session cognitive–behavioral program offered to women recently diagnosed with early-stage breast or gynecological cancer and their partners. The six sessions include an initial session with the woman and five conjoint sessions with the couple. We conducted a randomized, controlled trial with 90 married women diagnosed with early-stage breast or gynecological cancer. Relative to either standard care or a cognitive–behavioral education program for the women alone, CanCOPE for couples produced significantly greater improvements in mood and greater reductions in long-term psychological morbidity (Scott, Halford, & Ward, 1998b).

The first session involves the woman alone, when she is approached at the treating hospital and offered the program. If she agrees to participate (approximately 90% of the women agree), we follow up with a telephone call to the woman and her partner. The program is explained in detail, and then we mail the couple an educational videotape on the particular cancer the patient has, plus a package of assessment materials. The couple is asked to review the videotape together and to complete the assessment package individually. Each subsequent session involves both the woman and her partner. (We currently are conducting a trial of a variant of CanCOPE for women working with a support person other than their partner, and we believe most of CanCOPE is appropriate when the support person is a family member or close friend.)

Couples usually are recruited into the program at the time of initial diagnosis, and the second session (a conjoint session with the couple) occurs before the woman undergoes surgery. This session is about 2 hours long. Subsequent sessions are typically 90 minutes long. In most of our work, we have held sessions in the couple's home. Sessions can be offered in a hospital or clinic, but given the stress on couples at the time of the program, the possibility of missed sessions is much higher when the couple needs to travel to attend them.

Key Content

The content of the first conjoint session involves reviewing and clarifying each partner's understanding of the patient's diagnosis and medical treatments. The core-partner support skills of supportive communication and helpful behaviors are introduced, and partners are assisted in providing these types of support. The physical, affective, behavioral, and cognitive aspects of the stress model also are explained. Each partner's current stress reactions are discussed, especially his or her cognitions and the role of cognitions in mediating responses and coping. Relaxation exercises are introduced as a way of managing anxiety and tension, and couples are instructed in a brief, guided relaxation exercise. The partners are asked to self-monitor self-talk associated with stressful cancer-related situations, practice relaxation exercises together, and conduct two conversations about cancer issues in which they discuss their feelings and concerns.

The next conjoint session is focused on coping training. The emphasis is on positive self-talk and stress management training. Using a self-regulation focus, we review each person's coping repertoire, and goals are set for expanding his or her range of coping options. The couple is taught how to review each other's self-talk and to promote positive coping cognitions. The impact of partner-support behaviors is reviewed, and supportive communication is encouraged as a means for tracking changes in support needs across the course of their disease experience. Each person is asked to practice positive coping self-talk and to review each other's progress. Partners are asked to share self-talk monitoring using supportive communication skills, to provide each other with constructive feedback, and to gently challenge negative self-talk.

The third conjoint session focuses on core beliefs and activities management. The vertical-arrow technique is used to explore core beliefs that may impede individual coping or undermine the quality of partner-support skills. The vertical-arrow technique involves the therapist first identifying negative thoughts and asking the patients the meaning of this cognition. Activities management is introduced as a component of stress management. Partners set individual and couple goals for the gradual return to activities and routines that may have been suspended because of medical treatments. This session also focuses on partner-support skills, especially the value of supportive communication and the insights gained through the shared thought-monitoring tasks for fostering empathic understanding and renewed emotional intimacy. Between sessions, partners reintroduce one individual and one couple activity into their weekly routine, continue to practice shared thought monitoring for stressful cancer situations, and maintain practice of their relaxation exercises.

The fourth conjoint session focuses on goal setting and prevention of sexual problems. Couples explore the existential challenges posed by their cancer experience and the impact it has had on them individually and on their relationship. They look beyond activities management to examine the effect of their experience on broader individual and relationship life goals. A goal-setting task may be used where appropriate. In addition, the couple discusses their goals for resumption of an intimate sexual life. The sensate focus technique is suggested as a way they can reintroduce intimacy into their relationship without provoking anxiety or causing pain. Sensate focus involves graduated sensual and sexual pleasuring to reduce anxiety and enhance sexual intimacy (Spence, 1997). Specific problems are identified, and couples are provided with advice, specific instructions, and reading materials. Where appropriate, referral for medical interventions is recommended.

The fifth conjoint session is a 20- to 30-minute telephone call to the couple, held with both partners about 3 months later. The conversation focuses on reviewing progress and identifying any problems that may have arisen. An appointment is made with the couple for the 6-month follow-up session, which is aimed to review progress with both individual and couple coping skills. Existential issues that may have arisen during the recovery and follow-up periods are discussed. The couple is helped to recognize the positive outcomes resulting from their experience and the implication of these outcomes for them as individuals and as a couple. Sexual functioning and intimacy also are discussed. Difficulties are problem solved using specific instructions, and sexual therapy techniques are taught. Future difficult cancer-related situations are identified, and strategies for managing these scenarios are planned. Finally, the main points of the session are summarized, and the positive gains the couple has identified are reaffirmed.

Assessment

Assessment serves two important functions. First, it provides the therapist with the opportunity to develop an empathic working relationship with the couple. Second, it allows assessment of the couple's current coping and helps identify their needs. Individuals' psychological functioning may subjectively bias self-reports of variables central to the objectives of couples-based intervention, such as perceptions of the adequacy of social support provision or coping. The combined use of interviews, self-report inventories, and behavioral observation maximizes the accuracy of data collected.

Assessment in CanCOPE typically consists of an initial conjoint interview with the couple, usually conducted before the patient has surgery. Patient and partner also complete a battery of self-report inventories. The answers to these inventories are reviewed in the first conjoint therapy session to clarify couple coping and identify areas of need. The key couple goals are then related to the general CanCOPE program, and particular areas needing emphasis are negotiated. For example, if the couple has difficulties in discussing highly emotional issues, then helping them to discuss issues around cancer is a goal for them.

Engaging the Couple

An important part of engaging the couple is to review and clarify each partner's understanding of medical information. Distress often stems from confusion about medical terminology and procedures. Myths about cancer or medical treatments also may be uncovered, such as the belief that "surgery exposes the cancer to air, thereby causing it to spread." These misapprehensions need to be gently challenged.

It is also important to help couples explore their feelings about diagnosis and treatment, especially newly diagnosed patients and their partners. These couples may feel overwhelmed by the many demands confronting them, such as undergoing diagnostic procedures and preparing for cancer treatment, and may feel they have had little opportunity to collect their thoughts.

Finally, hospital and treatment settings often focus solely on the patient, and the adjustment and coping of the partner are not routinely explored, leading some partners to feel excluded. Many patients also worry about their partner's adjustment and feel he or she needs support (Scott, Halford, & Ward, 1998a). Thus, attending to the partner's thoughts and feelings legitimizes her or his role in the process of coping with cancer. It builds rapport with both individuals and sends the implicit message that the therapeutic focus is on helping the couple cope with cancer rather than on helping a patient cope.

The Initial Interview

Table 5.1 lists topics that should be covered in an initial interview. The sequence presented is one that seems to make the interview flow well most of the time, although it is not a rigid order. In conducting the interview, the therapist should emphasize providing empathy for the distress most patients and partners feel in the initial period after diagnosis.

Conducting a conjoint interview enables the therapist to observe the couple's support for each other when discussing cancer-related issues. To enhance the value of this observational opportunity, the therapist should seat the couple close to each other. For example, sit them beside each other on a couch or on chairs placed close together and angled toward each other. The therapist should position him- or herself so as to be equidistant between the partners and so as to allow eye contact with each person. As the interview proceeds, the therapist should attend to the manner in which each partner responds to upset or distress in the other. In some couples, the partner will respond with physical comforting (e.g. a hug or stroking of the arm), whereas other couples may gently soothe each other. However, in some couples, the partner will look discomforted by the upset and either minimizes the issues verbally (e.g., "it will all be okay, don't cry, you can't let this get to you") or withdraws from the interaction. The reactions of the couple to each other in the interview situation may differ somewhat from private interactions when only the couple is present. However, the couple interaction in the interview does help the therapist generate hypotheses about the strengths and weaknesses in how the partners support each other.

Note that the interview begins with how the couple is coping with the current crisis of cancer diagnosis and treatment and moves to consideration of coping with previous life stresses. An individual's experience and success in coping with previous life stresses predict the manner with which she or he copes with the challenges posed by cancer (Rowland, 1990). Hence, it is useful to explore how the partners coped with events with similar ongoing emotional demands to cancer, such as divorce, bereavement, or serious illnesses in the self or loved ones. A history of coping through reliance on avoidant coping strategies, such as abuse of drugs, alcohol, or prescription medication, suggests increased risk for impaired coping with cancer. Past psychological problems are also predictive of poor adjustment to cancer. Individuals with a history of psychiatric disorders, depression, anxiety, phobias, or PTSD are at increased risk for poor adjustment (Cella, Jacobsen, & Lesko, 1990).

Self-Report Inventories

Table 5.2 lists self-report inventories that are helpful in assessing couples. Asking partners to complete these assessment inventories often prompts patients to think about their current difficulties and how they are coping. For example, completing the Psychosocial Adjustment to Illness Scale (PAIS) often prompts patients and spouses to reflect on their current functioning and to identify areas in which they need help.

We do not ask couples to complete all of the inventories in Table 5.2. We routinely ask patients and their spouses each to complete the PAIS to assess global level of adjustment. If the initial interview suggests that sexual functioning is a problem, the Sexual Interaction Inventory, a comprehensive assessment of partner current sexual behaviors and preferences, is used. The Dyadic Adjustment Scale (DAS) is an assessment of global relationship satisfaction. Low scores on the DAS predict poorer adjustment in patients after cancer treatment, and more specifically, low scores predict couples not engaging together in emotionally supportive discussion about the cancer (Scott et al., 1998a). Scores below 100 are indicative of relationship distress. Couples in which either partner scores below 100 may have difficulty in supporting each other, and it may be that someone other than the spouse is better suited to be the support person for the patient in these couples.

The Ways of Coping Questionnaire (WOC) and the Cancer Behavior Inventory (CBI) are both assessments of aspects of individual coping. The WOC is a global measure of coping strategies, whereas the CBI is a measure of self-efficacy in coping with specific cancer situations and challenges. These scales are generally useful. The Constructed Meaning Scale assesses the meaning associated with the experience of having a serious illness. This scale is most useful for prompting patients to reflect on the cancer experience after the initial crisis of diagnosis and treatment is resolved.

Behavioral Observation

We have already pointed out the opportunities to observe couples' support for each other during the conjoint assessment interview. It also is useful to have the couple talk directly to each other about the cancer experience and to observe this discussion. We ask the couples to discuss the following topic: "how is [patient's name]'s diagnosis of cancer and treatment affecting the two of you, how are you coping, and how might you support each other in the future?" During such discussions, therapists should physically distance

TABLE 5.1
Areas to Assess During Initial Interview

Specific questions	Implications for therapy
Current reactions and concerns	
How did you react when you found out you had cancer? What effects is the stress having on you now?	Assess current level of distress and need for specific coping strategies to cope with severe distress.
Cancer knowledge and beliefs	
What is the couple's understanding and knowledge of the cancer?	Some people have memories of caring for a loved one with cancer. The
What are their beliefs about the efficacy of cancer treatments generally and for the cure of their or their partner's cancer?	nature of these memories and how they relate to their adjustment and coping with their or their partner's diagnosis need to be thoroughly
What are the origins of their beliefs about cancer? For example, whom else do they know who has had cancer, and what involvement did they have with that person during the course of treatment? Was that person cured?	explored. Some individuals have been adversely affected by their experiences, which they generalize to their current situation. Other individuals find their experiences are a source of emotional strength and inspiration for coping with their own or their partner's cancer.
Couple communication about cancer	
To what extent has the couple discussed their emotions and feelings about the diagnosis and treatment? Have they also discussed how they might support each other?	Resistance to practicing supportive communication about cancer can stem from prior attempts that one or both partners perceive as aversive or unsuccessful. The circumstances surrounding prior efforts and the
How are their impressions of each other's adjustment and coping formed? Do they rely on "mind reading" to determine each other's thoughts and feelings?	reasons why they consider the outcome a failure or disappointment need to be addressed.
Other current stresses	
Are there other stressful situations with which the individual or couple are also coping (e.g., financial difficulties, caring for an elderly or ill relative, behavior problems or illness in a child)?	An individual's resources for coping with cancer may be diminished by her or his efforts to cope with a number of stressful life events. Some couples may benefit from assistance in generalizing stress management skills to situations.
Past stressful life events	
What other significant life stresses has the person with cancer faced? Pay particular attention to protracted stressful events, such as chronic illnesses, or those involving strong emotions, such as bereavement.	Client's self-efficacy for coping with cancer or for practicing core program skills may be impeded by negative appraisals of his or her prior coping.

Specific questions	Implications for therapy
What strategies did each partner use to cope, and how helpful did they find them? Explore for overreliance on avoidant coping strategies, such as abuse of alcohol or other drugs.	Analogies drawn from other stressful times in their life can be used in therapy to introduce the rationale for the core skills of the program.
What is each partner's subjective appraisal of his or her own coping during past challenges? What responses or actions does she or he consider indicative of good coping?	Appraisal of their partner's coping and supportiveness in the past may affect their expectations for partner support with cancer.
What are each partner's perceptions and satisfaction with support from the other during past stressful times?	
History of psychological disorders	
Are there psychological and psychiatric problems, such as affective, adjustment, or eating disorders, and how are these problems managed or treated?	Preexisting psychological problems can increase vulnerability to adjustment difficulties after diagnosis and treatment. Symptoms of comorbidity in either partner may impede his or her ability to cope and to support the partner and need to be addressed. In cases where premorbid psychosocial difficulties are mild, mastery of cancer coping skills can motivate self-efficacy for coping with other problems and issues.
Are there difficulties that may have been subclinical, never treated or more general, such as low self-esteem or unassertiveness?	
Sexual functioning	
What is the etiology of any premorbid or current sexual difficulties, especially organic problems caused by cancer or other illnesses and treatment?	Sometimes diagnosis and treatment interrupt a couple's sexual life. During therapy, their wishes and expectations for the resumption of sexuality and intimacy in their relationship need to be addressed.
What is their usual range of sexual practices and their satisfaction with their sexual life?	

themselves from the couples by sitting as far away as possible and directing the couple to talk to each other.

There is no correct interpersonal style for couples to support each other in the crisis of cancer treatment. But there are some generally useful responses that, if couples do not use them, are associated with poorer adjustment and less perceived support from the couple discussion (Scott et al., 1998a). In research, we code the behaviors of couples using highly trained

TABLE 5.2

Self-Report Assessment Measures in Psycho-oncology

Measure	Description	Scores produced	Reference
		Psychosocial functioning	
Psychosocial Adjustment to Illness Scale	46-item multidimensional scale examining 7 psychosocial–quality-of-life domains. Normative data for cancer patients available	Provides total adjustment score from 7 subscales scores: Health Care Orientation, Vocational and Domestic, Environment, Extended Family Relations, Sexual Relationship, and Psychological Distress	Derogatis (1986); Derogatis and Lopez (1983)
Impact of Event Scale	15-item measure of subjective distress indicated by frequency of avoidant and intrusive thoughts	Total score from 2 subscale scores: Intrusion and Avoidance	Horowitz, Wilner, and Alvarez (1979)
		Sexual functioning and body image	
Sexual Interaction Inventory	102 items, 17 heterosexual behaviors rated for frequency and satisfaction across 6 dimensions	Provides profile of couple's functioning across 11 scales with means of 50 and standard deviations of 10	LoPiccolo and Steger (1974)
		Partner support	
Dyadic Adjustment Scale	32 items assessing areas of satisfaction and conflict in relationship	Total score and 4 subscales scores: Consensus, Satisfaction, Cohesion, and Affection Expression	Spanier (1976)

Measure	Description		Reference
Partner Support Inventory	Ratings of provision and extent of helpfulness of 32 behaviors performed by male partner	Designed for clinical use. Aims to help couples achieve a shared view of the helpfulness of specific support behaviors	Unpublished measure available on request from authors
Coping strategies			
Ways of Coping Questionnaire (Cancer version)	49 items assessing cognitive and behavioral coping strategies	Total score and subscales scores for five types of strategies: seek and use social support, cognitive escape–avoidance, distancing, focus on the positive, and behavioral escape–avoidance	Dunkel-Schetter, Feinstein, Taylor, and Falke (1992)
Cancer Behavior Inventory	Self-efficacy for coping with 40 cancer-specific situations–challenges	Total score and five factor scores for coping with or maintaining activity–independence, treatment-related side effects, positive attitude–accepting cancer, medical information, and affect regulation	Merluzzi and Martinez-Sanchez (1997)
Existential issues			
The Constructed Meaning Scale	Eight items assessing the concept of meaning within the context of adapting to a life-threatening illness	A high score is indicative of positive meaning of the illness for one's self and one's future	Fife (1995)

raters, but in clinical work, it is possible to use the coding categories used in research in a less exact manner to describe the way in which the couple talks and to identify targets for therapeutic change. We watch as the couple talks and identify the most common responses used, and from this we formulate goals for promoting more supportive couple communication. For example, use of self-disclosure of feelings, active and empathic listening, and verbal and physical comforting in response to distress would all be seen as positive responses. Withdrawal, nonattending, criticizing, and minimizing concerns would all be seen as potentially negative communication behaviors.

Treatment

Medical Information Access and Informed Decision Making

Most patients experience severe distress when told of their diagnosis of cancer, are understandably upset when discussing their treatment, and find it hard to concentrate and to retain the information provided by medical staff (Sardell & Trierweiler, 1993; Woodward & Parmies, 1992). Some details of the medical aspects of care, such as treatment options, side effects of treatment, and prognosis, are beyond the expertise of psychologists. However, psychologists who understand the essential elements of treatments for common cancers can help patients access important information. For example, we often help women and their partners generate lists of questions that they wish to pose of their medical treatment team.

Psychological considerations are important in helping patients make informed choices about treatment and recovery, and psychologists can make an influential contribution here (Andersen & Golden-Kreutz, 1998). For example, as noted earlier, there is substantial data that women with breast cancer who undergo lumpectomy rather than mastectomy have fewer sexual difficulties and body image concerns after treatment (Margolis et al., 1990). In a similar manner, men with prostate cancer who undergo radiation treatment rather than surgery report fewer problems with erectile dysfunction or ejaculation (Andersen & Lamb, 1995). The psychological impact of these outcomes needs to be discussed with patients, to assist them in making an informed decision about which treatment to choose.

Couples in CanCOPE are provided with educational materials that explain medical aspects of their particular cancer and common diagnostic and treatment procedures. Many cancer organizations produce videotapes and written materials, and couples often find that reviewing these resources helps demystify medical information. In some cases, the woman or her partner may be fearful of reviewing educational material and avoid doing this. Suggest to the couple that you sit with them and review the package together. When showing a videotape, pause the tape at various points and integrate the discussion of reactions and concerns about the material. Once the material has been reviewed, the couple's understanding of the diagnosis and recommended treatment should be systematically explored and clarified. The couple is asked open-ended questions, such as, Why do you think the lymph nodes in your armpit will be removed as part of your surgery? What are your feelings about the type of treatment that you are to receive? Unrealistic concerns or misunderstandings are gently challenged, and couples are reassured that they are not alone.

The extent and the accuracy of patients' knowledge about aspects of their disease also depend, in part, on their ability to communicate effectively with medical professionals. Being appropriately assertive with health care professionals, asking questions and, if need be, asking for explanations to be repeated using lay terminology can be difficult. The couple is prompted to use the task of information seeking as an opportunity for mutual support. They work together to generate a list of questions they wish to clarify with their treating doctor or other members of their medical team. If required, role-playing and rehearsals are used to help them practice asking questions. It is suggested that they attend consultations together when seeking to discuss their concerns because they can aid each other's recall and provide one another with support.

Partner Support

Positive social support for people with cancer is beneficial (Manne, Taylor, Dougherty, & Kemeny, 1997; Rook, 1984), and promoting that support is associated with better psychological adjustment (Fawzy et al., 1990). Therefore, one goal of the couple intervention is to promote support from the patient's partner in coping with cancer. Because partners also have psychological adjustment difficulties in coping with cancer, the development of mutual support is highly desirable.

Social support is multidimensional in nature (Bloom & Spiegel, 1984) and can include emotional support, instrumental support (e.g. practical help with chores or attending treatment), provision of information, and assistance in decision making about treatment options (Cohen, 1988). Patients seek different types of support from different people. Emotional support is most frequently desired from partners by cancer patients, is rated the most helpful type of support, and has the strongest links with long-term adjustment (Helgeson & Cohen, 1996). Practical support also is an important aspect of support sought from the spouse. Hence, development of emotional and practical support between partners is a key goal of the intervention.

Although almost all couples report wanting to support each other emotionally during their experience with cancer, about 50% of couples 1 week after diagnosis of cancer have not discussed their emotional responses to cancer (Scott et al., 1998a). During periods of high stress involving confronting situations and strong emotions, couples' communication skills often are strained (Halford, Kelly, & Markman, 1997). In our experience, this strain can be extreme after diagnosis of cancer. Many couples avoid talking about the cancer for fear of distressing themselves or each other. Partners also are sometimes uncertain how to initiate a discussion and unsure what they can say that is helpful. However, the use of some basic communication skills, such as high rates of empathy, self-disclosure, and active positive listening, are associated with greater perceived support, reduced immediate distress in both partners, and better long-term adjustment to cancer (Pistrang & Barker, 1995; Pistrang, Barker, & Rutter, 1997; Scott et al., 1998a). Hence, one goal of our intervention is to promote supportive communication.

The available research is clear that perceptions of practical support behaviors by partners are associated with better adjustment to cancer treatment (Manne et al., 1997). However, almost all research has assessed global ratings of perceived support, and it is hard to identify specific behaviors that partners do that help each other. It is clear that undergoing cancer treatment interrupts couples' usual daily routines (Manne, Alfieri, Taylor, & Dougherty, 1999). For example, some patients are physically unable to perform some of their usual household or work duties, and partners need to adjust to new roles. Partners asked to rate the occurrence and helpfulness of specific behaviors during diagnosis and cancer treatment show low levels of agreement (Scott et al., 1998a). In our experience, many couples find it hard to know how best to support each other, with partners sometimes doing too much, too little, or missing the crucial help needed. Hence, promotion of effective mutual support behaviors is another goal of the intervention.

The therapist introduces the notion of supportive communication by suggesting that cancer can be a difficult topic to discuss, even for couples with good communication skills (Scott et al., 1998a). Common communication difficulties and the reasons why these may occur are explored. The couple is encouraged to examine their own communication, and any issues that may prevent them from talking to each other about cancer are normalized and challenged. For example, although partners frequently look to each other for clues to how to behave and support one another, many avoid direct discussion of these issues.

Supportive communication involves the speaker–listener skills of empathic listening, summarizing, validation, self-disclosure of thoughts and feelings, use of "I" statements, and indications of what the listener might do or say that is helpful. Empathic listening involves attending to the emotional significance or personal meaning of what is said by the speaker. Partners are taught they do not have to feel the same way as the speaker but that it is important to accept and acknowledge their feelings. Sometimes partners feel concerned that there is nothing they can do, in response to the speaker's concerns, that will be helpful. They are told they do not have to solve the issues raised for the speaker to find a discussion helpful. In fact, during therapy, many partners discover that using supportive communication is doing something useful (Scott et al., 1998b).

Empathic listening skills are modeled by the therapist while having each partner describe her or his reactions to diagnosis and treatment to the therapist. The therapist then has the couple speak directly to each other about these experiences. The therapist prompts and reinforces use of self-disclosure and active listening skills. Weekly homework tasks involve the couple spending 20 minutes practicing the supportive communication skills, taking turns "nominating" a cancer-related issue, and alternating speaker and listener roles. Talking about the cancer to the exclusion of all other things in their life can be draining and depressing. They need to balance their discussion about cancer with time spent talking about other topics and doing enjoyable activities together.

Undergoing cancer treatments temporarily interrupts couples' daily lifestyle and routines. Partner support involves behaviors that couples can do to help each other cope more effectively. Couples review behaviors listed on the Partner Support Checklist, a 32-item, cancer-specific measure designed for clinical use with couples coping with cancer (Scott et al., 1998a). The patient and spouse each identify actions that their partner could do that they would find helpful. The most helpful behaviors tend to change over time. As patients recover from treatments, they need less practical assistance and seek to resume activities that they may have stopped, some of which their partner may have been doing for them. Patients often value resuming tasks because they signify that they are coping well or that things are "back to normal." Partners, on the other hand, may become overprotective and seek to prevent the patient from attempting some activities, perhaps through fear they are doing too much too soon. The nature of the emotional support preferred by patients and partners may also change according to variations in the situational demands confronting them.

Active Coping Skills

Given that the use of active coping skills predicts better outcome in patients with cancer (Grassi & Rosti, 1996: Heim et al., 1997), we aim to promote active coping efforts. More specifically, we teach the patients and their partners relaxation training, engagement in positive activities, and cognitive restructuring as means to promote effective coping. This content is drawn from several structured educational interventions that improve psychosocial adjustment in cancer patients with nonmetastatic disease (Fawzy et al., 1990; Heinrich & Schag, 1985; Moorey & Greer, 1989; Telch & Telch, 1986).

Couples are taught about the components of the stress response model and the link between their thoughts and feelings. Each person's physical, behavioral, emotional, and cognitive responses to cancer are reviewed. This provides the partners with understanding of their own responses to cancer.

It also affords them a deeper understanding of the phenomenology of their partner's experiences and gives them insight into the cognitions and behaviors that enhance their partner's coping.

Next, couples are introduced to the rationale and steps for monitoring cognitions associated with stressful cancer-related situations. The high concordance between patient and partner's adjustment may in part be accounted for by the manner in which they influence each other's threat appraisals and choice of coping options (Folkman et al., 1986; Manne, 1999; Scott et al., 1998a). For this reason, we use a shared-thought self-monitoring homework exercise to utilize the process of cognitive contagion in a positive way. For example, partners may be thinking so negatively that they are unable to encourage helpful thinking in one another. They may reinforce each other's distress by agreeing with and accepting any negative or irrational thoughts that are verbalized. With the shared thought-monitoring approach, couples use their supportive communication skills to help each other review one another's thought-monitoring forms, identify and challenge negative thoughts, and practice more helpful self-talk statements that enhance coping.

Sometimes patients or partners encounter persistent irrational cognitions or schema that may impede or undermine their ability to cope and support each other effectively. Some themes evolve from prior or current relationships with significant others and mold the person's understanding about the nature of support provision or receipt in interpersonal relationships (Snyder, 1998). Relationship themes particularly relevant for couples' adjustment include the durability and dependability of relationships in times of duress, the value of emotional intimacy as a form of support, appraisals of self-worth and support entitlement, and the behavioral indicators of good couple or individual coping (Snyder, 1998).

Distorted relationship themes can create unrealistic expectations for support or misinterpretations of partner support and coping behaviors and adversely affect the acquisition of partner-support skills. Other negative self-referent schema may impair a person's ability to use or benefit from support provision. Core beliefs such as "I am not worthy of love," "I will be abandoned," or "I cannot rely on anyone" are sometimes expressed by individuals who have experienced neglect, abuse, or rejection during formative years, especially from a caregiver such as a parent. These beliefs color their interactions with others during their cancer experience. They may be hypervigilant or overly sensitive to comments and actions from their partner or doctor that they construe as signs of rejection. Close relationships are perceived as highly fragile and vulnerable. An individual may avoid making specific support requests in case these annoy their partner and she or he forsakes them.

Core issues are addressed with the couple by using the vertical arrow approach, to help each person systematically explore underlying maladaptive core beliefs. In a process akin to affect reconstruction in couples therapy (e.g., Halford, in press; Snyder, 1998), individuals are helped to identify relationship themes and to link these with current patterns in their individual coping strategies or their support transactions as a couple.

Sexual Difficulties

Sexual difficulties often result after cancer treatment, due to both the iatrogenic effects of cancer treatments and the psychological concerns of the couple about altered body image and sexual functioning. We provide education and support to promote the couple's reengaging in a mutually satisfying sexual relationship. A sensate focus (Masters & Johnson, 1970; Spence, 1997) approach to the reintroduction of sexual intimacy is taken, with the focus on the couple becoming reacquainted and relaxed with each others' bodies rather than on the immediate resumption of sexual intercourse. Couples where medical treatments have altered one partner's sexual responsiveness or anatomy also are given advice and specific instructions about sexual positions that may reduce the likelihood of pain during lovemaking.

Existential Issues

Many people find that the experience of diagnosis and treatment for cancer alters their sense of life meaning and values. For some couples, this is a profound and positive experience, leading them to place greater emphasis on core life values. For others, the experience is profoundly unsettling, destroying their preexisting sense of safety and predictability of their world. One goal of our program is to explore with the couple their individual and joint sense of meaning of the cancer experience.

This therapy component focuses on helping partners examine the impact cancer has had on their lives and on their relationship. The therapist encourages couples to reflect on experiences during cancer treatment and recovery and what has been learned. Issues often of relevance include people's sense of meaning and purpose in their lives, the importance of relationships, and their future goals.

Relapse Prevention

After cancer treatment, many patients fear recurrence of the disease. For example, some patients misattribute minor aches and pains to cancer, and this can be very distressing. We discuss the common concerns around this issue and help the couple make realistic appraisals of the likelihood of future problems. Two follow-up sessions are conducted, involving a telephone call at 3 months and a booster session at 6 months after medical treatment is completed. These sessions are designed to review the progress of both individuals' and couples' coping skills. This includes a review of the existential issues that may have arisen or been realized during the recovery and follow-up periods.

Issues relevant to being a cancer survivor or the partner of a survivor, such as resurgence of cancer memories in response to media stories about cancer, also are discussed. Difficult cancer-related situations that might occur in the future are identified and problem solved. For example, many patients find attending a routine medical checkup an aversive and anxiety-provoking experience. Helping couples plan for these situations and rehearse appropriate coping strategies increases the likelihood that they will implement these skills to alleviate their distress in the future.

CONCLUSIONS AND FUTURE DIRECTIONS

CanCOPE is a couples-based intervention to help women recently diagnosed with early-stage cancer and their partners to support each other through the processes of diagnosis, treatment, and recovery. CanCOPE has the goals of promoting knowledge about the treatment process, supporting effective decision making, promoting mutual support between partners, promoting effective and active coping, and preventing sexual problems or future relapse. A controlled trial has shown that the treatment was effective and better than individual support provided to the women patients alone. These findings are consistent with research demonstrating the crucial role of intimate support in coping with cancer (Helgeson & Cohen, 1996; Manne, 1999).

A number of important research directions need to be pursued. First, replication of the research on the effects of CanCOPE on women's adjustment after treatment for breast or gynecological cancer is desirable. Adaptations of CanCOPE can assist men with prostate and other cancers and their partners with coping. However, there may be gender differences in the utility of partner support in promoting better coping. We are beginning work evaluating the usefulness of couple-based interventions for male cancer patients. In addition, many patients do not have a partner or choose to use someone other than a partner for support. CanCOPE also might be adapted to assist people other than partners (e.g., other relatives or close friends) to provide support through cancer diagnosis and treatment.

CanCOPE involves one individual and five couple sessions for all patients diagnosed with early-stage cancer, and this potentially is expensive to provide in an era of increasing health service delivery cost. Given that a substantial number of patients cope reasonably well with cancer when receiving standard care, the need for routine use of an intensive intervention like CanCOPE may be questionable. However, most women do have substantial short-term psychological adjustment problems, and a briefer education program might reduce these problems. For patients at higher risk of long-term problems, an intensive intervention like CanCOPE may be necessary (Andersen, 1993; Watson, 1983). Our research team is exploring matching the intensity of interventions to patients' level of risk for adaptation problems. In this way, we hope to maximize the cost-effectiveness of support provided to patients and their partners.

Psychologists working with patients with cancer and their partners face a number of challenges. In addition to professional skills as a clinical psychologist, considerable knowledge is needed about the diagnosis and treatment of cancer and psychological reactions to diagnosis and treatment. Liaison with other health professionals is crucial to providing quality services. Useful information for psychologists, patients, and their families can be obtained from a number of excellent web sites, such as the American Cancer Society at www.cancer.org, the British Association of United Cancer Patients at www.cancerbacup.org.uk, and the Anti-Cancer Council of Victoria in Australia at www.accv.org.au.

The diagnosis of cancer and its treatment pose a major challenge to all patients and their loved ones. Effective mutual partner support throughout the process promotes better psychological adaptation. The evidence on the effects of psychological adjustment on cancer survival holds out the intriguing possibility that good mutual couple support might provide greater quantity, as well as quality, of life in cancer patients.

***

Looking back now I think the whole thing brought us closer together, made us realize how important family and friends really are. We got through this as a team. We are definitely even closer now than before. (Michael, looking back 12 months after his wife's operation for uterine cancer)

REFERENCES

Abramson, L. Y., Seligman, M. E., & Teasdale, J. D. (1978). Learned helplessness in humans: Critique and reformulation. *Journal of Abnormal Psychology, 87,* 49–74.

Andersen, B. L. (1993). Predicting sexual and psychologic morbidity and improving the quality of life for women with gynecologic cancer. *Cancer, 71*(Suppl. 4), 1678–1690.

Andersen, B. L. (1996). Stress and quality of life following cervical cancer. *Journal of the National Cancer Institute Monographs, 21,* 65–70.

Andersen, B. L., Anderson, B., & deProsse, C. (1989a). Controlled prospective longitudinal study of women with cancer: Psychological outcomes. *Journal of Consulting and Clinical Psychology, 57,* 692–697.

Andersen, B. L., Anderson, B., & deProsse, C. (1989b). Controlled prospective longitudinal study of women with cancer: Sexual functioning outcomes. *Journal of Consulting and Clinical Psychology, 57,* 683–691.

Andersen, B. L., & Golden-Kreutz, D. M. (1998). Cancer. In A. S. Bellack & M. Hersen (Eds.), *Comprehensive clinical psychology: Vol. 8. Health psychology* (pp. 217–236). Oxford, England: Elsevier Science.

Andersen, B. L., & Jochimsen, P. R. (1985). Sexual functioning among breast cancer, gynecologic cancer, and healthy women. *Journal of Consulting and Clinical Psychology, 53,* 25–32.

Andersen, B. L., Kiecolt-Glaser, J. K., & Glaser, R. (1994). A biobehavioral model of cancer stress and disease course. *American Psychologist, 49,* 389–404.

Andersen, B. L., & Lamb, M. A. (1995). Sexuality and cancer. In G. P. Murphy, W. Lawrence, & R. E. Lenhard (Eds.), *American Cancer Society textbook of clinical oncology* (2nd ed., pp. 699–713). Atlanta, GA: American Cancer Society.

Andersen, B. L., Woods, X. A., & Copeland, L. J. (1997). Sexual self-schema and sexual morbidity among gynecologic cancer survivors. *Journal of Consulting and Clinical Psychology, 65,* 221–229.

Baider, L., Koch, U., Esacson, R., & Kaplan De-Nour, A. (1998). Prospective study of cancer patients and their spouses: The weakness of marital strength. *Psychooncology, 7,* 49–56.

Bartelink, H., van Dam, F., & van Dongen, J. (1985). Psychological effects of breast conserving therapy in comparison with radical mastectomy. *International Journal of Radiation Oncology, Biology, Physics, 11,* 381–385.

Baum, A., & Posluszny, D. M. (1999). Health psychology: Mapping biobehavioral contributions to health and illness. *Annual Review of Psychology, 137,* 1–19.

Beck, J. S. (1995). *Cognitive therapy: Basics and beyond.* New York: Guilford Press.

Bloom, J. R. (1982). Social support, accommodation to stress and adjustment to breast cancer. *Social Science and Medicine, 16,* 1329–1338.

Bloom, J. R., & Spiegel, D. (1984). The relationship of two dimensions of social support to the psychological well being and social functioning of women with advanced breast cancer. *Social Science and Medicine, 19,* 831–837.

Bremer, B. A., Moore, C. T., Bourbon, B. M., Hess, D. R., & Bremer, K. L. (1997). Perceptions of control, physical exercise, and psychological adjustment to breast cancer in South African women. *Annals of Behavioral Medicine, 19,* 51–60.

Burgess, C., Morris, T., & Pettingale, K. W. (1988). Psychological response to cancer diagnosis—II. Evidence for coping styles (Coping styles and cancer diagnosis). *Journal of Psychosomatic Research, 32,* 263–272.

Burman, B., & Margolin, G. (1992). Analysis of the association between marital relationships and health problems: An interactional perspective. *Psychological Bulletin, 112,* 39–63.

Carlsson, M., & Hamrin, E. (1994). Psychological and psychosocial aspects of breast cancer and breast cancer treatment. *Cancer Nursing, 17,* 418–428.

Carver, C. S., Pozo, C., Harris, S. D., Noriega, V., Scheier, M. F., Robinson, D. S., Ketcham, A. S., Moffat, F. L., Jr., & Clark, K. C. (1993). How coping mediates the effect of optimism on distress: A study of women with early stage breast cancer. *Journal of Personality and Social Psychology, 65*, 375–390.

Cassileth, B. R., Lusk, E. J., Miller, D. S., Brown, L. L., & Miller, C. (1985). Psychosocial correlates of survival in advanced malignant disease. *New England Journal of Medicine, 312*, 1551–1555.

Cassileth, B. R., Lusk, E. J., Strouse, T. B., Miller, D. S., Brown, L. L., & Cross, P. A. (1985). A psychological analysis of cancer patients and their next-of-kin. *Cancer, 55*, 72–76.

Cella, D. F., Jacobsen, P. B., & Lesko, L. M. (1990). Research methods in psycho-oncology. In J. C. Holland & J. H. Rowland (Eds.), *Handbook of psycho-oncology: Psychological care of the patient with cancer* (pp. 737–749). New York: Oxford University Press.

Cella, D. F., & Tross, S. (1986). Psychological adjustment to survival from Hodgkin's disease. *Journal of Consulting and Clinical Psychology, 54*, 616–622.

Chandra, R. K. (1983). Numerical and functional deficiency in T helper cells in protein energy malnutrition. *Clinical and Experimental Immunology, 51*, 126–132.

Christensen, A. J., Wiebe, J. S., Smith, T. W., & Turner, C. W. (1994). Predictors of survival among hemodialysis patients: Effect of perceived family support. *Health Psychology, 13*, 521–525.

Classen, C., Koopman, C., Angell, K., & Spiegel, D. (1996). Coping styles associated with psychological adjustment to advanced breast cancer. *Health Psychology, 15*, 434–437.

Cohen, S. (1988). Psychosocial models of the role of social support in the etiology of physical disease. *Health Psychology, 7*, 269–297.

Cordova, M. J., Andrykowski, M. A., Kenady, D. E., McGrath, P. C., Sloan, D. A., & Redd, W. H. (1995). Frequency and correlates of posttraumatic-stress-disorder-like symptoms after treatment for breast cancer. *Journal of Consulting and Clinical Psychology, 63*, 981–986.

Derogatis, L. R. (1986). The Psychosocial Adjustment to Illness Scale (PAIS). *Journal of Psychosomatic Research, 30*, 77–91.

Derogatis, L. R., & Lopez, M. C. (1983). *The Psychosocial Adjustment to Illness Scale (PAIS & PAIS–SR): Administration, scoring and procedures manual—I.* Baltimore: Clinical Psychometric Research.

Derogatis, L. R., Morrow, G. R., Fetting, J., Penman, D., Piasetsky, S., Schmale, A. M., Henrichs, M., & Carnicke Jr., C. L. M. (1983). The prevalence of psychiatric disorders among cancer patients. *Journal of the American Medical Association, 249*, 751–757.

Dunkel-Schetter, C., Feinstein, L. G., Taylor, S. E., & Falke, R. L. (1992). Patterns of coping with cancer. *Health Psychology, 11*, 79–87.

Ell, K., Nishimoto, R., Morvay, T., Mantell, J., & Hamovitch, M. (1989). A longitudinal analysis of psychological adaptation among survivors of cancer. *Cancer, 63*, 406–413.

Epping-Jordan, J. E., Compas, B. E., & Howell, D. C. (1994). Predictors of cancer progression in young adult men and women: Avoidance, intrusive thoughts, and psychological symptoms. *Health Psychology, 13*, 539–547.

Epping-Jordan, J. E., Compas, B. E., Osowiecki, D. M., Oppedisano, G., Gerhardt, C., Primo, K., & Krag, D. N. (1999). Psychological adjustment in breast cancer: Processes of emotional distress. *Health Psychology, 18*, 315–326.

Eskola, J., Ruuskanen, O., Soppi, E., Vilijanen, M. K., Jarvinen, M., Toivonen, H., & Kouvalainen, K. (1978). Effect of sport stress on lymphocyte transformation and antibody formation. *Clinical and Experimental Immunology, 32*, 339–345.

Fallowfield, L. J., Baum, M., & Maguire, G. P. (1986). Effects of breast conservation on psychological morbidity associated with diagnosis and treatment of early breast cancer. *British Medical Journal, 293*, 1331–1334.

Fawzy, F. I., Kemeny, M. E., Fawzy, N. W., Elashoff, R., Morton, D., Cousins, N., & Fahey, J. L. (1990). A structured psychiatric intervention for cancer patients: II. Changes over time in immunological measures. *Archives of General Psychiatry, 50*, 681–689.

Felten, D. L., Felten, S. Y., Bellinger, D. L., Carlson, S. L., Ackerman, K. D., Madden, K. S., Olschowki, J., & Livnat, S. (1987). Noradrenergic sympathetic neural interactions with the immune system: Structure and function. *Immunology Review, 100*, 225–260.

Fife, B. L. (1995). The measurement of meaning in illness. *Social Science and Medicine, 40*, 1021–1028.

Folkman, S., Lazarus, R. S., Dunkel-Schetter, C., De Longis, A., & Gruen, R. J. (1986). Dynamics of a stressful encounter: Cognitive appraisal, coping, and encounter outcomes. *Journal of Personality and Social Psychology, 50*, 992–1003.

Friedman, L. C., Baer, P. E., Nelson, D. V., Lane, M., Smith, F. E., & Dworkin, R. J. (1988). Women with breast cancer: Perception of family functioning and adjustment to illness. *Psychosomatic Medicine, 50*, 529–540.

Friedman, L. C., Nelson, D. V., Baer, P. E., Lane, M., & Smith, F. E. (1990). Adjustment to breast cancer: A replication study. *Journal of Psychosocial Oncology, 8*, 27–40.

Glanz, K., & Lerman, C. (1992). Psychosocial impact of breast cancer: A critical review. *Annals of Behavioral Medicine, 14*, 204–212.

Gotay, C. C. (1984). The experience of cancer during early and advanced stages: The views of patients and their mates. *Social Science and Medicine, 18*, 605–613.

Gottschalk, L. A., & Hoigaard-Martin, J. (1986). The emotional impact of mastectomy. *Psychiatry Research, 17*, 153–167.

Grassi, L., & Molinari, S. (1988). Pattern of emotional control and psychological reactions to breast cancer: A preliminary report. *Psychological Reports, 62*, 727–732.

Grassi, L., & Rosti, G. (1996). Psychosocial morbidity and adjustment to illness among long-term cancer survivors: A six-year follow-up study. *Psychosomatics, 37*, 523–532.

Greer, S., Morris, T., & Pettingale, K. W. (1994). Psychological responses to breast cancer: Effect on outcome. In A. Steptoe & J. Wardle (Eds.), *Psychological processes and health* (pp. 393–399). Cambridge: Cambridge University Press.

Greer, S., Morris, T., Pettingale, K. W., & Haybittle, J. L. (1990). Psychological response to breast cancer and 15 year outcome. *Lancet, 335,* 49–50.

Halford, W. K. (in press). *Brief couples therapy: Helping partners manage change.* New York: Guilford Press.

Halford, W. K., Kelly, A., & Markman, H. J. (1997). The concept of a healthy marriage. In W. K. Halford & H. J. Markman (Eds.), *Clinical handbook of marriage and couples intervention* (pp. 3–12). Chichester, England: Wiley.

Halldorsdottir, S., & Hamrin, E. (1996). Experiencing existential changes: The lived experience of having cancer. *Cancer Nursing, 19,* 29–36.

Heim, E., Augustiny, K. F., Schaffner, L., & Valach, L. (1993). Coping with breast cancer over time and situation. *Journal of Psychosomatic Research, 37,* 523–542.

Heim, E., Valach, L., & Schaffner, L. (1997). Coping and psychosocial adaptation: Longitudinal effects over time and stages in breast cancer. *Psychosomatic Medicine, 59,* 408–418.

Heinrich, R. L., & Schag, C. C. (1985). Stress and activity management: Group treatment for cancer patients and spouses. *Journal of Consulting and Clinical Psychology, 53,* 439–446.

Helgeson, V. S., & Cohen, S. (1996). Social support and adjustment to cancer: Reconciling descriptive, correlational, and intervention. *Health Psychology, 15,* 135–148.

Herbert, T. B., & Cohen, S. (1993). Stress and immunity in humans: A meta-analytic review. *Psychosomatic Medicine, 55,* 364–379.

Hilton, B. A. (1989). The relationship of uncertainty, control, commitment, and threat of recurrence to coping strategies used by women diagnosed with breast cancer. *Journal of Behavioral Medicine, 12,* 39–53.

Hislop, T. G., Waxler, N. E., Coldman, A. J., Elwood, J. M., & Kan, L. (1987). The prognostic significance of psychosocial factors in women with breast cancer. *Journal of Chronic Diseases, 40,* 729–735.

Holland, J. C., Korzun, A. H., Tross, S., Cella, D. F., Norton, L., & Wood, W. (1986). Psychosocial factors and disease-free survival in stage II breast cancer [Abstract]. *Proceedings of the American Society of Clinical Oncology, 5,* 237.

Horowitz, M. Wilner, N., & Alvarez, W. (1979). Impact of Event Scale: A measure of subjective stress. *Psychosomatic Medicine, 41,* 209–218.

Hoskins, C. N. (1995). Patterns of adjustment among women with breast cancer and their partners. *Psychological Reports, 77,* 1017–1018.

Hoskins, C. N. (1997). Breast cancer treatment-related patterns in side effects, psychological distress, and perceived health status. *Oncology Nursing Forum, 24,* 1575–1583.

House, J. S., Robbins, C., & Metzner, H. L. (1982). The association of social relationships and activities with mortality: Prospective evidence from the Tecumseh Community Health Study. *American Journal of Epidemiology, 116,* 123–140.

Hughes, J. (1982). Emotional reactions to the diagnosis and treatment of early breast cancer. *Journal of Psychosomatic Research, 26*, 277–283.

Hughson, A. V. M., Cooper, A. F., McArdle, C. S., & Smith, D. C. (1988). Psychosocial consequences of mastectomy: Levels of morbidity and associated factors. *Journal of Psychosomatic Research, 32*, 383–391.

Irvine, D., Brown, B., Crooks, D., Roberts, J., & Browne, G. (1991). Psychosocial adjustment in women with breast cancer. *Cancer, 67*, 1097–1117.

Jerrells, T. R., Marietta, C. A., Bone, G., Weight, F. F., & Eckardt, M. J. (1988). Ethanol-associated immunosuppression. *Advances in Biochemical Psychopharmacology, 44*, 173–185.

Kemeny, M. M., Wellisch, D. K., & Schain, W. S. (1988). Psychosocial outcome in a randomized surgical trial for treatment of primary breast cancer. *Cancer, 6*, 1231–1237.

Kosenvuo, M., Kaprio, J., Kesaniemi, A., & Sarna, S. (1980). Differences in mortality from ischemic heart disease by marital status and social class. *Journal of Chronic Diseases, 33*, 95–106.

Landis, S. H., Murray, T., Bolden, S., & Wingo, P. A. (1998). Cancer statistics, 1998. *CA: A Cancer Journal for Clinicians, 48*, 6–29.

Lasry, J. M., Margolese, R. G., Poisson, R., Shibata, H., Fleischer, D., Lafleur, D., Legault, S., & Taillefer, S. (1987). Depression and body image following mastectomy and lumpectomy. *Journal of Chronic Diseases, 40*, 529–534.

Lavery, J. F., & Clarke, V. A. (1996). Causal attributions, coping strategies, and adjustment to breast cancer. *Cancer Nursing, 19*, 20–28.

Lee, M. S., Love, S. B., Mitchell, J. B., Parker, E. M., Rubens, R. D., Watson, J. P., Fentiman, I. S., & Hayward, J. L. (1992). Mastectomy or conservation for early breast cancer: Psychological morbidity. *European Journal of Cancer, 28A*, 1340–1344.

Litt, M. D. (1988). Self-efficacy and perceived control: Cognitive mediators of pain tolerance. *Journal of Personality and Social Psychology, 54*, 149–160.

LoPiccolo, J., & Steger, J. C. (1974). The Sexual Interaction Inventory: A new instrument for assessment of sexual dysfunction. *Archives of Sexual Behaviour, 3*, 585–595.

Manne, S. L. (1999). Intrusive thoughts and psychological distress among cancer patients: The role of spouse avoidance and criticism. *Journal of Consulting and Clinical Psychology, 67*, 539–546.

Manne, S. L, Alfieri, T., Taylor, K. T., & Dougherty, J. (1999). Spousal negative responses to cancer patients: The role of social restriction, spouse mood and relationship satisfaction. *Journal of Consulting and Clinical Psychology, 67*, 352–361.

Manne, S. L., Taylor, K. L., Dougherty, J., & Kemeny, N. (1997). Supportive and negative responses in the partner relationship: Their association with psychological adjustment among individuals with cancer. *Journal of Behavioral Medicine, 20*, 101–125.

Margolis, G., Goodman, R. L., & Rubin, A. (1990). Psychological effects of breast-conserving cancer treatment and mastectomy. *Psychosomatics, 31*, 33–39.

Masters, W. H., & Johnson, V. E. (1970). *Human sexual inadequacy*. Boston: Little, Brown.

Mendelsohn, G. A. (1990). Psychosocial adaptation to illness by women with breast cancer and women with cancer at other sites. *Journal of Psychosocial Oncology, 8*, 1–25.

Merluzzi, T. V., & Martinez-Sanchez, M. A. (1997). Assessment of self-efficacy and coping with cancer: Development and validation of the Cancer Behavior Inventory. *Health Psychology, 16*, 163–170.

Moorey, S., & Greer, S. (1989). Adjuvant psychological therapy: A cognitive behavioural treatment for patients with cancer. *Behavioural Psychotherapy, 17*, 177–190.

Morris, T., Greer, H. S., & White, P. (1977). Psychological and social adjustment to mastectomy: A two-year follow-up study. *Cancer, 40*, 2381–2387.

Moyer, A., & Salovey, P. (1996). Psychosocial sequelae of breast cancer and its treatment. *Annals of Behavioral Medicine, 18*, 110–125.

Murphy, G. P., Lawrence, W., & Lenhard, R. E. (1995). *American Cancer Society textbook of clinical oncology* (2nd ed.). Atlanta, GA: American Cancer Society.

Noguchi, M., Saito, Y., Nishijima, H., Koyanagi, M., Nonmura, A., Mizukami, Y., Nakamura, S., Michigishi, T,. Ohta, N., Kitagawa, H., Earashi, M., Thomas, M., & Miyazaki, I. (1993). The psychological and cosmetic aspects of breast conserving therapy compared with radical mastectomy. *Surgery Today, 23*, 598–602.

Northouse, L. L. (1988). Social support in patients' and husbands' adjustment to breast cancer. *Nursing Research, 37*, 91–95.

Northouse, L. L. (1989). The impact of breast cancer on patients and husbands. *Cancer Nursing, 12*, 276–284.

Northouse, L. L., Dorris, G., & Charron-Moore, C. (1995). Factors affecting couples' adjustment to recurrent breast cancer. *Social Science and Medicine, 41*, 69–76.

Northouse, L. L., Templin, T., Mood, D., & Oberst, M. (1998). Couples' adjustment to breast cancer and benign breast disease: A longitudinal analysis. *Psychooncology, 7*, 37–48.

O'Leary, A., Shoor, S., Lorig, K., & Holman, H. R. (1988). A cognitive–behavioral treatment for rheumatoid arthritis. *Health Psychology, 7*, 527–544.

Omne-Ponten, M., Holmberg, L., Bergstrom, R., Sjoden, P. O., & Burns, T. (1993). Psychosocial adjustment among husbands of women treated for breast cancer: Mastectomy versus breast-conserving surgery. *European Journal of Cancer, 29A*, 1393–1397.

Orr, E. (1986). Open communication as an effective stress management method for breast cancer patients. *Journal of Human Stress, 12*, 175–185.

Palmblad, J., Petrini, B., Wasserman, J., & Akerstedt, T. (1979). Lymphocyte and granulocyte reactions during sleep deprivation. *Psychosomatic Medicine, 41*, 273–278.

Palmer, A. G., Tucker, S., Warren, R., & Adams, M. (1993). Understanding women's responses to treatment for cervical intra-epithelial neoplasia. *British Journal of Clinical Psychology, 32*, 101–112.

Pensiero, L. (1995). Stage IV malignant melanoma: Psychosocial issues. *Cancer, 75,* 724–747.

Peterson, C., & Seligman, M. E. (1987). Explanatory style and illness. *Journal of Personality, 55,* 237–265.

Pettingale, K. W., Burgess, C., & Greer, S. (1988). Psychological response to cancer diagnosis—I. Correlations with prognostic variables. *Journal of Psychosomatic Research, 32,* 255–261.

Pistrang, N., & Barker, C. (1995). The partner relationship in psychological response to breast cancer. *Social Science and Medicine, 40,* 789–797.

Pistrang, N., Barker, C., & Rutter, C. (1997). Social support as conversation: Analysing breast cancer patients' interactions with their partners. *Social Science and Medicine, 45,* 773–782.

Psychological Aspects of Breast Cancer Study Group. (1987). Psychological response to mastectomy: A prospective comparison study. *Cancer, 59,* 189–196.

Ptacek, J. T., Pierce, G. R., Dodge, K. L., & Ptacek, J. J. (1997). Social support in spouses of cancer patients: What do they get and to what end? *Personal Relationships, 4,* 431–449.

Ren, X. S. (1997). Marital status and quality of relationships: The impact on health perception. *Social Science and Medicine, 4,* 241–249.

Rook, K. S. (1984). The negative side of social interaction: Impact on psychological well-being. *Journal of Personality and Social Psychology, 46,* 1097–1108.

Rowland, J. H. (1990). Intrapersonal resources: Coping. In J. C. Holland & J. H. Rowland (Eds.), *Handbook of psycho-oncology: Psychological care of the patient with cancer* (pp. 44–57). New York: Oxford University Press.

Sardell, A. N., & Trierweiler, S. J. (1993). Disclosing the cancer diagnosis. *Cancer, 72,* 3355–3365.

Schain, W. S., d'Angelo, T. M., Dunn, M. E., Lichter, A. S., & Pierce, L. J. (1994). Mastectomy versus conservative surgery and radiation therapy. *Cancer, 73,* 1221–1228.

Schover, L. R., Fife, M., & Gershenson, D. M. (1989). Sexual dysfunction and treatment for early stage cervical cancer. *Cancer, 63,* 204–212.

Schover, L. R., Yetman, R. J., Tuason, L. J., Meisler, E., Esselstyn, C. B., Hermann, R. E., Grundfest-Broniatowski, S., & Dowden, R. V. (1995). Partial mastectomy and breast reconstruction. *Cancer, 75,* 54–64.

Scott, J. L., Halford, W. K., & Ward, B. (1998a). *Helping each other through the night: Behavioural assessment of intimate social support in couples where the woman has cancer.* Manuscript submitted for publication.

Scott, J. L., Halford, W. K., & Ward, B. (1998b). *We can cope: The efficacy of couple supportive psychoeducation in helping women with breast and gynaecological cancer and their partners.* Manuscript submitted for publication.

Silberfarb, P. M. (1984). Psychiatric problems in breast cancer. *Cancer, 53*(Suppl. 3), 820–824.

Snyder, D. K. (1998, July). Beyond behavioral couples therapy: Affective reconstruction of relationship dispositions. In W. K. Halford (Chair), *Beyond traditional behavioral couples therapy: New directions in the treatment of relationship problems*. Symposium conducted at the World Congress of Behavioral and Cognitive Therapies, Acapulco, Mexico.

Spanier, G. B. (1976). Measuring dyadic adjustment: New scales for assessing the quality of marriage and similar dyads. *Journal of Marriage and the Family, 38*, 15–28.

Spence, S. H. (1997). Sex and relationships. In W. K. Halford & H. J. Markman (Eds.), *Clinical handbook of marriage and couple interventions* (pp. 73–106). Chichester, England: Wiley.

Spencer, S. M., Lehman, J. M., Wynings, C., Arena, P., Carver, C. S., Antoni, M. H., Derhagopian, R. P., Ironson, G., & Love, N. (1999). Concerns about breast cancer and relations to psychosocial well-being in a multiethnic sample of early-stage patients. *Health Psychology, 18*, 159–168.

Spiegel, D. (1995). Commentary. *Journal of Psychosocial Oncology, 13*, 115–121.

Stanton, A. L., Estes, M. A., Estes, N. C., Cameron, C. L., Danoff-Burg, S., & Irving, L. M. (1998). Treatment decision-making and adjustment to breast cancer: A longitudinal study. *Journal of Consulting and Clinical Psychology, 66*, 313–322.

Stanton, A. L., & Snider, P. R. (1993). Coping with a breast cancer diagnosis: A prospective study. *Health Psychology, 12*, 16–23.

Steinberg, M. D., Juliano, M. A., & Wise, L. (1985). Psychological outcome of lumpectomy versus mastectomy in the treatment of breast cancer. *American Journal of Psychiatry, 142*, 34–39.

Tang, C. S., Siu, B., Lai, F. D., & Chung, T. K. H. (1996). Heterosexual Chinese women's sexual adjustment after gynecologic cancer. *The Journal of Sex Research, 33*, 189–195.

Taylor, S. E., Lichtman, R. R., & Wood, J. V. (1984). Compliance with chemotherapy among breast cancer patients. *Health Psychology, 3*, 553–562.

Telch, C. F., & Telch, M. J. (1986). Group coping skills instruction and supportive group therapy for cancer patients: A comparison of strategies. *Journal of Consulting and Clinical Psychology, 54*, 802–808.

Timko, C., & Janoff-Bulman, R. (1985). Attributions, vulnerability and psychological adjustment: The case of breast cancer. *Health Psychology, 4*, 521–544.

Vinokur, A. D., Threatt, B. A., Caplan, R. D., & Zimmerman, B. L. (1989). Physical and psychosocial functioning and adjustment to breast cancer. *Cancer, 63*, 394–405.

Watson, M. (1983). Psychological intervention with cancer patients: A review. *Psychological Medicine, 13*, 839–846.

Weisman, A. D., & Worden, J. W. (1976). The existential plight in cancer: Significance of the first 100 days. *International Journal of Psychiatry in Medicine, 7*, 1–15.

Wingate, P., & Wingate, R. (1988). *The Penguin medical encyclopedia* (3rd ed.). London: Penguin.

Wolberg, W. H., Romsaas, E. P., Tanner, M. A., & Malec, J. F. (1989). Psychosexual adaptation to breast cancer surgery. *Cancer, 63,* 1645–1655.

Woodward, L. J., & Parmies, R. J. (1992). The disclosure of the diagnosis of cancer. *Primary Care, 19,* 657–663.

6

COUPLES WITH HIV/AIDS

SETH C. KALICHMAN

Couples affected by AIDS face a plethora of challenges, some of which are common to many life-threatening illnesses and others of which are unique to AIDS. HIV infection is in many ways a disease of couple relationships. Today, nearly all adults living with HIV infection in industrialized nations became infected with the virus through interpersonal relations, by either a sexual or syringe-sharing partner. In many cases, the relationship within which a person became HIV infected dissolves, only to be followed by new relationships. Partners of people living with HIV/AIDS may or may not themselves be HIV infected. Couples living with HIV/AIDS therefore are complex in terms of psychological and social challenges. In this chapter, I discuss the factors associated with couples living with HIV/AIDS and how these factors interact with HIV/AIDS disease-related processes. Issues facing couples in which both partners are HIV positive as well as mixed-HIV-status couples are discussed. Two case vignettes also are included to illustrate the issues facing many couples with HIV/AIDS. Finally, this chapter provides an overview of psychologically assessing and treating couples affected by AIDS

National Institute of Mental Health Grant R01-MH57624 and Center Grant P30 MH52776 supported the preparation of this chapter.

and concludes with suggested areas for further research. First, however, I review the history of HIV/AIDS and its association to relationships.

BACKGROUND

In 1981, the U.S. Centers for Disease Control (now Centers for Disease Control and Prevention) reported on five young men who had rare medical conditions, all of which involved seriously compromised immune systems. Disease investigators quickly learned that these men were sexually involved with other men and, as it turned out, they shared a common lineage of sex partners. This cluster of cases was among the first to be diagnosed with what would later become known as AIDS. Since then, more than 700,000 people have been diagnosed with AIDS in the United States, where there are an estimated 1 million people living with HIV infection (Centers for Disease Control and Prevention [CDC], 1999). AIDS has been diagnosed in more than 10 million people worldwide, with greater than 30 million people thought to be HIV infected. HIV/AIDS has spread rapidly, with AIDS affecting people of all walks of life. Men and women of every ethnic background and sexual orientation are represented among the people living with HIV/AIDS.

In the United States, 3 out of 4 people with AIDS became infected through sexually transmitted HIV; most others become infected from shared injection-drug equipment. HIV transmission therefore occurs in the context of what are often our most personal and intimate relationships. Partners of people living with HIV, who themselves may be HIV infected, often become caregivers. When HIV transmission has occurred within a relationship, the person who was more recently infected will very likely end up caring for his or her partner because of their less advanced HIV disease state. Thus, often, a person will provide care to a partner who served as the source for her or his HIV infection.

Like everything else about AIDS, the course of HIV infection and how it wreaks havoc on the immune system is constantly changing. HIV infection results from a cascade of biological events that initiate when cells that are vulnerable to HIV, those that bear the molecule CD4 on their surface membrane, are exposed to HIV-virus particles. The principal targets of HIV infection are T-helper lymphocyte cells, which serve as control and coordinating centers for immune reactions. Once established in T-helper cells, HIV rapidly disseminates throughout the body, multiplying at a rate of a billion new virus particles each day and doubling the number of virus particles every 2 days (Ho, 1996).

The HIV replication cycle is a complicated process, primarily because the usual direction of biological events is reversed: The flow of genetic information moves from RNA to DNA rather than vise versa. HIV's genetic material is reverse transcribed to a DNA copy in the host cell. The virus serves to produce new HIV particles by controlling the functions of infected cells. As shown in Figure 6.1, the HIV replication cycle depends on several enzymes to orchestrate cellular events. The figure shows the major elements, including the viral envelope and genetic core of free HIV, the attachment of HIV to the surface of a CD4 cell, the viral RNA in a cell that produces the enzyme reverse transcriptase, which in turn transforms the viral RNA into viral DNA. The enzyme integrase combines the viral DNA with the cell DNA. Now under the control of the virus, the cell produces proteins that are spliced by the protease enzyme and new viral RNA that is repackaged into new virus particles. The HIV replication cycle is prone to error and therefore propagates with multiple mutations. There are usually numerous distinct variants of HIV within a given individual. The great genetic diversity of HIV enables the virus to rapidly adapt to pressures in its environment, including developing resistance to viral-suppressing treatments.

The earliest period of HIV infection, or primary HIV infection, may be accompanied by mild to moderate symptoms, such as fever, fatigue, and swollen lymph glands. Primary HIV infection occurs as a person develops antibodies against the virus. Unfortunately, the usual immune reactions set in motion to fight infection are ineffective at suppressing HIV. Primary HIV infection is followed by a long progression of disease advancement that occurs over years, most of which are relatively symptom free.

HIV destroys the immune system by systematically eliminating T-helper lymphocyte cells. The rate of T-helper cell loss in untreated persons

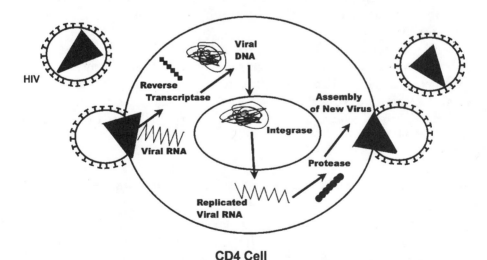

CD4 Cell

Figure 6.1. HIV replication process and three critical enzymes in HIV infection: reverse transcriptase, integrase, and protease. From *Understanding AIDS: Advances in Treatment and Research* (p. 108), by S. C. Kalichman, 1998, Washington, DC: American Psychological Association. Copyright 1998 by the American Psychological Association. Adapted with permission.

occurs at approximately 50 cells per unit of blood each year. There are roughly 1,000 T-helper cells/mm³ in the non-HIV-infected, healthy immune system. Therefore, 10 years of untreated HIV infection at a rate of 50 cells lost per year result in T-helper cell counts below 500 cells/mm³, bringing vulnerability to illnesses that people with healthy immune systems are usually protected against. Early symptoms of HIV infection therefore begin to appear when T-helper cell counts drop below 500 cells/mm³, and when a person has 200 cells/mm³ or less, he or she is diagnosed with AIDS. It is when a person has AIDS that he or she is most susceptible, or already has acquired, life-threatening, opportunistic illnesses. A person with AIDS, of course, has an immune system too disabled to combat these otherwise rare disease-causing agents.

The length of time between contracting HIV infection and developing AIDS is, however, lengthening because of increasingly more effective treatment regimens. For people who are diagnosed as HIV positive sooner, as opposed to later, after they have become infected, new treatments are reducing the rate of T-helper cell loss. Since 1995, the number of people dying of AIDS-associated causes, as well as the number of people dying of AIDS-related conditions, has steeply declined (CDC, 1999). This decline in deaths coincides with the availability of protease-inhibitor medications and their use in combination with reverse transcriptase inhibitors; protease and reverse transcriptase are two enzymes with essential roles in the replication of HIV. By simultaneously targeting two enzyme systems, HIV's ability to mutate and become treatment resistant is sharply hampered. Hospitalizations of people with HIV/AIDS have declined since new treatments have become available, accompanied by improved health, longer life expectancies, and revitalized hope.

The trajectory of HIV disease has therefore changed in recent years; progression of HIV infection is interrupted by periods of effective antiviral treatments as well as improved treatments for opportunistic illnesses. However, along with the welcome and long-awaited advances in treating people with HIV/AIDS have come increasingly urgent challenges to people affected by AIDS, particularly issues that arise in relationships.

ASSOCIATION OF ILLNESS WITH COUPLE FACTORS

Social losses and isolation are common experiences among people living with HIV. As a result of HIV/AIDS, many people withdraw from relationships and, in doing so, can increase their emotional vulnerability. Not surprisingly, people with HIV infection are prone to disruptions in their most intimate relationships. In a study of HIV-infected gay men, for example, Crystal and Jackson (1989) found that 31% had been rejected by at least one family member and that friends had abandoned 38%. Even more apparent are the disruptions that HIV/AIDS causes in relationships. For example, Pergami et al. (1993) found that 27% of women living with HIV/AIDS experienced changes in their intimate relationships after notification of HIV infection and that nearly two thirds suffered severe disruptions to their sexual relationships. Turner, Hays, and Coates (1993) found similar relationship conflicts in the lives of gay men with HIV infection, particularly among family members who were previously unaware of the men's sexual orientation. People with HIV/AIDS commonly turn to non–family members who are aware of their having practiced socially unaccepted behaviors that subsequently led to their becoming HIV infected. For persons with AIDS who are in committed relationships, their partner is often their sole source of support and daily assistance. When present, relationship partners therefore play unique roles in the lives of people living with HIV/AIDS.

HIV/AIDS as a Couple's Disease

With transmission of HIV via contaminated blood transfusions becoming rare and the occurrence of perinatal HIV transmission becoming less frequent, the vast majority of HIV infections now result from intimate acts in private relationships. HIV infection at its most basic level is therefore a disease rooted in relationships. In fact, people are known to take far fewer precautions against becoming HIV infected in their most trusted and closest relationships. It is therefore one of the many ironies of AIDS that people are frequently infected with HIV by those they love and care for the most (Misovich, Fisher, & Fisher, 1997). However, the relationship within which HIV transmission occurs often is short-lived, and many if not most people living with HIV/AIDS are not in long-term, committed relationships. For example, a community-based study of people living with HIV/AIDS found that only 9% of men and 25% of women reported having been in a committed relationship for at least 6 months (Kalichman, 1998).

The lack of long-term relationships found among people living with HIV/AIDS is at least in part attributable to the characteristics of subpopulations most affected by AIDS. There are few social structures that facilitate and support long-term relationships among gay or bisexual men. Studies of HIV-positive gay or bisexual men mirror those of HIV-negative gay or bisexual men, finding that about 70% are not in committed relationships (Kalichman, Kelly, & Rompa, 1997; Kalichman, Roffman, Picciano, & Bolan, 1997). Thus, regardless of HIV-infection status, durable gay male relationships are more the exception than the rule. Similarly, the general instability that accompanies chronic substance abuse interferes with maintaining long-term relationships in many HIV-affected couples. Commercial sex work and young age are additional facets of HIV/AIDS-affected populations that are barriers to long-term relationships even without introducing HIV infection into the picture.

Unfortunately, within relationships, HIV infection creates an added burden. For example, women living with HIV/AIDS experience relationship disturbances brought on by the disease that complicate other sources of relationship stress (Price & Murphy, 1996). Perhaps most important in affecting the quality of an HIV-positive person's relationship is the HIV serostatus of his or her partner. In some cases, both partners have HIV infection, referred to as *HIV-seroconcordant* couples, whereas other couples are composed of mixed infected and uninfected partners, or *HIV-serodiscordant* couples. The issues facing HIV-seroconcordant and HIV-serodiscordant couples are distinct and are briefly outlined in the sections below.

HIV-Seroconcordant Couples

There is wide variation in the composition and characteristics of couples in which both partners are HIV infected. Seroconcordant couples may consist of persons who became infected within her or his current relationship, meaning that the source of infection for one partner is their current partner. Both partners may have been aware of the potential risks for HIV transmission in that the source partner had previously tested HIV positive and had disclosed this information to their partner. On the other hand, people who have tested HIV positive do not always disclose their HIV-infection status to their partner, who subsequently becomes infected. Therefore, uninfected partners are not always aware of their risks. Finally, seroconcordant couples also can be composed of persons who have not tested HIV positive and unknowingly put their partners at risk.

As the population of people living with HIV/AIDS has grown, it has become increasingly common for couples to come together after each partner had been infected in previous relationships. People living with HIV/AIDS often meet through shared life experiences, such as support groups, AIDS-related services, volunteer organizations, clinic waiting rooms, or mutual friends. The life-defining issues of HIV/AIDS offer multiple opportunities for people to become connected. Many barriers to establishing relationships, including stigmas, fears, and stresses of HIV infection, can actually foster bonding. The burdens people face in having to disclose their HIV status and the strain of potentially infecting an HIV-negative partner are also relieved when both partners are infected.

Caregiving is an important dimension to seroconcordant relationships. Depending on their stages of illness, both partners will require support and assistance related to accessing services, adhering to complicated treatments, and managing the progression of HIV infection. Folkman, Chesney, Cooke, Boccellari, and Collette (1994) found that HIV-seropositive caregivers experienced more burden in assisting their HIV-infected partners than did HIV-negative caregivers. Seropositive caregivers were also more likely than their HIV-negative counterparts to use emotion-focused coping strategies, such as spiritual practices, positive reappraisal, and escape–avoidance behaviors. Using emotion-focused rather than problem-focused coping can be of concern when stressors can be managed with individual action. Thus, having HIV infection clearly adds to the burden of providing care to an HIV-positive partner in seroconcordant relationships.

HIV-Serodiscordant Couples

Similar to seroconcordant couples, there is great diversity among couples with mixed HIV serostatuses. Although serodiscordant couples can include those in which one partner is HIV infected but has not yet tested HIV positive, the term is typically reserved for those couples in which the infected partner and usually both partners have been tested and are aware of their HIV status. In addition to the many challenges that HIV/AIDS brings to relationships, HIV-serodiscordant couples must manage the potential for transmission in their sexual intimacies and must face the necessity of practicing safer sex. Demands placed on couples to practice safer sex can interfere with establishing and maintaining emotional attachments. Harmon and Volker (1995) reported that sexual satisfaction and emotional intimacy between partners are seriously limited by the threat of HIV transmission and demands to practice safer sex. In addition, Remien, Carballo-Dieguez, and Wagner (1995) reported qualitative research findings that further support the adverse effects of HIV-transmission fears on relationship satisfaction.

The roles of partners in serodiscordant couples must be redefined as HIV disease progresses. Uninfected partners may assume greater responsibility as primary caregivers, a role that can carry considerable stress (Hackl, Somlai, Kelly, & Kalichman, 1997). The need for HIV-positive partners to accept care is also a source of relationship stress. On the other hand, the sense of obligation to provide care, which uninfected partners can experience, as well as the HIV-infected partner's increasing dependence for care, can serve to keep couples together. The long-term outlook for the infected partner's health therefore influences the interdependence of serodiscordant partners. As noted by Rabkin and Ferrando (1997), the promise of new HIV treatments for improved long-term prognosis has brought many couples to reconsider their relationship. As people live healthier and longer, they are inclined to reassess their lives, including their relationships. Ending a relationship can be the source of many feelings, including relief, regret, and grief. In addition, the long-term outlook for anti-HIV therapies is variable, so ending a relationship can leave a person without a caregiver.

Stress and Coping With HIV/AIDS

Research has shown that committed relationships can buffer stress and improve coping with illness. Although there is limited research to confirm these associations in couples with HIV infection, a recent study supports the benefits of having a relationship partner in coping with HIV infection. In a survey conducted with 220 HIV-infected men and women in Atlanta, Kalichman (1998) found that individuals who were in relationships for at least 6 months reported significantly less use of coping strategies that distanced themselves from the source of stress as well as fewer attempts to escape stressful situations. Although there were no differences in the use of problem-focused coping strategies, less use of avoidance coping might indicate more use of effective coping strategies. This study also found that persons in relationships reported significantly less symptoms of somatic distress than those without partners. Relationship partners quite likely buffer emotional distress by providing both tangible and emotional social support (Kalichman, 1998). Thus, relationships may offer some protection from the emotional distress of living with HIV/AIDS.

There are many sources of stress for couples living with HIV/AIDS. For individuals, illness-associated events are particularly disturbing, including anniversary dates for testing HIV positive; first experience with HIV symptoms; being admitted to the hospital for HIV-related problems for the first time; and symptoms, illnesses, and deaths of friends and family with HIV/AIDS. Couples face additional stress that stems from the nature of being in an intimate relationship. For example, it is common for HIV-affected couples to experience stress in sexual intimacy. Safer sex can become a burden, particularly for couples of mixed HIV statuses, where there are obvious concerns for infecting the uninfected partner. On the other hand, in seroconcordant couples, there are the risks of transmitting other sexual pathogens that can have disastrous effects on an impaired immune system as well as the uncertainties of reinfection with different strains of HIV, including those that may be resistant to anti-HIV drugs. Financial problems also can be a significant stress in seroconcordant relationships because of the costs of HIV-related medical care and the loss of income experienced from disability.

Disclosure of HIV infection holds a special status among potential HIV/AIDS-related stressors. Concealing HIV infection decreases the availability of social support (Herek, 1990). Stress caused by efforts to conceal a positive HIV serostatus is due in part to the necessity of structuring interactions to minimize risks of disclosure. Selective disclosure of HIV infection tends to divide one's world into those who know and those who do not know. Living a "double life" can involve lying about recurrent illnesses, hiding medications, and covering up symptoms (Siegel & Krauss, 1991). In a study of Hispanic men living with HIV infection, Marks, Richardson, Ruiz, and Maldonado (1992) found disclosure of HIV status to be a selective process, where disclosure increased as HIV disease advanced. Men also disclosed to their sexual partners and close friends more often than to their families. Disclosure of HIV serostatus and communicating about HIV infection with friends and family can lead to greater satisfaction with the social support one receives (Turner et al., 1993).

Considerable differences exist in patterns of disclosing within various types of relationships. For example, Mason, Marks, Simoni, Ruiz, and Richardson (1995) found that Latino and White men disclosed their HIV serostatus to their mothers more often than to their fathers. In addition, White men were more likely to disclose to parents than were English-speaking Latinos, who in turn were more likely to disclose than Spanish-speaking Latinos. In related research, Simoni et al. (1995) found that HIV-seropositive persons were about equally as likely to disclose to their mothers and fathers.

Likewise, HIV-seropositive parents can find it painful to disclose their serostatus to their children. Parents may fear that their children will suffer harm from the stigmatization of having a parent with HIV/AIDS (Armistead & Forehand, 1995; Pliskin, Farrell, Crandles, & DeHovitz, 1993). Parents are more likely to disclose their HIV status to older children and when the HIV-infected parent becomes seriously ill (Armistead, Klein, Forehand, & Wierson, 1997). Families have expressed concerns about revealing an HIV-seropositive family member, more so because of risk behavior histories such as sexual activity and drug use than HIV/AIDS itself. Related to these fears, families report greater emotional distress about family members with HIV/AIDS than family members with other serious illnesses (Brown, 1996). The social baggage of AIDS, particularly attitudes toward HIV-transmission-related behaviors, also complicates familial disclosure. Disclosing that one is HIV positive can mean having to come out with one's sexual orientation, sexual history, or drug use history. Thus, having HIV/AIDS can reveal personal aspects of individuals that they prefer to keep private.

People living with HIV/AIDS who are in sustained relationships do not always disclose their HIV serostatus to their main relationship partner. Marks, Richardson, and Maldonado (1991), for example, found that 31% of HIV-seropositive men who reported having only one current sex partner had not disclosed to their partner. Failing to disclose one's HIV status to partners can be motivated by fears of abandonment, abuse, or violence. For example, research has shown that many women living with HIV/AIDS fear that they will be abused if they disclose their HIV serostatus and that many women actually experience such abuse (Rothenberg & Paskey, 1995). Like other sexually transmitted diseases, disclosing HIV infection to relationship partners can bring about feelings of resentment and betrayal.

Couples Living With HIV/AIDS: Two Cases

The full range of issues experienced by couples living with HIV/AIDS cannot be fully appreciated through research reports alone; there is no substitute for the stories of couples affected by AIDS in understanding their life situations. To provide greater depth of discussion, I present two brief case vignettes that depict couples living with HIV/AIDS. The two case examples are taken from a clinical interview study that did not include clinical assessment or therapy. Therefore, the two cases were not taken from a clinical practice and therefore may represent some of the more typical issues facing couples with HIV/AIDS. The first case involves an HIV-seroconcordant couple in which both partners only recently learned of their HIV-infection status. The second couple is HIV serodiscordant and have been together as a serodiscordant couple for years. Although not universal, many of the issues described in these relationships are common to couples living with HIV/AIDS. Most of the details of these cases are retained as they were reported in the interviews, with names and other identifying information changed to protect identities.

Dan and Leslie

Dan and Leslie were both in their mid-20s, White, and of lower-to-middle incomes. They had been friends for more than 4 years before they started dating. Together for nearly 2 years as a couple, Dan and Leslie had been living together for almost a year and were planning to be married. Dan worked in construction, and Leslie was an elementary school teacher. For as long as they had known each other, Dan and Leslie had been active and had enjoyed good health, that is, until Dan fell ill with chronic diarrhea. He lost 20 pounds before he reluctantly went to a doctor. Dan was diagnosed with having cryptosporidium, an intestinal parasite that he contracted through contaminated drinking water. When his symptoms persisted for several weeks, Dan's doctor tested him for HIV, and his results were positive. But Dan was only somewhat surprised. He had been sexually involved with men in his late teens, behavior that he described as sexual experimentation. Uncomfortable with his past sexual relations, Dan had never shared them with anyone, including Leslie.

Dan was emotionally devastated when he learned his HIV-test results and felt that he had no one to turn to except Leslie. But because she herself was at risk because of a past she was unaware of, Dan could not face her. Dan resorted to calling Leslie on the telephone to tell her that he had seen a doctor and was infected with HIV. Leslie had been very concerned about Dan's weight loss and had fleeting thoughts that he might have AIDS, but she had never seriously considered that possibility. Leslie was shocked. She was convinced that she too had become infected and immediately went to her doctor to be tested. Leslie and Dan supported each other as she waited 2 weeks for her test results, and she had agreed not to discuss Dan's HIV status with anyone until she received her own results. Leslie's worst fears were confirmed when she received her own HIV-positive test results. Unlike Dan, Leslie decided to tell everyone in her family about her condition. Although Leslie felt her family loved her and supported her, they blamed Dan for her condition and refused to see him again. Leslie also felt betrayed by Dan for not warning her of his risks. Leslie, her family, and her friends felt that she was a victim of Dan and his past. However, Leslie also felt badly for the man that she loved because he had became ill so quickly, and she wanted to care for him. These conflicting feelings were difficult for Leslie to reconcile. Nevertheless, Leslie was committed to staying with Dan, in part because she loved him and in part because she felt that she was "damaged goods"—that no one else would ever want her.

HIV/AIDS entirely changed Dan and Leslie's relationship. Dan was burdened by guilt for not having owned the truth of his sexuality and for not accepting the risks of his own behavior. He too blamed himself for Leslie's contracting HIV, and Leslie often acted out her anger by feeding his guilt with comments and innuendos. As Dan's illness progressed, Leslie became increasingly involved in his care. They both eventually stopped working and started receiving disability benefits. In terms of their HIV care, Dan and Leslie were each other's sole source of support. Time healed the pain from learning that they were HIV infected, and they became closer through their mutual support and care for each other.

Mark and Phil

Mark and Phil had both been formerly involved with other people. Mark was 30 years old and had been married to a woman for 6 years before acknowledging his attraction to men. Phil was 25 years old and had been in and out of relationships with men. The two had met through a mutual gay friend, and their interest in each other was instantaneous. They became friends, then sex partners, and then committed in a relationship. Both Mark and Phil were well aware of AIDS. On entering their relationship, they agreed to get tested for HIV together. Because he had tested HIV negative only 6 months earlier, Mark was shocked to learn that he was HIV infected. He had taken risks in the past, but Mark had sex with men who he had felt sure were not infected with HIV. He also felt that he had done his part to prevent himself from becoming infected by getting tested every 6 months. Phil tested HIV negative. Both men had seen many people live with and die of AIDS. Their mixed HIV serostatus did not drive them apart. They had come to accept AIDS as a reality in their lives and their community—a reality that was now in their home.

Mark and Phil had an active sex life throughout their relationship. Both had made a commitment to practice safe sex to protect Phil from becoming infected. However, practicing safe sex all of the time was difficult. Despite the risks that unsafe sex posed to him, Phil was usually the one who pressured Mark to have sex without using a condom. Phil believed that as long as they did not ejaculate inside of each other, the risk for HIV transmission was acceptable. Although Mark usually resisted Phil's urging for unsafe sex, there were times when Mark gave in, usually after they both had been drinking. In fact, Phil came to use alcohol as a way to loosen up Mark's guard and get him to have unsafe sex. Phil came to believe that he would rather take what he thought were minimal risks for getting infected in exchange for a more fulfilling relationship with the man he loved. Unsafe sex caused a great deal of tension in their relationship, but neither of them was taking steps to change this pattern.

Mark and Phil enjoyed a great deal of support from both their HIV-positive and their HIV-negative friends. They were active in their community and well-known in gay social circles. Phil tended bar at a local gay club, and Mark managed rental properties. Mark's health was generally good, and he did not require much in the way of health care. However, both Mark and Phil were concerned that should Mark's health deteriorate, Phil would not make a very good caregiver. In fact, Mark's greatest fear was that Phil would abandon him if he became ill. It was easy for both of them to deal with HIV when it was concealed by good health. Despite Mark's concerns, Phil felt committed to Mark and knew that he would see him through the difficult times to come. Fortunately, Mark's health suggested that it would be some time before they crossed those bridges.

ASSESSMENT

Psychological assessment and treatment of couples affected by AIDS are complicated by two major issues: the characteristics of populations most represented in the HIV epidemic and the uncertain course of HIV disease. The populations most affected by AIDS, for example, raise questions about how scores from many clinical instruments should be interpreted. In North America and Europe, the majority of AIDS cases have occurred among gay and bisexual men, whereas assessment instruments are inherently biased toward heterosexual relationships. In addition, racial and ethnic minorities account for a significant number of AIDS cases in the United States, with the relative proportion of minorities with AIDS increasing each year. Thus, instruments may yield invalid results when they do not take into account cultural differences in relationship structures, roles, and language. Another important factor in assessing couples with HIV/AIDS is the diversity of family systems found in populations most affected by AIDS. Nontraditional families, including same-sex partnerships and single-parent homes, are common in gay and bisexual men and ethnic minorities. Assessing couples and families therefore requires consideration of the diversity of family structures represented in the AIDS epidemic.

Clinical assessment of persons with HIV infection and their partners must also consider potential cultural differences when evaluating scores against existing norms. Populations most affected by the HIV epidemic have also been the most underrepresented in normative samples. Cultural and gender differences in symptom expression and subpopulation base rates of psychological distress must be considered in clinical evaluations. These issues underscore the importance of collecting convergent and divergent sources of clinical information when evaluating persons with HIV infection.

Screening for clinical depression and anxiety with most standardized inventories may result in high false-positive rates. Several aspects of HIV disease must also be considered when persons with HIV infection are clinically assessed. The overlapping relationships among symptoms of chronic medical illnesses, medication side effects, and physical symptoms of emotional distress that can be manifested in couples experiencing relationship problems, such as depression and anxiety, have been well recognized. HIV disease and emotional distress share several physical symptoms, and comorbid symptoms pose problems in assessing clinical depression. For example, 7 of the 21 items on the Beck Depression Inventory (BDI; Beck & Steer, 1993) reflect symptoms of depression that are also characteristic of HIV infection. Overlap occurs for problems in mental concentration and decision making, negative changes in physical appearance, increased difficulty in social and occupational functioning, sleep disturbances, increased fatigue, loss of appetite, and excessive weight loss (Kalichman, Sikkema, & Somlai, 1995). Additional items on the BDI and other measures of depression reflect worries about physical health and physical attractiveness, declining sexual interests, and excessive guilt, all of which may be a part of HIV/AIDS-related experiences. Similarly, the *Diagnostic and Statistical Manual of Mental Disorders* (American Psychiatric Association, 1994) criteria for major depression rely heavily on physical symptoms. For a diagnosis with major depression, a person must exhibit five of nine symptoms, five of which overlap with symptoms of HIV disease: significant weight loss, insomnia, fatigue, diminished ability to think or concentrate, and psychomotor retardation. Diagnostic criteria for dysthymia reflect similar overlapping physical symptoms. Thus, both paper-and-pencil and interview diagnostic assessments of depression include physical symptoms that overlap with symptoms of HIV infection.

Similar problems exist in assessing anxiety. The Trait Anxiety subscale of the State–Trait Anxiety Inventory (Speilberger et al., 1983), for example, includes items that reflect fatigue and cognitive confusion. In addition, the Hamilton Anxiety Scale (Hamilton, 1959; Riskind, Beck, Brown, & Steer, 1987) has several items related to autonomic reactivity, including gastrointestinal distress and fatigue, symptoms that may also be indicative of progressing HIV infection. Thus, affective disturbances that frequently accompany relationship problems are confounded in nature with HIV-disease symptomatology.

Clinical assessment of couples with HIV infection by means of tests that do not include physical symptoms as benchmarks for depression and anxiety can reduce the potential problems of disease–distress symptom overlap. For example, the Hospital Anxiety and Depression Scale (Zigmond & Snaith, 1983) was developed to avoid physical symptom overlap with medical illnesses by emphasizing affective and cognitive processes. Another strategy is to assess clinical constructs that are closely associated with clinical depression and anxiety but do not reflect physical symptomatology, such as hopelessness, optimism, guilt, anger, and obsessive thoughts. Such corollary assessments may therefore be used in combination with clinical depression and anxiety inventories to support or question other test results. In assessing couples, partner reports of mood and activity can help clarify whether symptoms of depression are related to or independent of health status.

Assessing couples with HIV infection almost necessarily demands integrative, multidimensional approaches. Biopsychosocial models may therefore be useful in conceptualizing evaluations of couples with HIV infection (Engel, 1980). Biological, psychological, and social systems of each partner interact to form a dynamic in the couple's relationship. The interrelated experiences of partners are reciprocally tied to physiological processes, emotional reactions, and behaviors. In assessing couples, therefore, it is essential to inquire about health status, physical symptoms of illness, beliefs about diagnosis and prognosis, and supportive resources available to the couple living with HIV/AIDS.

TREATMENT

Given the stress that serious illnesses bring to relationships, couples can benefit from supportive and therapeutic interventions. Counseling and therapy for couples living with HIV/AIDS, however, present several unique challenges. Kain (1996) identified a number of themes that arise in counseling HIV-affected couples, again emphasizing the distinctions between issues facing HIV-seroconcordant and HIV-serodiscordant couples. Challenges facing serodiscordant couples include trying to deal with one partner being HIV positive and the other partner HIV negative. The very nature of a serodiscordant relationship can lead to both partners feeling misunderstood. Fear of HIV transmission, either through sexual contact or perhaps irrational fears of casual contagion, impede intimacy in serodiscordant relationships. Additional fears that both partners may experience include those of dependency, loss, or abandonment.

For HIV-seroconcordant couples, Kain (1996) found that questioning who was the source of each partner's infection is an important issue for many couples. In addition, seroconcordant couples are concerned with which partner has the more advanced stage of illness, who requires more care, and who may or may not be responding to medical treatment. Couples in which both partners are HIV positive must also determine caregiver roles. Finally, HIV-seropositive partners can serve as constant reminders of one's

HIV disease, mirroring HIV to each other throughout the course of their relationship.

There is, unfortunately, little empirical research on mental health services for people living with HIV/AIDS and even less of relevance to couples. Many of the themes in counseling couples with HIV/AIDS, however, may not differ much from those identified in treating individuals with HIV infection, including planning for the future, managing substance abuse, treating a history of trauma and abuse, maintaining a meaningful sexual relationship, managing financial declines, and redefining relationship roles. The sections below provide brief overviews of these themes as they may arise in treating couples with HIV/AIDS.

Planning for the Future

Couples with HIV infection become acutely aware of mortality and recognize that their time is limited. The goals that a couple sets will therefore require attention to both short-term and long-term time lines. Couples must face the reality of AIDS while also recognizing the great hope offered by increasingly effective HIV treatments. For serodiscordant couples, planning requires attention to how the role of the HIV-negative partner will change as HIV infection progresses. Some partners function well as caregivers, whereas others do not. Similar issues arise for seroconcordant couples, but with the uncertainty for which partner will advance more rapidly toward AIDS. The uncertain health of an HIV-positive partner is therefore a central source of stress in couples with HIV/AIDS.

Managing Substance Abuse

Substance abuse is common among people living with HIV/AIDS. Kalichman, Kelly, & Rompa (1997), for example, found high rates of alcohol and other drug abuse in a sample of HIV-positive men who had sex with men. Of particular concern was the finding that HIV-positive men who practiced unprotected anal intercourse were likely to have used substances during sex and that their partners were also more likely to use drugs during sex. Couples where at least one partner has a history of injecting drugs may be particularly difficult to treat because of the strong addictive qualities of these drugs and issues related to potential transmission of HIV in association to their use. Substance use can also become an integral part of the emotional, social, and economic lives of couples. All types of substance use, including that of alcohol, can function as avoidance coping strategies and can also raise the risk for engaging in HIV transmission behaviors. Treatment can assist couples living with HIV who are motivated to stop using substances by helping them replace drug use with adaptive coping behaviors.

However, specialized treatment may be necessary for substance-abusive clients, often requiring drug-treatment referrals.

Treating a History of Trauma and Abuse

Research has suggested that many people living with HIV/AIDS have a history of trauma, including sexual abuse as children and adults. For example, as many as 1 in 4 gay and bisexual men report a history of childhood sexual abuse, and over 20% of men with a history of abuse may be HIV infected (Jinich et al., 1998). In a study of HIV-seropositive women, Vlahov et al. (1998) showed that over 40% had a history of childhood sexual abuse. Because of the long-term effects of child sexual abuse, particularly with regard to establishing intimate relationships, therapy for couples living with HIV/AIDS must assess abuse histories and treat the residual symptoms of trauma.

Maintaining a Meaningful and Satisfying Sexual Relationship

The risks for transmitting mutant variants of HIV and other sexually transmitted pathogens place a couple's sexual relationship in an entirely new context. The challenge for serodiscordant couples is to protect the uninfected partner from contracting HIV infection while maintaining a sexually meaningful relationship. Padian, O'Brien, Chang, Glass, and Francis (1993) reported that couples counseling could significantly reduce HIV transmission risks for serodiscordant couples. In this study, counseling focused on the couple exploring and practicing safer sex while building on the strengths of their relationship. For seroconcordant couples, the necessity of practicing safer sex is more controversial because it is unproven whether a person already infected with HIV can become reinfected. Although other sexually transmitted diseases pose a clear and serious threat to people with HIV infection, truly monogamous couples will rightfully view the risks as minimal.

Managing Financial Losses

HIV disease is a progressive and disabling condition. Treatment with combination therapies has shifted the expense of HIV infection from the later stages to the earlier ones (Kalichman, Ramachandran, & Ostrow, 1998). The cost of drug therapies alone can reach over $15,000 per year. Because the majority of people with later stage HIV infection will stop working to access disability benefits, the economic effects of HIV/AIDS on couples can be devastating. Finances are often the source of stress in relationships even when both partners have a steady income. Thus, the tolls of financial stress on couples are amplified when one or both are required to live on public assistance. Adjustments in lifestyle and strategies for managing financial stressors are therefore a common theme in HIV-related couples therapy. Budgeting, planning, and decisions of when to stop working, as well as the possibility of going back to work, all are fruitful topics for couples therapy.

Reframing Relationships and Roles

The ever changing effect of HIV/AIDS on a person's health creates parallel changes in a relationship. As HIV progresses, partners become caregivers and care recipients. The nature of support that people require also changes as HIV disease progresses, with emotional and informational support being more important early in the disease process and tangible assistance becoming more important at later stages. Changes in quality of life demand that couples readjust their expectations and redefine the meaning of relationship quality. The trajectories of HIV disease require continued reassessment of physical, emotional, and relationship functioning. Reframing the effects of HIV as a force that challenges the growth of a couple can assist couples in adjusting to the progression of HIV/AIDS.

CONCLUSIONS AND FUTURE DIRECTIONS

As evidenced by the lack of empirical studies included in the current chapter, there is a great need for research on couples facing HIV infection. The little research that has been reported focuses on HIV-serodiscordant couples, mostly concerning their sexual practices as related to protecting the uninfected partner. We know little about the emotional and social functioning of HIV-affected couples. Research is needed to identify the key stresses facing couples living with HIV/AIDS and how these couples are coping. How couples provide support within their relationships and how they determine when to seek outside support also are important. Research should be directed at identifying the major milestones along the continuum of HIV infection in the context of serodiscordant and seroconcordant couples. HIV-affected couples must become a high priority in AIDS prevention and care research agendas. Some critical questions include, At what points will couples face their greatest challenges? What are the characteristics of couples who are most resilient and those who are most vulnerable? What interventions are most likely to succeed in assisting couples living with HIV/AIDS, and at what point in a couple's development? These and other fundamental questions will become increasingly pressing as more people living with HIV infection live healthier and longer lives and therefore establish and maintain relationships.

Advancing research on issues facing couples with HIV/AIDS will require innovative research designs. Most important, studies are needed that investigate the emotional, social, and relationship functioning of HIV-seroconcordant and HIV-serodiscordant couples, where couples are treated as the unit of analysis. Couple characteristics may well predict individual adjustment to HIV/AIDS. Research can therefore help inform the strength and resiliency of couples who remain intact through major HIV-related events, such as onset of symptoms, first hospitalizations, and declining physical functioning. Interventions for HIV-affected couples are also in need of study, again using designs that allow for treating couples as the unit of randomization and analysis. Measures of dyadic adjustment, interpersonal communication, relationship satisfaction, and other relationship-oriented constructs will require adaptation and adjustments for use with same-sex and ethnic minority couples.

REFERENCES

American Psychiatric Association. (1994). *Diagnostic and statistical manual of mental disorders* (4th ed.). Washington, DC: Author.

Armistead, L., & Forehand, R. (1995). For whom the bell tolls: Parenting decisions and challenges faced by mothers who are HIV seropositive. *Clinical Psychology: Science and Practice, 2,* 239–250.

Armistead, L., Klein, K., Forehand, R., & Wierson, M. (1997). Disclosure of parental HIV infection to children in the families of men with hemophilia: Description, outcomes, and the role of family process. *Journal of Family Psychology, 11,* 49–61.

Beck, A. T., & Steer, R. A. (1993). *BDI: Beck Depression Inventory manual.* New York: Psychological Corporation.

Brown, W. A. (1996). Is interpersonal psychotherapy superior to supportive psychotherapy? *American Journal of Psychiatry, 153,* 1509–1510.

Centers for Disease Control and Prevention. (1999). *HIV/AIDS surveillance report: Mid-year edition, 1999.* Atlanta, GA: U.S. Department of Health and Human Services.

Crystal, S., & Jackson, M. M. (1989). Psychosocial adaptation and economic circumstances of persons with AIDS and ARC. *Family and Community Health, 12,* 77–88.

Engel, G. L. (1980). The clinical application of the biopsychosocial model. *American Journal of Psychiatry, 137,* 535–544.

Folkman, S., Chesney, M. A., Cooke, M., Boccellari, A., & Collette, L. (1994). Caregiver burden in HIV-positive and HIV-negative partners of men with AIDS. *Journal of Consulting and Clinical Psychology, 62,* 746–756.

Hackl, K. L., Somlai, A., Kelly, J. A., & Kalichman, S. C. (1997). Women living with HIV/AIDS: The dual challenges of being a medical patient and a primary caregiver. *Health and Social Work, 22,* 53–62.

Hamilton, M. (1959). The assessment of anxiety states by rating. *British Journal of Medical Psychology, 32*, 50–55.

Harmon, L., & Volker, M. (1995). HIV-positive people, HIV-negative partners. *Journal of Sex and Marital Therapy, 21*, 127–140.

Herek, G. (1990). Illness, stigma, and AIDS. In G. M. Herek, S. M. Levy, S. Maddi, S. Taylor, & D. Wertlieb, *Psychological aspects of chronic illness: Chronic conditions, fatal diseases, and clinical care* (pp. 7–60). Washington, DC: American Psychological Association.

Ho, D. D. (1996). Therapy of HIV infections: Problems and prospects. *Bulletin of the New York Academy of Medicine, 73*(1), 37–45.

Jinich, S., Paul, J., Stall, R., Acree, M., Kegeles, S., Hoff, C., & Coates, T. (1998). Childhood sexual abuse and HIV risk-taking among U.S. adults 18–49 years. *AIDS and Behavior, 2*, 41–52.

Kain, C. (1996). *Positive: HIV affirmative counseling.* Alexandria, VA: American Counseling Association.

Kalichman, S. C. (1998). *Understanding AIDS: Advances in treatment and research* (2nd ed.). Washington, DC: American Psychological Association.

Kalichman, S. C., Kelly, J. A., & Rompa, D. (1997). Continued high-risk sex among HIV seropositive men. *Health Psychology, 16*, 369–373.

Kalichman, S. C., Ramachandran, B., & Ostrow, D. (1998). Protease inhibitors and the new AIDS combination therapies: Implications for psychological services for people living with HIV–AIDS. *Professional Psychology: Theory, Research, and Practice, 29*, 349–356.

Kalichman, S. C., Roffman, R., Picciano, J., & Bolan, M. (1997). Sexual relationships and sexual risk behaviors among human immunodeficiency virus (HIV) seropositive gay and bisexual men seeking risk reduction services. *Professional Psychology: Research and Practice, 28*, 355–360.

Kalichman, S. C., Sikkema, K., & Somlai, A. (1995). Assessing persons with human immunodeficiency virus (HIV) infection using the Beck Depression Inventory: Disease processes and other potential confounds. *Journal of Personality Assessment, 64*, 86–100.

Marks, G., Richardson, J. L., & Maldonado, N. (1991). Self-disclosure of HIV infection to sexual partners. *American Journal of Public Health, 81*, 1321–1323.

Marks, G., Richardson, J., Ruiz, M., & Maldonado, N. (1992). HIV-infected men's practices in notifying past sexual partners of infection risk. *Public Health Reports, 107*, 100–105.

Mason, H., Marks, G., Simoni, J., Ruiz, M., & Richardson, J. (1995). Culturally sanctioned secrets? Latino men's nondisclosure of HIV infection to family, friends, and lovers. *Health Psychology, 14*, 6–12.

Misovich, S. J., Fisher, J. D., & Fisher, W. A. (1997). What's love got to do with it? Evidence for increased AIDS risk behavior in close relationships and possible underlying psychological processes. *General Psychology Review, 1*, 72–107.

Padian, N. S., O'Brien, T. R., Chang, Y. C., Glass, S., & Francis, D. P. (1993). Prevention of heterosexual transmission of human immunodeficiency virus through couple counseling. *Journal of Acquired Immune Deficiency Syndromes, 6,* 1043–1048.

Pergami, A., Gala, C., Burgess, A., Durbano, F., Zanello, D., Riccio, M., Invernizzi, G., & Catalan, J. (1993). The psychosocial impact of HIV infection in women. *Journal of Psychosomatic Research, 37,* 687–696.

Pliskin, M., Farrell, K., Crandles, S., & DeHovitz, J. (1993). *Factors influencing HIV positive mothers' disclosure to their non-infected children.* State University of New York Health Science Center, Brooklyn, NY.

Price, G., & Murphy, S. (1996). HIV seropositivity and the breakdown of heterosexual relationships in northwest London. *International Journal of STD- and AIDS, 7,* 146.

Rabkin, J. G., & Ferrando, S. (1997). A "second life" agenda: Psychiatric research issues raised by protease inhibitor treatments for people with human immunodeficiency virus or the acquired immunodeficiency syndrome. *Archives of General Psychiatry, 54,* 1049–1053.

Remien, R. H., Carballo-Dieguez, A., & Wagner, G. (1995). Intimacy and sexual behavior in serodiscordant male couples. *AIDS Care, 7,* 429–438.

Riskind, J. H., Beck, A. T., Brown, G., & Steer, R. A. (1987). Taking the measure of anxiety and depression. Validity of the reconstructed Hamilton scales. *Journal of Nervous and Mental Diseases, 175,* 474–479.

Rothenberg, K. H., & Paskey, S. (1995). The risk of domestic violence and women with HIV infection: Implications for partner notification, public policy, and the law. *American Journal of Public Health, 85,* 1569–1576.

Siegel, K., & Krauss, B. (1991). Living with HIV infection: Adaptive tasks of seropositive gay men. *Journal of Health and Social Behavior, 32,* 17–32.

Simoni, J. M., Mason, H. R. C., Marks, G., Ruiz, M. S., Reed, D., & Richardson, J. L. (1995). Women's self-disclosure of HIV infection: Rates, reasons, and reactions. *Journal of Consulting and Clinical Psychology, 63,* 474–478.

Speilberger, C. D., Gorsuch, R., Lushene, P., Crane, P., Jacobs, G., & Marden, T. (1983). *Manual for the State–Trait Anxiety Inventory.* Palo Alto, CA: Consulting Psychologists Press.

Turner, H. A., Hays, R. B., & Coates, T. J. (1993). Determinants of social support among gay men: The context of AIDS. *Journal of Heath and Social Behavior, 34,* 37–53.

Vlahov, D., Wientge, D., Moore, J., Flynn, C., Schuman, P., Shoenbaum, E., & Zierler, S. (1998). Violence among women with or at risk for HIV infection. *AIDS and Behavior, 2,* 53–60.

Zigmond, A. S., & Snaith, R. P. (1983). The Hospital Anxiety and Depression Scale. *Acta Psychiatrica Scandanavia, 67,* 361–370.

7

COUPLES AND CHRONIC PAIN

LAUREN SCHWARTZ AND DAWN M. EHDE

Chronic pain is defined as recurrent or persistent pain that is present for greater than 6 months. The definition of chronic pain also includes pain that persists beyond expected healing time (Loeser, 1991). There are at least three subtypes of chronic pain. Some people may have an identified, ongoing disease process that results in pain (e.g., chronic pancreatitis or cancer). Others may have clear evidence of pathology directly involving peripheral tissue damage or injury to the peripheral or central nervous system (e.g., causalgia or postamputation pain). Finally, for many persons with chronic pain, the pathophysiology is either undetectable by current diagnostic procedures or the level of organic pathology cannot fully explain the pain symptoms or level of disability. Examples of this third subtype include chronic low back pain, fibromyalgia, and chronic headache. This subtype is by far the most perplexing to the health care field and to persons experiencing this type of pain. As such, much of the psychological research in the area of pain has focused on this large subgroup of patients with pain. Therefore this chapter focuses primarily on research and clinical interventions conducted with this subgroup.

BACKGROUND

Functioning

Chronic pain is frequently accompanied by changes in physical, emotional, social, and vocational functioning. For example, individuals with chronic pain often experience changes in their lifestyle, such as severe physical deconditioning and decreased participation in social activities (Fordyce, 1990; Gatchel & Turk, 1996). Chronic pain also has been associated with psychiatric disorders (Gatchel & Turk, 1996; Merskey, 1990; Polatin, Kinney, Gatchel, Lillo, & Mayer, 1993; Romano & Turner, 1985; Ward, 1990). In a sample of 200 persons with chronic low back pain, Polatin et al. found that 59% had current symptoms and 77% met lifetime criteria for at least one psychiatric diagnosis. Major depressive disorder, substance abuse, and anxiety disorders were the most commonly experienced disorders in this sample. Over half of the sample (51%) also met criteria for at least one personality disorder. These prevalence rates are clearly greater than base rates for the general population (Polatin et al., 1993; Reiger et al., 1988; Ward, 1990). Chronic pain can interfere with vocational functioning as well. For example, one study reported that over 14% of all Americans missed at least 1 day of work per year because of pain (J. Taylor & Curran, 1985). In many cases, biomedical interventions have provided minimal or no success in reducing the person's pain and disability.

Epidemiology

It has been estimated that one third of the U.S. population experiences chronic pain (Bonica, 1990; Osterweis, Kleinman, & Mechanic, 1987). Chronic pain accounts for over 80% of all physician visits (Turk, 1996). Back pain is the most prevalent type of chronic pain and the second leading symptom prompting physician visits (Deyo & Tsui-Wu, 1987). Chronic pain is a significant public health problem, costing society over $70 billion each year in health care costs, disability benefits, and decreased work productivity (Turk, 1996). Chronic pain is one of the greatest health care problems challenging patients, their families, and health care providers in the 20th century.

Models

Three conceptual models of chronic pain warrant discussion (see Gatchel & Turk, 1996, for a review). The *biomedical* model assumes that pain results from a specific disease-state process. In this model, diagnosis is confirmed by objective tests, with treatment directed toward correcting the organic dysfunction. Psychosocial factors are viewed as reactions to pain rather than as contributing factors. This dualistic model assumes that symptoms are either psychogenic or organic despite no empirical evidence for this dichotomy. This model has long been criticized for not recognizing psychosocial variables in chronic pain or the interactional influence of these variables with pathophysiology (Engel, 1977).

The *gate control* theory of pain (Melzack & Wall, 1965) conceptualizes pain as a multidimensional phenomenon with affective, cognitive, and sensory–physiological components, all of which have potentiating or moderating effects on pain perception. This model includes psychological factors as well as central nervous system mechanisms and provides a physiological basis for psychological factors in pain perception. This model radically changed the way that researchers and clinicians thought about pain. Most significantly, the gate control theory emphasizes that there is not a one-to-one relationship between organic pathology or tissue damage and pain symptoms.

The *biopsychosocial* model, often considered an extension of the gate control theory, conceptualizes chronic pain as the result of the complex interaction of biological, psychological, and social variables. Within this model, these factors interact in a dynamic process, affecting a person's experience of pain. This model accounts for the diversity often seen in persons' expression of and responses to pain. This model incorporates cognitive–behavioral psychological approaches with medically based treatments.

ASSOCIATION OF CHRONIC PAIN AND COUPLE FACTORS

Effects of Chronic Pain on the Couple

In the event of a chronic medical condition, family members are often forced to take on increased responsibilities, and family roles are altered. The demands for increased emotional support and physical assistance can create distress even in highly functioning families. This may be particularly true for chronic pain, where there is often uncertainty about the cause of the pain and course of recovery. Research in this area highlights that chronic pain can take a significant toll on the relationship, as well as on the partner (Basolo-Kunzer, Diamond, Maliszewski, Weyerman, & Reed, 1991; Flor, Turk, & Rudy, 1987; Flor, Turk, & Scholz, 1987, Roy, 1982; A. G. Taylor, Lorentzen, & Blank, 1990).

Relationship and sexual dissatisfaction are frequent complaints of patients with chronic pain and their partners. Two comprehensive literature reviews have concluded that patients with chronic pain and their partners have poor relationship adjustment as compared with control groups (Payne & Norfleet, 1986) and higher than average marital dissatisfaction (Turk, Flor, & Rudy, 1987). Rates of relationship dissatisfaction in couples with chronic pain range from 35% to 60% depending on the measure used and sample characteristics (community vs. specialty clinic based; Turk et al., 1987). Maruta and Osborne (1978) found among couples reports of decreased sexual activity and satisfaction secondary to chronic pain. Sexual activity decreases may be due to increased pain during or after sexual activity, deconditioning secondary to pain, effects of medications, or psychological or relationship distress. Note that all of the studies in this area are retrospective, thus it is unclear whether relationship–sexual difficulties were premorbid or due to the chronic pain. Clinicians' observations suggest that in approximately half of the couples presenting with relationship or sexual difficulties, the problems are secondary to the chronic pain. Other couples have a history of relationship–sexual difficulties that predate the pain problem and are exacerbated by chronic pain. These couples, however, may initially report that the difficulties followed the chronic-pain problem, although further assessment often uncovers premorbid problems in these areas.

Some research suggests that chronic pain may take a greater toll on the relationship for the partner than for the patient. Maruta, Osborne, Swanson, and Hallwig (1981) found that partners reported greater relationship dissatisfaction than the person with chronic pain. Romano, Turner, and Jensen (1997) found a trend in their study of family environments and chronic pain for partners to report greater marital dissatisfaction as compared with the patients. Gender may also be a mediating factor in relationship adjustment to chronic pain. In a sample of 88 patients with chronic low back pain, Romano, Turner, and Clancy (1989) found that female partners tended to be more distressed and have higher levels of relationship dissatisfaction as compared with male partners. However, Taylor et al. (1990) found no difference for gender in their study of the impact of chronic pain on the partner, with similar scores for male and female partners on the Somatization, Depression, and Anxiety subscales of the Symptom Checklist (SCL–90).

Living with someone who has chronic pain can take a significant emotional toll on the partner. Substantial additional demands are often placed on partners who have to cope with major life changes (e.g., entering the work force for the first time) and financial strains, as well as trying to be supportive to the person in pain. Studies of emotional functioning of partners have shown that 20% to 50% of a sample of partners may be experiencing at least mild depressive symptoms, as rated on standard self-report measures (Ahern, Adams, & Follick, 1985; Ahern & Follick, 1985; Flor, Turk, & Scholz, 1987; Schwartz & Slater, 1991). This is higher than community control samples (Comstock & Helsnig, 1976). However, many of the previous studies lacked control groups. Also, it is not known how depressive symptomatology for partners of patients with chronic pain compares with that of partners of persons with other chronic medical conditions. Finally, although rates of clinical depression or major depressive episode (MDE) in patients with chronic pain are approximately 30% to 40%, three to four times higher than the general population, no published studies have been conducted on rates of MDE in the partners.

Rowat and Knafl (1985) found that for their chronic-pain sample, the partner's perceived control over their situation was an important moderating factor in whether they experienced distress. Another study showed that higher levels of pain and anger in men with chronic pain were associated with higher depressive symptoms in their female partners (Schwartz & Slater, 1991). Relationship satisfaction was also a significant predictor of depressive symptoms in this study. Such partners may be caught in an approach–avoidance conflict, in that they are drawn to a patient who is suffering with high levels of pain but then are pushed away by the patient's irritability and anger. These partners may then avoid interaction with the patient, which may produce feelings of guilt, decreased control, and helplessness. A study that used a qualitative approach to examining families with chronic pain found that the extent to which chronic pain negatively affected a family member was related to how well the family as a whole was coping (Snelling, 1994). Given the above studies, it appears that intrapsychic as well as interpersonal factors are associated with depression in partners. Most studies have not found that patients' level of disability due to pain is associated with their partners' depressive symptoms.

Several studies have examined the potential effects of living with someone with chronic pain on the physical health of the partner (Flor, Turk, & Scholz, 1987; Rowat & Knafl, 1985). Partners were found to have more pain-specific symptoms, but not more general physical symptoms, as compared with a sample of spouses of patients with diabetes. Flor, Turk, and Scholz (1987) also found that poorer physical health in the partner was strongly associated with her or his level of depressive symptomatology.

The following case illustrates the impact of chronic pain on a patient and his wife. Martin, a 37-year-old construction worker, has had pain for 3 years since an on-the-job injury. He and his wife, Molly, have been married for 10 years and have two children. Martin has not worked since the accident. He rarely sleeps at night and spends the majority of his day in bed or on the couch due to pain. He is always fatigued and frequently irritable with his family. Molly is frustrated with the doctors for not "fixing" her husband's pain problem. She is overwhelmed with her responsibilities at home and with the children. She receives no help from Martin with chores or the children. Molly also had to take on a part-time job for the first time in her life due to the financial strain of her husband's unemployment and unpaid medical bills. Molly reports that at times she feels that Martin is upset at her for working. He complains when she comes home from work that the house is not clean and the children are being neglected. She reports feeling angry at her husband as well as guilty because she knows he is suffering. She tries not to express her negative feelings toward him and to keep the children quiet around her husband. Molly reports that she has been sleeping poorly for the past 6 months, has little appetite, has some aches and pains in her back and legs, and feels "jumpy" a lot. She thinks she is ill herself or just overtired, but she has no time to see her own doctor.

Effects of Couple Factors on Chronic Pain

One of the most well known models of chronic pain, a *behavioral–operant model*, which is strongly linked to the biopsychosocial model, strongly emphasizes the role of the partner and the social context of pain (Fordyce, 1976). This model focuses on the way the partner responds to the patient's displays of pain (i.e., *pain behaviors*), which may affect the display of future pain behaviors. Pain behaviors are verbal and nonverbal behaviors that communicate that a person is in pain, such as grimacing, guarding, or limping. The belief is that these pain behaviors come under the control of reinforcing consequences in the environment (e.g., attention or sympathy from a partner, avoidance of stress or conflict, financial gains) and may be maintained by such consequences. This process is thought to explain prolonged disability and dysfunction in some patients with chronic pain, particularly those in which organic pathology is minimal but disability levels are high (Fordyce, 1976, 1990). Family members, as well as health care providers, are thought to be primary sources of reinforcement for pain behaviors, as well as potential providers of discouragement for patient *well behaviors* (e.g., increased activity, exercise, or returning to work).

Within this model, there are three types of partner responses believed to affect the functioning of the patient with chronic pain: *solicitous, negative,* and *facilitative.* Many research studies have shown that the spouse's or partner's attentive responses (i.e., solicitousness) to the patient's pain behaviors are associated with increased pain reports and disability (Block, Kremer, & Gaylor, 1980; Flor, Kerns, & Turk, 1987; Kerns, Haythornthwaite, Southwick, & Giller, 1990; Lousberg, Schmidt, & Groenman, 1992; Romano et al., 1995; Schwartz, Jensen, & Romano, 1996). In an important observational study, Romano et al. (1992) found that patient pain behaviors (e.g., "Oh, that hurts" or grimacing) and spouse solicitous responses (e.g., "I'll do that; you rest now" or "You should not be doing that; you'll pay for it later") sequentially followed one another, thus providing significant support for an operant–behavioral model of chronic-pain behavior. There are some data to suggest that relationship satisfaction may moderate the impact of such partner responses on patient functioning. Flor, Kerns, and Turk (1987) found that solicitous partner responses were more highly associated with patient pain reports if the couple was satisfied with their relationship.

Partners' negative responses (e.g., irritation or criticism) to patient pain behaviors also have been shown to potentially influence patient functioning. Behavioral models posit that aversive responses from a partner are "punishers" and reduce the frequency of pain behaviors, and several studies have found this (Flor, Kerns, & Turk, 1987). However, at least two studies have found that negative partner responses are associated with higher pain reports (Schwartz, Slater, & Birchler, 1996) and greater disability (Schwartz, Slater, & Birchler, 1996; Sullivan, Katon, Russo, Dobie, & Sakai, 1994). The most consistent finding in this area is that aversive partner responses to patient pain behaviors are associated with greater psychological distress in the patient (Kerns et al., 1990; Schwartz, Jensen, & Romano, 1996; Schwartz, Slater, & Birchler, 1996; Turk, Kerns, & Rosenberg, 1992). The general marital literature suggests that the association between negative partner behaviors and poorer functioning in the other partner exists mostly for distressed couples (Beach, Sandler, & O'Leary, 1990). It is not known if relationship satisfaction moderates the impact of negative partner responses in chronic pain. Further research in this arena is warranted.

Partners also can play an important role in encouraging better physical functioning in the patient by reinforcing well behaviors. Well behaviors involve engaging in some kind of functional activity, such as working, exercising, family activity, or household chores. Research demonstrates that patient activity levels increase and reports of pain decrease when praise and attention are given in response to increases in patient activity (Cairns & Pasino, 1977). Similarly, increases in patient activity and decreases in pain behaviors and medication usage are seen when patients' pain behaviors are ignored (Cinciripini & Floreen, 1982; Fordyce et al., 1973). An interesting study by White and Sanders (1986) found that paying attention to pain patients' "well talk" and ignoring "pain talk" were associated with decreased pain intensity reports. These studies were mostly conducted in pain treatment programs, with staff representing the partner. Little research has been conducted on the specific effects of partner responses to well behaviors on patient functioning. Schwartz, Jensen, and Romano (1996) conducted a recent study that found that partners' facilitative or encouraging responses to the patient well behaviors were significantly correlated with better physical and psychological functioning in the patient. Patrick and D'Eon (1996) found that patients with pain did not find partner encouragement of increases in physical activity alone reinforcing. Patients whose partners were more emotionally supportive while the patient was being active had higher activity scores. Thus, partner expressions of support, particularly in response to patient well behaviors but also in a more general fashion, may be important for helping patients to be more active. Providing task-related encouragement may not be as useful.

In a related area of research, positive support from the partner in response to patient pain behaviors may buffer against patient depression (Goldberg, Kerns, & Rosenberg, 1993; Paulsen & Altmaler, 1995). It may be that these partners are considered generally supportive to a variety of patient behaviors, which tends to decrease patients' distress. However, these presumably positive partner responses to patient pain behaviors (e.g., solicitousness), in particular, may also inadvertently contribute to higher patient pain intensity reports and behavior frequency (Kerns et al., 1990). The issue of general partner support versus solicitous partner responses (i.e., pain-contingent support) has only received brief attention in the literature (Turk et al., 1992). This is likely to be an exciting area of research in the future.

The following excerpt from a clinical case highlights some of the above points. Anita has had total body pain for 2 years since a car accident. She currently takes prescription narcotic medication for pain. Her significant other, Carlos, is in charge of doling out her medications because he fears that she will become addicted, like his mother, who also had a pain problem, did. If Anita needs a pain pill, she asks Carlos. He only wants her to take medication when her pain is severe. Carlos states he can tell by looking at Anita if she needs medication. Anita reports that she is happy with this arrangement and feels that it is evidence of Carlos's love and caring for her well-being. Anita is also going to physical therapy and has a home exercise–stretch program. She does the home exercises only when Carlos can watch her, to make sure she is not "overdoing it." Carlos tells Anita to stop the exercise if he thinks it may cause her pain, even though the physical therapist has specified how many of each she should do and that it is safe for her to do the exercises. Carlos is concerned that Anita will injure herself doing these exercises or activities around the house. He does not believe that her physical therapist or doctor understands this.

Three Models for Understanding Chronic Pain and Couple Factors

Behavioral–Operant Model

As mentioned above, this model posits that the maintenance and exacerbation of chronic pain behaviors and disability are thought to be linked to positive or negative reinforcement after displays of pain. This model has received the most attention over the past three decades. The majority of pain treatment programs have been modeled on behavioral–operant theory. Central to this model is the belief that observable pain behaviors (e.g., activity limitations, grimacing, limping, complaining of pain, taking medications) may be maintained through pain-behavior-contingent social reinforcement or discouragement of patient well behaviors, most notably from the partner. Research supports these proposed relationships, although findings are not consistent (Block et al., 1980; Flor, Kerns, & Turk, 1987; Kerns & Turk, 1984; Romano et al., 1992, 1995). The operant approach does not take into account the impact on the family system but focuses on the role of the family, namely, the partner, in the development and maintenance of pain behavior and disability in the patient.

Cognitive–Behavioral Model

In recent years, the cognitive–behavioral model has received a lot of attention (Turk, Michenbaum, & Genest, 1983). Most chronic-pain treatment programs now include a cognitive therapy component in addition to behavioral strategies. This model emphasizes the impact of chronic pain on the patient and the couple as well as the way the couple or family copes with the associated life changes. This model adds to the behavioral–operant model by including the role of cognitive appraisal and other cognitive processes (e.g., patient and partner beliefs, attributions, and expectations regarding patient or couple-related pain interactions). There is a need to apply this model more specifically to couple processes, but at this time, this is limited because of lack of appropriate cognitive-assessment devices. Kerns and Payne (1996) have proposed a cognitive–behavioral transactional model for understanding the role of the family in chronic pain. This model can be conceptualized as an extension of a diathesis–stress model applied to chronic pain. It incorporates the family's response to the pain problem and how the pain's effects impact interpretations of stress and challenges in the future.

Family Systems Model

It has been suggested that a person's health may be affected not only by traumatic or significant life events but also by dysfunctional family interactional patterns. Such processes may be associated with the development and maintenance of physical symptoms (Ehde, Holm, & Metzger, 1991; Turk et al., 1987). In chronic pain, it has been suggested that the pain is being maintained to enable the couple to avoid confronting other problems that might threaten the relationship (Hanson & Gerber, 1990; Roy, 1985; Waring, 1977). Although this theory is considered somewhat controversial, there is general agreement in the field that illness can significantly affect a family and that there are likely to be relationships among a person's physical health, illness behavior, family interaction patterns, and stressful events. Specifically, in the area of couples with chronic pain, Roy (1985) has suggested that the symptom of pain can serve as a substitute for intimacy or as a means of avoiding conflict.

Some previous research in chronic pain may provide support for a family systems perspective. Faucett and Levine (1991) found that negative couple interactions may decrease in the presence of patient pain behaviors. Schwartz, Slater, and Birchler's (1996) study indicated that patients with chronic pain and their partners reported that the patient responded to relationship conflict with increases in pain behaviors. Given these findings, it has been hypothesized that such couples may then avoid conflictual situations as a means of decreasing pain behaviors. Bringing behavioral concepts to these findings, Rowat and Knafl (1985) found that a solicitous partner may attempt to minimize tension or conflict in the household to decrease patient pain behaviors. In general, there are many clinical observations and a few studies, but strong empirical support for a family systems model, as it applies to chronic pain, is currently lacking. However, it is generally believed that viewing the maintenance of chronic pain through a family systems perspective can be helpful for a subset of chronic-pain couples. Often these cases will not be successfully treated with a solely behavioral or self-management treatment approach and require longer term couple or family therapy to promote improved functioning in the patient with pain.

ASSESSMENT AND INTERVENTION

Assessment Strategies

It is generally accepted practice to evaluate the partner as part of a comprehensive assessment of chronic pain. In fact, many clinics or programs often will not conduct a patient evaluation unless the partner is also willing to participate.

One assessment approach is to ask a series of pain-related questions during a structured clinical interview with the partner. The following are examples of some useful questions:

- What do you believe is the cause of your partner's pain?
- How have your activities changed as a result of your partner's pain?
- How can you tell when your partner is having pain (i.e., what are the pain behaviors)?
- What do you do or say to your partner when he or she is having pain (i.e., what is the partner's response to the pain behaviors—solicitous, negative, neutral)?
- What do you do or say to your partner when she or he is engaging in activity or work (i.e., what is the partner's response to the well behaviors—encouraging, negative, neutral)?
- Discuss briefly your partner's premorbid psychological, physical, and vocational functioning.

There are several standardized questionnaires that also can be used when assessing couple issues related to chronic pain both in research and clinical settings:

- The West Haven–Yale Multidimensional Pain Inventory (WHYMPI; Kerns, Turk, & Rudy, 1985) is a frequently used measure of significant-other responses to patients' pain behaviors and pain's interference in their life, given to persons with pain and their partners. The Spouse Response subscales from the WHYMPI measure three types significant-other responses to patient pain behavior (solicitous, punishing, and distracting). A number of research studies have confirmed the validity of this questionnaire and its clinical utility (Kerns & Jacob, 1992). The WHYMPI does not assess partner responses to patient well behaviors.

- The Spouse Response Inventory (SRI; Schwartz, Jensen, & Romano, 1996) is a recently developed questionnaire to assess partner responses to patient pain and well behaviors. Part I consists of two subscales assessing significant-other solicitous and negative responses to a patient's displays of pain. In Part II, two subscales assess significant-other facilitative and negative responses to a patient's well behaviors (e.g., exercising, doing chores, working).

- The SCL–90 (Derogatis, Rickels, & Rock, 1976) assesses psychological distress and has been used for both patients with pain and their partners. The subscales assess nine dimensions, including depressive symptoms, anxiety, and somatization—all potentially useful for evaluating the chronic-pain couple.

- The Dyadic Adjustment Scale (DAS) is a commonly used, 32-item self-report instrument measuring relationship satisfaction (Spanier, 1976). The DAS has high reliability and validity (Spanier, 1976). Subscale scores may be particularly useful for highlighting potential areas of difficulty (e.g., sexual relationship).

- The Family Environment Scale (FES; Moos & Moos, 1986) assesses the functioning of families and couples in several areas, including level of conflict, cohesiveness, independence, and control. Romano et al. (1997) summarized this literature by stating that chronic-pain patients view their families as higher in conflict and lower in cohesion as compared with control patients. Other research has shown that patients with pain whose families score highly on Control and Disorganization scales may have difficulty responding to pain treatment (Tota-Faucette, Gil, Williams, Keefe, & Goli, 1993).

- The Roland Disability Scale (Roland & Morris, 1983) is derived from the Sickness Impact Profile—Physical Disability subscale (Bergner, Bobbitt, Carter, & Gilson, 1981). The Roland scale, widely used for individuals with pain to assess self-report of disability, has been shown to be a reliable and valid measure of physical disability in individuals with chronic pain (Jensen, Strom, Turner, & Romano, 1992; Roland & Morris, 1983).

When assessing couples issues, it is important to obtain a measure of the person with pain's level of disability.

Current Interventions

At this time, there is no single curative treatment for chronic pain (Turk, 1996). The most commonly accepted treatment approach is multidisciplinary and is based on a biopsychosocial model of chronic pain (Loeser, Seres, & Newman, 1990). Interventions grounded in this model address the pathophysiologic processes as well as the psychological, social, and behavioral factors that empirically have been associated with pain, emotional distress, and disability. Treatment goals typically involve modifying affective, behavioral, cognitive, and sensory symptoms associated with the person's disability and suffering with pain and, ultimately, to increase the functioning of the person with pain. Considerable evidence exists on the efficacy of multidisciplinary pain programs in improving psychological and physical functioning, although the impact on pain intensity reports is variable (e.g., Guck, Skultety, Meilman, & Dowd, 1985; Jensen, Turner, & Romano, 1994; Mellin, Harkapaa, Hurri, & Jarvikoski, 1990; Mellin, Hurri, Harkapaa, & Jarvikoski, 1989; Turner & Clancy, 1988).

The multidisciplinary treatment approach, while comprehensive, often requires the individual with chronic pain to make significant behavioral changes that are likely to affect the couple. For example, a person with chronic pain may be expected to engage in a daily exercise regimen, perform regular relaxation exercises, and attend treatment sessions, all of which may interfere with his or her ability to perform other household responsibilities. Similarly, a person learning alternative coping strategies for managing pain may be encouraged to minimize discussion of his or her pain problem. This may represent a significant change for the couple. Although it has been shown that chronic pain affects the couple and couples are often involved in the assessment of individuals with chronic pain, to date, partners often have limited involvement in most chronic-pain treatment programs.

Couple Strategies

Despite extensive support in the literature for the role of the partner in the development and maintenance of chronic pain and the availability of theory-driven models for understanding the relationships between chronic pain and couple factors, there is a paucity of empirical research on couple interventions in chronic pain. Discussions of couple interventions in the chronic-pain literature are usually brief and nonspecific. Only a few detailed descriptions exist in the literature that specifically discuss intervention strategies targeting couples coping with chronic pain (e.g., Kerns & Payne, 1996; Schwartz & Slater, 1991).

Two studies have examined the impact of including the partner in the chronic-pain treatment process. Moore and Chaney (1985) evaluated the effects of including the partner in an outpatient cognitive–behavioral group treatment for chronic pain ($N = 43$). Participants with a variety of chronic-pain problems were assigned to patient-only group treatment, couples group treatment, or a waiting-list control condition. Both the patient and couples treatment groups consisted of eight 2-hour sessions, which included education about the gate control theory of pain, problem-solving skills, relaxation training, assertiveness, and suggestions for changing contingencies for patient pain and well behaviors. Both treatment groups improved significantly on measures of pain severity, pain behavior, somatization, and community adjustment. However, partner participation in the group did not appear to improve patients' response to treatment. This study has been criticized for the lack of couples focus in the treatment groups and small sample size. In a sample of 59 adults with rheumatoid arthritis, Radojevic, Nicassio, and Weisman (1992) compared behavior therapy without family involvement, behavior therapy with family involvement, and a family education group with a no-treatment control group. Significant improvement was found in the two behavior therapy groups in the areas of pain level, disease activity, and psychological functioning at 2 months postintervention, but family participation in treatment did not appear to significantly improve the patient's response to treatment. However, the literature suggests that couple issues may not be as salient for this pain population as compared with other chronic-pain samples, such as in chronic low back pain (Williamson, Robinson, & Melamed, 1997).

A series of three studies have examined the efficacy of couples therapy in the treatment of chronic low back pain (Saarijarvi, 1991; Saarijarvi, Alanen, Rytokoski, & Hyyppa, 1992; Saarijarvi, Rytokoski, & Alanen, 1991). The therapy consisted of five sessions based on family systems theory and was described as "active questioning" with the couple ($n = 63$). Couples were followed for 5 years. The only significant finding reported was that at the 5-year follow-up ($n = 56$), psychological distress had decreased in the person with pain in the couples treatment condition as compared with those in the control condition. The authors concluded that the couples therapy had a beneficial impact on the mental well-being of people with chronic low back pain. There was a significant amount of attrition in the study.

Given the small number of intervention studies available, it is premature to make conclusions regarding the efficacy of any specific couple interventions in chronic pain. Because of the lack of detailed and empirically supported couple interventions in the chronic-pain literature, many of the following treatment recommendations are based on theoretically driven interventions from the general couples literature, as well as research on partner responses and patient pain functioning and the authors' clinical experiences working in this area.

Interventions Targeting the Partner

Most pain treatment programs attempt to include partners and families in some way. However, the level of partner involvement is often limited, with most programs inviting partners to attend one to two educational sessions. Occasionally, more intensive interventions are done with the partner, although these usually focus on supporting the patient's treatment gains. For many couples, however, it is likely to be important to have partners incorporated into the overall treatment plan by providing education and training in behavioral techniques in a variety of formats, such as written educational materials and groups specifically for partners.

Education for partners should include information on the physiology and anatomy of chronic pain, problems of deconditioning due to pain, medication issues, and behavioral principles for managing pain and lifestyle changes (Schwartz & Slater, 1991). This information should parallel what the patient is learning in his or her own treatment program. Clinical interventions for partners should also be aimed at correcting inaccurate beliefs about the pain (e.g., "My husband will end up in a wheelchair someday because of his pain" or "My partner's pain is due to a serious problem that the doctors have missed"). It is also important for all partners to understand that some increases in pain are expected if the person with pain is participating in a rehabilitation program focused on gradually increasing the patient's physical capacities. Partners should be strongly encouraged to observe the patient in physical therapies and participate in skills-building sessions with the patient (e.g., relaxation and coping-skills training sessions). All partners should also be taught specific skills for encouraging or supporting healthy patient behaviors (e.g., exercising, relaxing, or working) and ways to decrease their attention to the person's pain and disability behaviors. As in other psychological therapies, learning to support positive patient behaviors is equally as important as ignoring undesired behaviors (i.e., pain behaviors). The above strategies are used, to varying degrees, in most multidisciplinary pain treatment programs. Finally, given that partners of persons with chronic pain may be at risk for psychological distress, it is important to screen partners for distress and depression and, when indicated, provide or recommend treatment.

Interventions Targeting the Couple

Cognitive–behavioral models, including the transaction model proposed by Kerns and Payne (1996), provide a good framework for couple interventions in the area of chronic pain. Goals of such therapy include changing patterns of interaction that may serve to reinforce patient pain behaviors, disability, and distress (including relationship distress) and promote adaptive couples functioning. Couples therapy can be a useful vehicle for encouraging the couple to collaborate on increasing both the patient's activity level and pleasurable couples activities. Increased engagement in enjoyable couples activities not only will indirectly encourage and reinforce patient well behaviors but also will enhance relationship satisfaction. It is important to target specific skills necessary to effectively manage the pain and its impact on the relationship (Kerns & Payne, 1996; Schwartz & Slater, 1991). For example, couples could work on developing a plan for managing pain flare-ups, such as the partner allowing and encouraging the patient to take time out to do a relaxation or stretch exercise. Another area that warrants particular focus is the couple's belief system regarding the patient's pain problem. Some couples will persist in the belief that the person with pain is doomed to only get worse. These couples will need cognitive therapy focusing on developing more accurate beliefs. Similarly, couples who are waiting for a "magic cure" for the pain, when there is not one forthcoming, will benefit from cognitive therapy to help them acquire more realistic beliefs about the pain problem and possible treatments.

Given that sexual dissatisfaction is a frequent complaint among couples with chronic pain, sex therapy may also be a useful adjunct to chronic-pain treatment. Many interventions for sexual dysfunction and dissatisfaction can be found in the literature (e.g., Carey, Wincze, & Meisler, 1993; Heiman, Epps-Hill, & Ellis, 1995). These techniques can be generalized to the couple in which one person has chronic pain.

Integrative behavioral couples therapy (IBCT; Cordova & Jacobson, 1993; Jacobson & Christensen, 1993) is one promising intervention for couples in which one person has chronic pain. Although never formally tested on chronic pain, it has been demonstrated to be an effective intervention for distressed relationships (Cordova & Jacobson, 1993). IBCT is a reformulation of behavioral couples therapy, which includes both behavior change and acceptance strategies. This therapy begins with an assessment to determine the appropriateness of treatment and the degree to which to emphasize change versus acceptance strategies. Depending on the clinician's conceptualization of the relationship problems, therapy is structured to promote behavior change, acceptance, or both. Examples of acceptance strategies include promoting empathic joining around the problem, turning the problem into a third entity separate from the relationship, and learning strategies for tolerating differences within the relationship. Behavior change strategies include behavior exchange, problem solving, and communication training. This therapeutic approach may prove useful for couples with chronic pain given the chronicity of the pain and the likelihood of the couple's need to accept the changes the pain has brought to their lives while also working on changing some of their behaviors and interactions regarding the pain. An excellent discussion of IBCT's theoretical underpinnings and implementation strategies can be found in Cordova and Jacobson (1993).

Example of a Multimodal Intervention for a Couple

Mary, age 34, has experienced chronic headaches since sustaining a whiplash injury in a motor vehicle accident 2 years ago. She has been living with her partner, Jim, who was driving the car at the time Mary was injured, for the past 5 years. At the time of her accident, Mary was in her third year of law school. She has not returned to school because of her headaches. Mary reports that when experiencing a headache, she is irritable, unable to concentrate, and will typically try to deal with her headache by resting in a dark room. She also frequently takes pain medication for her headaches, and she has noticed that she needs more medication to have the same pain relief. She believes that physical exertion, stress, and sexual activity trigger her headaches and attempts to avoid them. Despite several medical workups, Mary is concerned that the headaches might be the result of an undetected neurological condition such as a tumor or aneurysm. Although Jim and Mary had enjoyed hiking and exercising before her accident, she is now reluctant to plan social and recreational activities out of fear that she will experience a headache. When interviewed, Jim reported that he has attempted to help Mary by creating a stress-free home environment. He has taken over all of the household chores, in addition to working 50 hours a week to pay their living expenses and Mary's student loans. Jim reports that he is often frustrated by their lack of sexual and social activities but does not discuss this directly with Mary out of fear of putting more pressure on her. He also expressed anger and sadness that the couple's plans to start a family have been put on hold indefinitely out of concerns that pregnancy might trigger additional headaches. Jim feels guilty about his anger as well as the fact that he was driving when the accident occurred. Lately, Jim has begun drinking more after work to "blow off steam." Mary reports feeling distressed about how her pain problem has affected the relationship and fears that Jim will leave her because of the toll that her headaches have taken on their life.

Because traditional medical interventions had failed to relieve Mary's pain, she was offered the opportunity to participate in a multidisciplinary pain program that included education about chronic pain, physical therapy to increase her physical conditioning, stress management training, pain coping-skills training, and tapering of her pain medication (which was thought to be increasing the frequency and severity of her pain through "rebound headaches"). When Mary's pain problem was assessed, it became clear that the problem was affected by relationship factors and was negatively affecting the couple's relationship. Thus, several interventions were implemented to address the relationship distress. In several of the educational groups that she attended, Mary learned about how her pain problem affected her relationship and Jim. Jim also attended several educational sessions to learn about chronic pain and observed Mary in her physical therapy. He also met several times with the team psychologist to learn strategies to encourage

Mary's progress and healthy behaviors. The couple participated in several couples therapy sessions to teach them how their interactions were quite likely reinforcing Mary's pain and contributing to relationship distress. For example, the couple came up with a plan to gradually shift some of the household responsibilities from Jim to Mary and to gradually increase social and recreational pursuits. Given their apparent difficulties in discussing emotions with one another, they also learned communication skills as part of their couples therapy. Out of concern for Jim's escalating use of alcohol, he was referred for individual counseling to assist him in finding alternative coping skills to alcohol.

CONCLUSIONS AND FUTURE DIRECTIONS

Research Implications

Most of the research examining the impact of chronic pain on couples has focused on the impact of the partner's behavior on the person with pain, as opposed to couples or relationship issues. This research has shown that solicitous responses on the partner, such as attention and affection, to the patient's displays of pain are correlated with greater patient pain behaviors, higher disability, and higher pain intensity reports. One observational study also has shown that solicitous partner responses and patient pain behaviors occur in a reciprocal fashion for some chronic-pain couples, which suggests that these behaviors may act as cues for one another. Other research has shown that partners' encouragement of patient well behaviors is associated with better functioning in the patient with pain. These findings are generally well supported and accepted in the chronic-pain literature. However, no study has specifically examined the impact of partner training regarding responses to patient pain and well behaviors on patient functioning. This is perplexing because, as mentioned above, the vast majority of the literature on relationship issues in chronic pain has focused on the importance of these interaction patterns in promoting or discouraging patient pain functioning. Whether these partner responses are modifiable and whether altering them has a significant impact on the functioning of the patient with pain have yet to be determined. This is the next important step for the field.

Although some attention has been paid to the impact of chronic pain on the partner and on the couple, there is more work to be done in this arena. Some studies have provided evidence of increased relationship dissatisfaction, sexual dysfunction, and emotional distress in partners, but these studies could be improved in several ways. First, most studies have not included control groups; there is a need to compare the functioning of partners and couples with chronic pain with other illness populations, as well as with healthy people. It is not clear whether the difficulties that couples and partners experience is specific to chronic pain or the result of having to deal with any chronic medical condition. In addition, there is a need to examine the above-mentioned relationships across different chronic-pain subgroups, such as low back pain versus headache versus fibromyalgia. Most studies have lumped together multiple chronic-pain conditions or have focused just on back pain. It is possible that there may be differential effects of the pain on the couple and partner depending on the type of pain, as has been seen with pain associated with arthritis.

At this time, the chronic-pain literature, for the most part, lacks empirical evaluation of interventions focused on couples. The handful of studies that do exist are limited to two types of interventions: (a) inclusion of a partner to standard chronic-pain treatment with very little or no emphasis on partner issues or changing partner behaviors or (b) a very brief couples therapy. In addition, there is great methodological variability among these few studies, making cross-study comparisons difficult. Descriptions of treatments used are often lacking in detail and not empirically driven, making replication difficult. Finally, many of the studies use pain intensity as the primary outcome variable, which is problematic given that pain intensity may not have a strong association with patient functioning or disability (Fordyce et al., 1973; Jensen et al., 1994). More relevant outcome variables would be changes in patient health care use, activity–disability levels, psychological distress, or return to or maintenance of work. These studies also have been limited by their sole focus on the impact of treatment on the patient with pain. This strategy can perpetuate the belief that pain does not affect the couple and the couple does not affect pain treatment outcome. Controlled trials of theoretically driven interventions are needed that examine the impact of both partner-specific interventions and couple-focused treatments.

Clinical Directions

Most treatments for chronic pain are based on behavioral–operant theory and use a multidisciplinary approach. This approach often requires the person with chronic pain to make profound behavioral changes that are likely to affect the couple. Although it has been shown that chronic pain affects the couple, to date, partners are often only minimally involved in most treatments. As mentioned above, the literature is unclear on whether involvement of the partner in treatment makes a significant impact on outcome for the patient with pain. It is likely that for some couples, relationship and partner responses to patient pain and well behaviors are especially salient but for others, they may be less important. Previous research has suggested that pain couples may fall into different subgroups. These subgroups may be characterized by spouse responses to patient pain behaviors or the level of relationship adjustment, both of which may differentially affect the patient's and the couple's adjustment to the pain problem and response to treatment. Romano et al. (1992) have found that significant sequential relationships between solicitous partner responses and patient functioning exist for only a subset of couples. Thus, working on altering partner responses to pain and well behaviors displayed by patients may be significantly clinically meaningful for only a portion of couples. However, clinical observations suggest that addressing such partner responses is probably useful, at some level, for most couples in which one person has chronic pain.

The issues related to couples in which one person has chronic pain are quite likely more complex than a strict behavioral–operant perspective would imply. On the one hand, partner attentiveness to patient pain behaviors may inadvertently contribute to patient disability. However, partner support regarding the pain issue, as well as being generally supportive, may also buffer the patient from depression, particularly when the person with pain is deactivated and socially isolated. Further, negative partner responses do not consistently punish patient pain behaviors (i.e., decrease displays of pain and disability levels), as an operant model would predict. Rather, negative partner responses often are associated with greater psychological distress in the patient. So the question remains of how much partner support in response to which patient behaviors and for which particular patients is likely to have the most influence on patient functioning. The answer to this question is not yet known.

In summary, lacking strong evidence to the contrary, it is important to have partners actively participate in the treatment of chronic pain. Specifically, partners should receive education regarding the nature of chronic pain and the steps that patients can take to regain control of their life (e.g., self-management strategies), as well as on the accuracy of the couple's perception about the cause of the pain and the prognosis. Partners should be taught ways to respond to the patient's pain and disability behaviors with decreased attention and minimizing taking over the patient's responsibilities while also being supportive of the patient's attempts to engage in well behaviors. In addition, it is important to evaluate the partner's mood and, if appropriate, encourage her or him to seek treatment. Depressed or anxious partners are likely to have difficulty engaging in positive interactions with the patient and may not appropriately reinforce positive patient behaviors, such as increases in activity, exercising, or working. Furthermore, several studies have suggested that focusing on decreasing critical partner responses to patient pain behaviors and encouraging partners to help the patient engage in joint projects and activities, even when in pain, may be important for promoting higher patient functioning. Finally, Patrick and D'Eon's (1996) study suggests that partner expressions of caring and affection related to patient activity may be more reinforcing to the patient than just encouragement to be more active. Thus, as mentioned above, encouraging well behaviors while also being supportive of the patient in general may promote the highest level of physical and psychological functioning in the patient with chronic pain.

Relationship issues specific to the patient's pain problem, as well as more general relationship issues, also need to be addressed. For many couples faced with chronic pain, addressing couple issues specifically related to the pain problem (e.g., anger or guilt about the patient's inability to work and support the family; sexual problems due to pain) may be sufficient. However, there is likely to be a subset of couples who will require more intensive couples therapy, as an adjunct to pain treatment, to resolve premorbid or secondary relationship difficulties, such as communication or conflict-resolution problems. Finally, it is important to provide all couples with specific instructions on how to increase positive family activities and for family members to be encouraged to work together to not behave in ways that may inadvertently encourage patient pain behaviors and disability.

The following is a summary of directions for further investigation and clinical study:

- What specific couple or partner interventions affect the patient's disability and functioning? These investigations should focus on the type of treatment (cognitive–behavioral, educational, or supportive), individual treatment for the partner versus couple treatment, couple treatment in a group versus the dyad, and the ideal length of treatment. Developing and testing partner-training protocols (e.g., specific strategies for decreasing attention to patient pain behaviors and encouraging well behaviors) are strongly warranted.
- Further evaluation both in clinical and research settings of the issue of partner solicitousness (i.e., pain-contingent responses) versus more general support from the partner and the relationships to patient-functioning variables is warranted. This might involve further defining the specific characteristics of supportive versus solicitous partner responses. This would quite likely need to be the first step, before developing a spouse-training protocol.
- More research is needed to develop psychometrically sound assessment devices to address areas specific to relationship issues in chronic pain, such as partner behaviors that promote better patient functioning and intervention devices to assess family interaction patterns and outcomes. This may also aid in the identification of pain couple subgroups that may be most affected by relationship–partner factors.
- There is a need to examine relationships between partner responses to pain and well behaviors and patient functioning across different chronic-pain subgroups (e.g., headache vs. back pain vs. fibromyalgia). Most studies have lumped together multiple chronic-pain conditions. It would also be interesting to

assess these relationship factors in other pain conditions, such as postamputation, phantom limb, or cancer. There has been little research done on couples issues in these pain groups.

- Further investigation is warranted to evaluate how partner responses (solicitous vs. negative vs. facilitative) may affect patient recovery from medical interventions for the pain, such as surgery, blocks, or medication trials.

REFERENCES

Ahern, D. K., Adams, A. E., & Follick, M. J. (1985). Emotional and martial disturbance in spouses of chronic low back pain patients. *Clinical Journal of Pain, 1,* 69–74.

Ahern, D. K., & Follick, M. J. (1985). Distress in spouses of chronic pain patients. *International Journal of Family Therapy, 7,* 247–257.

Basolo-Kunzer, M., Diamond, S., Maliszewski, M., Weyerman, L., & Reed, J. (1991). Chronic headache patients' marital and family adjustment. *Issues in Mental Health Nursing, 12,* 133–148.

Beach, S. R. H., Sandler, E. E., & O'Leary, K. D. (1990). *Depression in marriage: A model for etiology and treatment.* New York: Guilford Press.

Bergner, M., Bobbitt, R. A., Carter, W. B., & Gilson, B. S. (1981). The Sickness Impact Profile: Development and final revision of a health status measure. *Medical Care, 19,* 787–805.

Block, A. R., Kremer, E. F., & Gaylor, M. (1980). Behavioral treatment of chronic pain: The spouse as a discriminant cue for pain behavior. *Pain, 9,* 243–252.

Bonica, J. J. (1990). General considerations of chronic pain. In J. J. Bonica (Ed.), *The management of pain: Vol. I* (2nd ed., pp. 180–196). Philadelphia: Lea & Febiger.

Cairns, D., & Pasino, J. (1977). Comparison of verbal reinforcement and feedback in the operant treatment of disability due to chronic low back pain. *Behavior Therapy, 8,* 621–630.

Carey, M. P., Wincze, J. P., & Meisler, A. W. (1993). Sexual dysfunction: Male erectile disorder. In D. H. Barlow (Ed.), *Clinical handbook of psychological disorders* (pp. 442–480). New York: Guilford Press.

Cinciripini, P. M., & Floreen, A. (1982). An outcome evaluation of a behavioral program for chronic pain. *Journal of Behavioral Medicine, 5,* 375–389.

Comstock, G. W., & Helsnig, K. J. (1976). Symptoms of depression in two communities. *Psychological Medicine, 6,* 551–563.

Cordova, J. V., & Jacobson, N. S. (1993). Couple distress. In D. H. Barlow (Ed.), *Clinical handbook of psychological disorders* (pp. 481–512). New York: Guilford Press.

Derogatis, L. R., Rickels, K., & Rock, A. F. (1976). The SCL–90 and the MMPI: A step in the validation of a new self-report scale. *British Journal of Psychiatry, 128,* 280–289.

Deyo, R. A., & Tsui-Wu, Y. J. (1987). Descriptive epidemiology of low-back pain and its related medical care in the United States. *Spine, 12,* 264–268.

Ehde, D. M., Holm, J. E., & Metzger, D. L. (1991). The role of family structure, functioning and pain modeling in chronic headache. *Headache, 31,* 35–40.

Engel, J. L. (1977). The need for a new medical model: A challenge for biomedical science. *Science, 196,* 129–136.

Faucett, J., & Levine, J. (1991). The contributions of interpersonal conflict to chronic pain in the presence or absence of organic pathology. *Pain, 44,* 35–43.

Flor, H., Kerns, R. D., & Turk, D. C. (1987). The role of spouse reinforcement, perceived pain, and activity levels of chronic pain patients. *Journal of Psychosomatic Research, 31,* 251–259.

Flor, H., Turk, D. C., & Rudy, T. (1987). Pain and families: II. Assessment and treatment. *Pain, 30,* 29–45.

Flor, H., Turk, D. C., & Scholz, O. B. (1987). Impact of chronic pain on the spouse: Marital, emotional and physical consequences. *Journal of Psychosomatic Medicine, 31,* 63–71.

Fordyce W. E. (1976). *Behavioral methods for chronic pain and illness.* St. Louis, MO: Mosby.

Fordyce, W. E. (1990). Learned pain: Pain as behavior. In J. J. Bonica (Ed.), *The management of pain: Vol. I.* (2nd ed., pp. 291–299). Philadelphia: Lea & Febiger.

Fordyce, W. E., Fowler, R., Lehmann, J., DeLateur, B. Sand, P., & Trieschmann, R. (1973). Operant conditioning in the treatment of chronic pain. *Archives of Physical Medicine and Rehabilitation, 54,* 399–408.

Gatchel, R. J., & Turk, D. C. (1996). *Psychological approaches to pain management: A practitioner's handbook.* New York: Guilford Press.

Goldberg, G. M., Kerns, R. D., & Rosenberg, R. (1993). Pain-relevant support as a buffer from depression among chronic pain patients low in instrumental activity. *The Clinical Journal of Pain, 9,* 34–40.

Guck, T. P., Skultety, F. M., Meilman, P. W., & Dowd, E. T. (1985). Multidisciplinary pain center follow-up: Evaluation with a no-treatment control group. *Pain, 21,* 295–306.

Hanson, R. W., & Gerber, K. E. (1990). *Coping with chronic pain.* New York: Guilford Press.

Heiman, J. R., Epps-Hill, P., & Ellis, B. (1995). Treating sexual desire disorders in couples. In N. S. Jacobsen & A. S. Gurman (Eds.), *Clinical handbook of couple therapy* (pp. 471–495). New York: Guilford Press.

Jacobson, N. S., & Christensen, A. (1993). *Couple therapy: An integrative approach.* New York: Norton.

Jensen, M. P., Strom, S. E., Turner, J. A., & Romano, J. M. (1992). Validity of the Sickness Impact Profile Roland Scale as a measure of dysfunction in chronic pain patients. *Pain, 50,* 157–162.

Jensen, M. P., Turner, J. A., & Romano, J. M. (1994). Correlates of improvement in multidisciplinary treatment of chronic pain. *Journal of Consulting and Clinical Psychology, 62,* 172–179.

Kerns, R. D., Haythornthwaite J., Southwick, S., & Giller, E. L. (1990). The role of marital interaction in chronic pain and depressive symptom severity. *Journal of Psychosomatic Research, 34,* 401–408.

Kerns, R. D., & Jacob, M. C. (1992). Assessment of the psychosocial context of the experience of chronic pain. In D. C. Turk & R. Melzack (Eds.), *Handbook of pain assessment* (pp. 235–253). New York: Guilford Press.

Kerns, R. D., & Payne, A. (1996). Treating families of chronic pain patients. In R. J. Gatchel & D. C. Turk (Eds.), *Psychological approaches to pain management: A practitioner's handbook* (pp. 283–304). New York: Guilford Press.

Kerns, R. D., & Turk, D. C. (1984). Depression and chronic pain: The mediating role of the spouse. *Journal of Marriage and the Family, 46,* 845–852.

Kerns, R. D., Turk, D. C., & Rudy, T. E. (1985). The West Haven–Yale Multidimensional Pain Inventory (WHYMPI). *Pain, 23,* 345–356.

Loeser, J. D. (1991). What is chronic pain? *Theoretical Medicine, 12,* 213–225.

Loeser, J. D., Seres, J. L., & Newman, R. I. (1990). Interdisciplinary, multimodal management of chronic pain. In J. J. Bonica (Ed.), *The management of pain: Vol. II.* (2nd ed., pp. 2107–2120). Philadelphia: Lea & Febiger.

Lousberg, R., Schmidt, A. J. M., & Groenman, N. H. (1992). The relationship between spouse solicitousness and pain behavior: Searching for more evidence. *Pain, 51,* 75–79.

Maruta, T., & Osborne, D. (1978). Sexual activity in chronic pain patients. *Psychosomatics, 19,* 531–537.

Maruta, T., Osborne, D., Swanson, D. W., & Hallwig, J. M. (1981). Chronic pain patients' and spouses' martial and sexual adjustment. *Mayo Clinic Procedures, 56,* 307–310.

Mellin, G., Harkapaa, K., Hurri, H., & Jarvikoski, A. (1990). A controlled study on the outcome of inpatient and outpatient treatment of low back pain: Part 4. Long-term effects on physical measurements. *Scandinavian Journal of Rehabilitation Medicine, 22,* 189–194.

Mellin, G., Hurri, H., Harkapaa, K., & Jarvikoski, A. (1989). A controlled study on the outcome of inpatient and outpatient treatment of low back pain: Part 2. Effects on physical measurements 3 months after treatment. *Scandinavian Journal of Rehabilitation Medicine, 21,* 91–95.

Melzack, R., & Wall, P. D. (1965). Pain mechanisms: A new theory. *Science, 150,* 971–979.

Merskey, H. (1990). Chronic pain and psychiatric illness. In J. J. Bonica (Ed.), *The management of pain: Vol. I* (2nd ed., pp. 320–327). Philadelphia: Lea & Febiger.

Moore, J. E., & Chaney, E. F. (1985). Outpatient group treatment of chronic pain: Effects of spouse involvement. *Journal of Consulting and Clinical Psychology, 53,* 326–334.

Moos, R. H., & Moos, B. S. (1986). *Family Environment Scale manual* (2nd ed.). Palo Alto, CA: Consulting Psychologists Press.

Osterweis, M., Kleinman, A., & Mechanic, D. (Eds.). (1987). *Pain and disability: Clinical, behavioral, and public policy perspectives*. Washington, DC: National Academy Press.

Patrick, L., & D'Eon, J. (1996). Social support and functional status in chronic pain patients. *Canadian Journal of Rehabilitation, 9*(4), 195–201.

Paulsen, J., & Altmaler, E. (1995). The effects of perceived versus enacted support the discriminative cue function of spouses for pain behaviors. *Pain, 60,* 103–110.

Payne, B., & Norfleet, M. (1986). Chronic pain and the family: A review. *Pain, 26,* 1–22.

Polatin, P. B., Kinney, R. K., Gatchel, R. J., Lillo, E., & Mayer, T. G. (1993). Psychiatric illness and chronic low back pain. *Spine, 18,* 66–71.

Radojevic, V., Nicassio, P. M., & Weisman, M. H. (1992). Behavioral intervention with and without family support for rheumatoid arthritis. *Behavior Therapy, 23,* 13–30.

Reiger, D. A., Boyd, J. H., Burke, J. D., Rae, D. S., Myers, J. K., Kramer, M., Robins, L. N., George, L. K., Karno, M., & Locke, B. Z. (1988). One-month prevalence of mental disorders in the United States. *Archives of General Psychiatry, 45,* 977–986.

Roland, M., and Morris, R. (1983). Development of a reliable and sensitive measure of disability in low back pain. *Spine, 8,* 141–144.

Romano, J. M., & Turner, J. A. (1985). Chronic pain and depression: Does the evidence support a relationship? *Psychological Bulletin, 97,* 18–34.

Romano, J. M., Turner, J. A., & Clancy, S. (1989). Sex differences in the relationship of pain patient dysfunction to spouse adjustment. *Pain, 39,* 289–295.

Romano, J. M., Turner, J. A., Friedman, L. S., Bulcroft, R. A., Jensen, M. P., Hops, H., & Wright, S. F. (1992). Sequential analysis of chronic pain behaviors and spouse responses. *Journal of Consulting and Clinical Psychology, 60,* 777–782.

Romano, J. M., Turner, J. A., & Jensen, M. P. (1997). The family environment in chronic pain patients: Comparison to controls and relationship to patient functioning. *Journal of Clinical Psychology in Medical Settings, 4,* 383–395.

Romano, J. M., Turner, J. A., Jensen, M. P., Friedman, L. S., Bulcroft, R. A., Hops, H., & Wright, S. F. (1995). Chronic pain patient–spouse behavioral interaction predict disability. *Pain, 63,* 353–360.

Rowat, K., & Knafl, K. (1985). Living with chronic pain: The spouse's perspective. *Pain, 23,* 259–271.

Roy, R. (1982). Pain-prone patient: A revisit. *Psychotherapy and Psychosomatics. 37,* 202–213.

Roy, R. (1985). Chronic pain and marital difficulties. *Health Social Workers, 10,* 199–207.

Saarijarvi, S. (1991). A controlled study of couple therapy in chronic low back pain patients: Effects on marital satisfaction, psychological distress, and healthy attitudes. *Journal of Psychosomatic Research, 35,* 265–272.

Saarijarvi, S., Alanen, E., Rytokoski, U., & Hyyppa, M. T. (1992). Couple therapy improves mental well-being in chronic low back pain patients: A controlled, five year follow-up study. *Journal of Psychosomatic Research, 36,* 651–656.

Saarijarvi, S., Rytokoski, U., & Alanen, E. (1991). A controlled study of couple therapy in chronic low back pain patients: No improvement of disability. *Journal of Psychosomatic Research, 35,* 671–677.

Schwartz, L., Jensen, M. P., & Romano, J. M. (1996). *Development of a measure to assess spouse responses to patient pain and well behaviors.* Paper presented at the National Center of Medical Rehabilitation Research Conference, Bethesda, MD.

Schwartz, L., & Slater, M. A. (1991). The impact of chronic pain on the spouse: Research and clinical implications. *Holistic Nursing Practice, 6,* 9–16.

Schwartz, L., Slater, M. A., & Birchler, G. R. (1996). The role of pain behaviors in the modulation of marital conflict in chronic pain couples. *Pain, 65,* 227–233.

Snelling, J. (1994). The effect of chronic pain on the family unit. *Journal of Advanced Nursing, 19,* 543–551.

Spanier, G. (1976). Measuring dyadic adjustment: New scales for assessing the quality of marriage and similar dyads. *Journal of Marriage and the Family, 38,* 15–28.

Sullivan, M., Katon, W., Russo, J., Dobie, R., & Sakai, C. (1994). Coping and marital support as correlates of tinnitus disability. *General Hospital Psychiatry, 16,* 259–266.

Taylor, A. G., Lorentzen, L. J., & Blank, M. B. (1990). Psychological distress in chronic pain suffers and their spouses. *Journal of Pain and Symptom Management, 5,* 6–10.

Taylor, J., & Curran, N. (1985). *The Nuprin pain report.* New York: Harris & Associates.

Tota-Faucette, M. E., Gil, K. M., Williams, D. A., Keefe, F. J., & Goli, V. (1993). Predictors of response to pain management treatment: The role of family environment and changes in cognitive processes. *Clinical Journal of Pain, 9,* 115–123.

Turk, D. C. (1996). Biopsychosocial perspective. In R. J. Gatchel & D. C. Turk (Eds.), *Psychological approaches to pain management: A practitioner's handbook* (pp. 3–32). New York: Guilford Press.

Turk, D. C., Flor, H., & Rudy, T. (1987). Pain and families: I. Etiology, maintenance and psychosocial impact. *Pain, 30,* 3–27.

Turk, D. C., Kerns, R. D., & Rosenberg, R. (1992). Effects of marital interaction on chronic pain and disability: Examining the downside of social support. *Rehabilitation Psychology, 37,* 259–274.

Turk, D. C, Michenbaum, D., & Genest, M. (1983). *Pain and behavioral medicine: A cognitive–behavioral perspective.* New York: Guilford Press.

Turner, J. A., & Clancy, S. (1988). Comparison of operant behavioral and cognitive–behavioral group treatment for chronic low back pain. *Journal of Consulting and Clinical Psychology, 58,* 573–579.

Ward, N. G. (1990). Pain and depression. In J. J. Bonica (Ed.), *The management of pain: Vol. I* (2nd ed., pp. 310–319). Philadelphia: Lea & Febiger.

Waring, E. M. (1977). Marital intimacy, psychosomatic symptoms, and cognitive therapy. *Psychosomatics, 21*, 595–601.

White, B., & Sanders, S. (1986). The influence on patients' pain intensity ratings of antecedent reinforcement of pain talk or well talk. *Journal of Behavior Therapy and Experimental Psychiatry, 17*, 155–159.

Williamson, D., Robinson, M. E., & Melamed, B. (1997). Pain behavior, spouse responsiveness, and marital satisfaction in patients with rheumatoid arthritis. *Behavior Modification, 21*, 97–118.

8

COUPLES AND PREMENSTRUAL SYNDROME: PARTNERS AS MODERATORS OF SYMPTOMS?

ANDREW JONES, VIOLET THEODOS, W. JEFFREY CANAR, TAMARA GOLDMAN SHER, AND MICHAEL YOUNG

For more than half a century, clinicians and researchers alike have been interested in the changes in mood, behavior, cognition, and physiology that precede the onset of menses (Rubinow & Roy-Byrne, 1984). However, despite the proliferation of interest and research regarding the origins, correlates, and consequences of this premenstrual syndrome (PMS), many basic questions about its definition and causes remain unanswered. In this chapter, we suggest a new way to understand PMS for both clinical and research applications, as well as offer a conceptualization of PMS that includes an intimate partner.

DEFINITION AND PREVALENCE OF PMS

The earliest reference to "premenstrual syndrome" has been credited to Hippocrates, who described the symptoms as a "headache" and "a sense of heaviness" (Simon, 1978, p. 273). Frank (1931) provided the first clinical description of PMS using the term *premenstrual tension*. Today, PMS refers to a constellation of somatic, affective, and cognitive symptoms that appear just before the onset of menses and then abate shortly thereafter (Backstrom & Hammarback, 1991; Parker, 1994). In addition to the temporal nature of the condition, PMS is also characterized as recurrent and sufficiently debilitating as to interfere with daily functioning (Backstrom & Hammarback, 1991; Parker, 1994; Schagen van Leeuwen, teVelde, Kop, van der Ploeg, & Haspels, 1993). Regardless of the problems inherent in defining PMS, most researchers today agree that for some women, there exists a menstrually related change in the way that they feel, and the subjective nature of the person's self-report of symptoms related to cyclical biological changes must be taken seriously.

Observed prevalence rates for PMS vary. Estimates of women who experience some level of symptomatology associated with menstruation range from 30% to 90% of menstruating women (Hargrove & Abraham, 1982; Logue & Moos, 1986; World Health Organization, 1981). This wide discrepancy in the incidence of PMS highlights at least two problems in the PMS literature. First, the PMS literature suffers from a lack of a clear, standardized definition of PMS, including its onset, characteristics of the population affected, and typical symptoms. For example, over 150 symptoms have been associated with PMS (Mortola, 1992; Rubinow & Roy-Byrne, 1984). These symptoms can range in intensity from mild to debilitating. In a large study of PMS symptom severity, investigators found that 49% of cases reported their severity of symptoms to be mild, 37% moderate, and 14% severe. Exhibit 8.1 lists some of the most common premenstrual symptoms (Futterman, Jones, Miccio-Fonseca, & Quigley, 1988). Second, investigators and clinicians use different approaches to the study of PMS, many of which do not seem intuitively obvious and do not reflect an approach that has been used with other similar conditions.

A TRADITIONAL MODEL OF PMS

Defining PMS, either for research or for clinical purposes, usually involves a dichotomous approach to the condition, that is, women are considered to have PMS or not to have PMS. This dichotomous conceptualization of PMS has been made for several reasons. One is that many people find that it is easier to think of a disorder as either present or absent. This approach is appealing to clinicians, where diagnosis is linked to treatment de-

EXHIBIT 8.1
Common Symptoms of Premenstrual Syndrome

Physical	Psychological
Fatigue	Isolation
Bloating	Anxiety
Breast tenderness	Depression
Acne	Oversensitivity
Headaches	Irritability
Gastrointestinal symptoms	Labile mood
Heart palpitations	Expressed anger
Hot flashes	Crying easily
Swelling	
Appetite changes (i.e., cravings)	
Forgetfulness	

cisions, which are essentially categorical. However, this approach can be an oversimplification that may distort treatment options as well as research findings. Another reason is that investigators and clinicians may consider PMS as present or absent because they believe that this is the nature of PMS. This view is consistent with the usual medical perspective and usually means one of two things: that the presenting syndrome is either present or absent or that the disorder is identified by a particular underlying pathology that is necessary (although rarely sufficient) for its occurrence (Rothman, 1976). This necessary factor is often thought of as the cause of the disorder or as the definition of the disorder itself. For example, an infection with the tubercle bacillus is considered to be the cause of tuberculosis or, alternatively, tuberculosis is an infection with the tubercle bacillus (Rothman, 1976).

Applying this analysis to PMS leads to two predictions: first that there is a distinct group of women who have the syndrome of PMS and, second, that there is a single, or at least necessary, underlying pathology present in women with PMS. The most obvious and most frequently examined such factor is an endocrine abnormality. We believe that the research providing evidence for these two predictions is lacking. As a result, we propose an alternative perspective based on the idea that PMS is not simply a dichotomous phenomenon. In addition, such a different conceptualization allows for more complex explanations for PMS that include multiple psychological components.

Is PMS Simply an Endocrine Disorder?

Although most believe that hormonal changes play a role in PMS, the mechanism of action is unclear. Symptoms of PMS occur in the late luteal phase of the menstrual cycle. Specifically, symptoms are reported approximately 1 week before the onset of menses. Most researchers believe that the hormonal changes of the luteal phase function as a trigger for physical and emotional symptoms of PMS. A biomedical model of PMS would suggest the presence of a physical abnormality in structure or function. The finding by some researchers that changes in ovarian steroids (estrogen and progesterone) play a role in PMS supports the abnormality hypothesis. For example, Muse, Cetel, Futterman, and Yen (1984) found that the use of a gonadotropin-releasing hormone agonist resulted in a decrease in physical and behavioral symptoms of PMS in 8 women. Both estrogen and progesterone were reduced to postmenopausal levels. However, other research has found contradictory results. Several studies reported a decrease in progesterone levels during the luteal phase (Abraham, Elsner, & Lucas, 1978; Backstrom & Carstensen, 1974; Monday, Brush, & Taylor, 1981). In addition, Rapkin, Chang, and Reading (1987) found that women with PMS who had progesterone administered during the luteal phase of their menstrual cycles did not benefit more than those receiving placebo.

Despite these findings, there is no direct evidence for a single biological causal factor for PMS. In a review of the biological contributions to PMS, Rubinow (1992) concluded that "both the levels of reproductive endocrine hormones . . . and their pattern of secretion over the menstrual cycle do not appear to be disturbed in PMS" (p. 1,909). This does not mean that the biology of the menstrual cycle is irrelevant to PMS. Rather, it means that menstrual biology is not the only contributing factor.

Is There a Distinct Group of Women With Clinically Significant PMS?

It is clear that many women experience some premenstrual symptoms and that for some women, these symptoms are severe and cause significant impairment in their daily functioning. However, little research has focused on the question of whether women with substantial symptomatology and impairment represent a qualitatively distinct group or are simply those that fall above an arbitrary (although perhaps clinically useful) cutoff.

Typically, epidemiological studies, such as those conducted in Sweden (Andersch, Wendestam, Hahn, & Ohman, 1986), Finland (Hargrove & Abraham, 1982; Widholm & Kantero, 1971), the United Kingdom (Gath et al., 1987), Iceland (Sveinsdottir & Marteinsdottir, 1991), and Switzerland (Merikangas, Foeldenyi, & Angst, 1993) have not presented data on whether there was a subgroup of women that appeared qualitatively different from the rest of their samples. Three studies specifically addressed this issue; all found evidence for continuous PMS severity. Futterman et al. (1988) found that severity of symptoms was "a matter of degree rather than type" in a sample of 878 generally recruited women (p. 19). In a similar study of 1,305 university women, investigators found that symptom-severity profiles of 10 symptoms increased continuously as a function of a total PMS score (Jorgenson, Rossignol, & Bonnlander, 1993). Sanders, Warner, Backstrom, and Bancroft (1983) examined daily ratings from three groups of women ($n = 55$): participants seen in clinic with PMS symptoms (clinic PMS+), participants not seen in clinic with PMS symptoms (non-clinic PMS+), and participants not seen in clinic without PMS symptoms (non-clinic PMS−). All three groups exhibited similar changes in somatic symptoms across the menstrual cycle (although the clinic PMS+ group had greater symptom severity throughout the cycle). For mood symptoms, the pattern of change across the cycle was similar in the three groups, but the magnitude of change was greatest in the clinic PMS+ group, intermediate in the non-clinic PMS+ group, and least in the non-clinic PMS− group. In summary, these studies suggest that PMS may exist across a continuum of severity in the population of menstruating women and that health care use is associated with greater symptom severity.

Psychological Factors

Because no clear biological factors have been found to explain PMS, increased attention has been directed to the psychological and social factors related to PMS. Most studies investigating the psychological etiology of PMS look to its co-occurrence with psychological distress, including affective disorders as well as personality or behavioral style.

Depression and PMS

Depressive symptoms are among the most frequently reported symptoms of PMS (Halbreich & Endicott, 1985; Hurt et al., 1992). Several studies have reported high incidence rates of affective disorders in women with PMS (DeJong et al., 1985; Endicott, Halbreich, Schacht, & Nee, 1981; Kashiwagi, McClure, & Wetzel, 1981). Classification systems have kept PMS and depressive disorders distinct. The criteria in the *Diagnostic and Statistical Manual of Mental Disorders* (American Psychiatric Association, 1994) for premenstrual dysphoric disorder diagnostically excludes those who evidence an exacerbation of symptoms related to another comorbid psychiatric disorder.

However, the connection between PMS and depressive disorders cannot be ignored. One interesting distinction between the two results from the identification of two groups of women who report depressive symptoms as part of PMS: those with pure PMS and those who have a premenstrual exacerbation of a subclinical affective disorder (Chisholm, Jung, Cumming, & Fox 1990; Endicott et al., 1981; Hallman, 1986). A lifetime history of depressive disorders was found in 70% of 140 participants seeking treatment for PMS in a study by Harrison, Endicott, Nee, Glick, and Rabkin (1989). Similarly, Mackenzie, Wilcox, and Baron (1986) reported that a history of an affective disorder was found among 45% of their 29 participants with premenstrual symptoms. Other researchers concluded that a history of depressive illness was associated with a tendency for premenstrual depression to be prolonged and with more severe depressive symptoms (Bancroft, Rennie, & Warner, 1994). Interestingly, Yonkers and White (1992) reported that PMS symptoms continued after successful treatment of major depression with antidepressants among 5 women identified with both major depression and PMS. These findings suggest that there is some covariance between PMS and depression but that the two can be considered to be independent syndromes.

Personality Correlates and PMS

Research on personality correlates and PMS has focused primarily on neuroticism. Neuroticism is a broad dimension that reflects individual differences in normal personality. It consists of "a tendency to experience negative, distressing emotions and to possess associated behavioral and cognitive traits such as fearfulness, irritability, low self-esteem, social anxiety, poor impulse control and helplessness" (Costa & McCrae, 1987, p. 301). It is recognized as a basic dimension of personality, even among authors who disagree about other aspects of the structure of personality. Neuroticism is distinguished from neurosis, which is a pathology concept. In addition, although neuroticism has some overlap with somatization, neuroticism is not defined in the psychoanalytic sense of converting psychological distress into physical symptoms or in terms of symptom perception in the total absence of somatic changes. Most studies have found a connection between neuroticism and PMS (Coppen & Kessel, 1963; Hallman, 1986; Levitt & Lubin, 1967), although there have also been negative results (Sampson & Jenner, 1977; Van den Akker & Steptoe, 1985). Specifically, Van den Akker and Steptoe found a significant association between trait anxiety and total scores on the Moos Menstrual Distress Questionnaire in 100 women ($p < .01$) for the follicular (.30), premenstrual (.31), and menstrual (.31) phases. Despite these inconsistent findings, the research has indicated several processes by which neuroticism affects the experience of PMS symptoms. Individuals who are described as neurotic attend more to bodily sensations and minor discomforts because of their tendency to be vigilant and internally focused. In addition, individuals high in neuroticism tend to interpret minor symptoms and sensations as painful or pathological. Thus, one can speculate that PMS severity and report of symptoms, or PMS illness behavior, increases as a function of neuroticism.

Biopsychosocial Explanations

Because neither psychological nor biological explanations of PMS have been found to be adequate, many investigators conceptualize PMS as resulting from a combination of both physiological and psychological factors. Bancroft et al. (1994) conceptualize PMS as consisting of three factors. The first is the *biogenic factor* related to the underlying hormonal cyclicity during the menstrual cycle. The second is a *menstruation factor* associated with the buildup and shedding of the endometrium. The third is a *vulnerability factor*, which refers to the woman's prior history, cognitions, and underlying mood, which affect her attributions and understanding of Factors 1 and 2. Thus, any woman's experience of PMS is thought to be a unique combination of her subjective experience of menses as well as underlying personality, affective, cognitive, and behavioral factors.

Similarly, PMS can be explained as resulting from a combination of PMS symptoms and the response to those symptoms by women. For example, Mechanic (1978) made the distinction between physiological changes and illness behavior, or the way that people perceive and react to physiological changes. Illness behavior itself can be subdivided into symptom perceptions, behavioral reactions, and cognitive evaluations of health status. Illness behavior is conceptualized on a continuum from avoiding, ignoring, or denying perceptions or behaviors to amplifying symptoms and behaviors (Whitehead et al., 1992). Thus, illness behaviors may be normal and appropriate or extreme and pathological.

The distinctions among symptom perception, impairment, and self-identification have been observed for PMS when they have been examined. One investigation found that 40% of a nonclinical sample of women who denied having PMS had daily ratings that indicated PMS symptoms. None of these women had sought treatment for PMS despite the fact that the somatic symptoms of this group were similar to those of confirmed-PMS treatment-seeking participants (Morse, Dennerstein, Varnavides, & Burrows, 1988). Similarly, Hart and Russell (1986) compared 31 women who did and 12 women who did not identify themselves as having PMS and found the severity of many symptoms to be the same in both groups. In addition, a significant correlation was found in the group identified as *high* PMS between baseline scores and premenstrual scores for all symptoms except irritability and breast tenderness. Thus, it has been proposed that treatment seeking represents an interaction of symptom severity and attitudes toward both premenstrual symptoms and available treatment (Scambler & Scambler, 1985) and might be another factor to consider when evaluating a woman's PMS severity.

In addition to underlying personality mechanisms, a variety of theories have sought to explain PMS as a learned illness-behavior response. Learning theory suggests that one's perceptions and behaviors are partly learned from others who model these behaviors. Despite frequent discussion about how women respond cognitively and behaviorally to menstrual and premenstrual symptoms (Clare, 1985), there have been few studies investigating the construct of learned illness behavior in relation to either menstrual or PMS symptoms. Whitehead et al. (1992) examined 340 participants' current menstrual illness behavior as a function of (a) each woman's mother's responses to the participant's menstrual illness behaviors during her adolescence (operant conditioning) and (b) her mother's own illness behavior in response to her own menstrual symptoms during the participant's adolescence (social learning). Results revealed that those menstrual symptoms that were rewarded were maintained in adulthood and became a focus of illness behavior. Furthermore, participants whose mothers exhibited menstrual illness behavior were more likely to engage in illness behavior themselves. Specifically, those participants encouraged to adopt a sick role for menstrual symptoms by their mother reported significantly more menstrual symptoms, clinic visits, and disability days for these symptoms as adults. Although this study did not ask specifically about premenstrual behavior, we believe the results could be generalized, in part because what participants reported as menstrual might have been premenstrual symptoms. In commenting on the Whitehead et al. studies, Woods (1992) noted that there has been little research on the effects of current modeling and conditioning. Clearly, future research that investigates the role of a woman's significant other in reinforcing this behavior is greatly needed.

A final consideration are the cognitive factors that influence the experience of PMS. A cognitive model of PMS suggests that cognitive processing differs among women with and without PMS (Reading, 1992). Specifically, this model states that women with PMS have a consistent set of beliefs regarding menstruation and PMS symptoms. These beliefs form an attribution that is often characterized as linking negative mood swings to menstruation. That is, women who think of themselves as having PMS symptomatology might link normal mood variation to menstrually related phenomena, especially in retrospective reports.

AN ALTERNATIVE MODEL OF PMS

Similar to an illness-behavior model, we propose that PMS be conceptualized as existing on a continuum, ranging from minimal menstrually related symptoms, unlikely to cause distress or impairment, to severe symptoms, likely to be accompanied by significant distress and impairment. That is, all menstruating women fall somewhere on this continuum.

One of the consequences of conceptualizing PMS on a continuum is the freedom to consider a variety of underlying mechanisms that might govern where on the continuum a given woman lies, that is, her PMS severity score. This score would be the result of the combination of a number of contributing factors, which may be present or absent or may occur in varying degrees across women. Furthermore, the factors may or may not be pathological by themselves; instead, two factors, such as behavioral reinforcement and neuroticism, may interact, so that in combination they increase symptom severity, whereas neither does alone.

This theory implies that what is pathological about PMS may not be a specific underlying disease state but rather the symptoms and impairment that result from a combination of underlying factors. Thus, the symptoms are not reflective of PMS pathology but *are* PMS.

This model closely approximates existing clinical practice. Typically, women with PMS complaints seek symptom relief, and clinicians offer pharmacological or behavioral treatments that may relieve their symptoms. Our model suggests omitting the categorization of women as "having PMS" or "not having PMS," using cutoffs with little empirical basis. Instead, the clinician can assess symptom severity for a given woman and individualize a treatment plan to match the particular symptoms presented. We expect that despite rigid diagnostic criteria, this is what most clinicians do most of the time.

This conceptualization also offers the freedom to individualize an understanding of PMS for individual women as we consider which biological, psychological, and relationship factors might play a role in her symptoms. What follows is one possible outcome of viewing PMS on a continuum and a product of multiple etiological factors.

ASSOCIATION OF PMS AND COUPLE FACTORS

When examining the relationship between intimacy and health or intimacy and illness, differences in physical health have been linked to relationship status and quality (Schmaling & Sher, 1997). But in the area of PMS research, more attention has been devoted to defining PMS and how symptom severity can affect a relationship. Keeping in mind the lack of empirical data specifically devoted to PMS and relationships, the following sections attempt to find an understanding of the impact a relationship has on PMS.

Relationship Status

Epidemiologic studies of PMS have typically dealt with the types of symptoms experienced as opposed to identifying and differentiating social attributes of those with PMS. The Epidemiologic Catchment Area Study (presented in Steege, Stout, & Rupp, 1988) asked symptom-related questions of a demographically representative sample of women but did not report any rates of PMS in single women versus women in relationships. Another survey of PMS symptom severity (217 women 17–29 years old and 25 women under 30 years old but older than the other group) determined that teenagers and young women report severe PMS as frequently as older women but that most women who seek treatment for PMS are in their 30s or 40s (Rivera-Tovar & Frank, 1990). Although one could speculate that a larger percentage of these women seeking treatment may be married, an adequate comparison of women in relationships and single women is necessary.

Although numerous investigations have posited that being unmarried is a risk factor for physical illness, most of these results apply to men only (House, Robbins, & Metzner, 1982; Reis, Wheeler, Kernis, Spiegel, & Nezlek, 1985). Also, divorced or separated persons have demonstrated poorer physical health than married or widowed persons (Kiecolt-Glaser et al., 1988), but both gender and the specific health problems also may affect health outcomes. However, an association between couple status and PMS has yet to be determined.

Relationship Satisfaction

Again, as with relationship status, a paucity of research has examined the effects of marital satisfaction on PMS symptom severity. Coughlin (1990) examined the sociopsychological variables of life event stressors, career, and career choice to see what part they may play in the symptomatology of PMS. Researchers used three groups of married women judged to vary in the intensity of their PMS symptoms from mild to moderate to severe. One hundred fifty women were sampled: 75 with a career outside of the home and 75 homemakers, all of whom were in their first marriage, were age 21 to 49 years, were White, had at least one child, were not pregnant, and had menstrual periods. Results demonstrated a significant association between scores on the Marital Satisfaction Inventory and the Menstrual Distress Questionnaire. Specifically, greater couple satisfaction was found to predict lower PMS symptom severity and vice versa ($r = -.26$, p $<$ .01). Future work needs to examine other correlates of PMS symptoms, such as whether married women seek more health-related help, thus leading to decreased symptom severity.

Siegel (1986) did find that 130 women with severe PMS had poor compatibility with their spouses in terms of background, activities, and goals ($r = .257$, $p = .004$). Quite possibly, being with an incompatible partner may lead to heightened PMS severity. Although the direction of cause cannot be determined in the Siegel (1986) study, this should be an avenue of future research.

How PMS Affects Relationships

Similar to the previous section, biopsychosocial research looking at relationships has focused more on chronic illness generally than on PMS specifically. Consistent findings, as reviewed in Schmaling and Sher (1997), suggest that the onset of chronic illness is often accompanied by adverse psychological reactions in both patients and their partners (Helgeson, 1993; Thompson & Cordle, 1988).

The diagnosis of PMS may impact relationships in various ways. Steege et al. (1988) have discussed how couples may attribute relationship difficulties to premenstrual emotional changes. Seeing PMS as a treatable, physical illness may allow couples to approach their differences constructively. Receiving a diagnosis of PMS could also have an opposite effect, reinforcing the woman's role as a scapegoat for problems with an etiology other than PMS. However, the use of a continuum model of PMS allows a woman, or a couple, to be given a PMS severity score that can then be examined in terms of both medical and psychosocial contributing variables.

The impact of PMS symptom severity on couples has received some attention. Researchers have begun to find an association between PMS and couple distress when measured in the luteal phase of the menstrual cycle. Brown and Zimmer (1985) have reported a significant correlation between the degree of PMS symptoms, and the quality of the marriage, family cohesiveness, and interference with the marital relationship. This study evaluated couples both pre- and postmenstrually, with the men and women evaluating their marriage more negatively during the premenstrual phase.

The work of Stout and Steege (1985) demonstrates another way in which stress created by PMS may have a negative impact on a couple. First, they found that almost half of the women with PMS in their sample of 100 women reported a significant level of couple distress, again establishing an association between PMS and couple satisfaction. The second finding of their study was that women viewed irritability during the premenstrual phase, especially that directed at their husbands, as "not like me," or different from the way that they normally view themselves.

One possible explanation of how PMS can lead to couple conflict is a shift in the roles that each person assumes within the relationship. McDaniels (1988) proposed a hypothesis concerning the power dynamic of a change in two disparate roles, described as *distancer* and *pursuer*, respectively. During a woman's premenstrual phase, she may assume a more domineering position and express her feelings in a way that the partner experiences as pursuing, angry, irrational, or pleading. Because of the role shift, the partner distances, causing both to feel misunderstood and needy. A power struggle and blame cycle ensue. This explanation is only a hypothesis, though, with no empirical support to date.

Ryser and Feinauer (1992) did set out to test two basic assumptions from systems theory about relationships among 64 couples in which women did or did not experience PMS: (a) The entire relationship system adjusts to the changes of one partner and (b) couple adjustment is related to the relative balance of positive and negative interaction at any given time. The researchers hypothesized that when PMS causes changes in one partner, and negative behaviors escalate or are introduced into the relationship, it is likely that these behaviors will be reciprocated and relationship adjustment will decrease. They assessed couples' level of distress during both luteal and follicular menstrual cycle phases, among couples in which the woman did or did not experience PMS. Results demonstrated that relationship adjustment during the follicular phase was similar across all couples. However, relationship adjustment during the luteal and follicular phases were similar only among couples in which the women did not have significant PMS symptoms. The luteal stage, when PMS symptoms were present, entailed poorer relationship adjustment for PMS couples. Whether these findings might be explained by McDaniels's (1988) distancer–pursuer hypothesis or possibly by a theory of negative reciprocity whereby negative behaviors elicit negative behaviors by the partner (Gottman, 1979) remains to be determined. This study is important, though, because it goes beyond the correlational work reported earlier, demonstrating an effect of PMS on relationship adjustment.

ASSESSMENT AND TREATMENT

The purpose of this section is to detail not how to assess and treat PMS per se, but how to assess and treat symptoms of PMS in the context of an intimate relationship. Readers who are interested in the clinical approach to evaluation and treatment of PMS should refer to Keye (1988) and Smith and Schiff (1993) for concise overviews. The assessment and treatment plan for couples in which a female partner has PMS is ideally multimodal and multidisciplinary. This plan includes as foci medical aspects of PMS; individual aspects of PMS, including both depression and neuroticism; and couples aspects of PMS.

Assessment of PMS Symptoms

The assessment of couples in which one person has PMS should necessarily begin with the assessment of PMS symptoms. An instrument such as the Moos (1969) Menstrual Distress Questionnaire (MDQ) can be used to gain an understanding of the nature and severity of PMS symptoms. The MDQ is perhaps the most widely used instrument for measuring changes of mood, behavior, concentration, pain, and physical symptoms in the menstrual cycle. Commonly, women are asked to recall their symptoms in previous cycles and rate the severity of 47 symptoms, although prospective report of symptoms is preferable. The majority of Moos's symptom subgroups focus on somatic changes, although emotional and behavioral changes also are included.

The MDQ also can be useful if given to the partner, with instructions to respond to each of the symptoms in terms of "what women sometimes experience" during three cycle phases. Parlee (1973) studied the MDQ when administered to men, finding that men and women responded in a similar manner, possibly reflecting stereotypic beliefs about menstruation. Clinically, giving the MDQ to both partners can highlight discrepancies in how each perceives the frequency and severity of symptoms.

Assessment of Individual Factors

Second, an assessment plan should evaluate both depression in a patient with PMS due to its high co-occurrence with PMS as well as personality variables shown to be related to PMS, such as neuroticism. Symptoms of depression should be evaluated on an ongoing basis with an easy-to-administer self-report measure such as the Beck Depression Inventory (BDI; Beck, Ward, Mendelson, Mock, & Erbaugh, 1961) or the Center for Epidemiologic Studies Depression Scale (CES–D; Radloff, 1977). Both were developed to measure depression in the general population and are easy to administer and score. Because the CES–D was developed to assess depressive symptomatology with an emphasis on the affective component (Radloff, 1977) and a de-emphasis on the vegetative components, we prefer its use for medical populations over the BDI.

In addition, the construct of neuroticism should be assessed, to understand its effect on current PMS symptomatology. A self-report measure such as the Eysenck Brief Inventory for Extraversion and Neuroticisim (Eysenck & Eysenck, 1964) is a 12-item scale commonly used for measuring neuroticism on the basis of decades of use by Eysenck and others.

Assessment of Couple Factors

Other necessary areas of assessment when dealing with couple issues include an overall assessment of the partners' satisfaction with their relationship, as well as the behaviors, thoughts, and emotions that each partner experiences. First, to obtain an overall idea of the couple's adjustment and frequencies of behaviors, the Dyadic Adjustment Scale (DAS; Spanier, 1976) could be used. The DAS is a self-report questionnaire completed by each partner, subscales of which include Affection, Cohesion, Consensus, and Satisfaction. The DAS can be evaluated on an item-by-item basis to clarify which content areas of the relationship are areas of disagreement for the couple.

Attributions, or thoughts about why events occur, are also an important type of cognition to assess because partners may have different ideas about why they are experiencing distress, including or not including PMS. The Marital Attitude Survey (MAS; Pretzer, Epstein, & Fleming, 1991) is a self-report questionnaire tapping into both attributions and *expectancies* (i.e., predictions of what will occur).

Finally, a self-report measure on the behavior of the couple around PMS symptoms should be included. The West Haven–Yale Multidimensional Pain Inventory (WHYMPI; Kerns, Turk, & Rudy, 1985) is a multifaceted instrument used to assess the behavioral responses of significant others to pain behaviors. The WHYMPI subscales include Distracting Responses Style, Punishing Responses Style, and Solicitous Responses Style of the partner toward PMS symptoms. It has been shown to be both reliable and valid with patients experiencing pain and has indicated a relationship between partner response to pain symptoms, couple satisfaction, and pain symptomatology. Canar, DeMarco, Sher, and Young (1998) modified Part II of the WHYMPI for use with women experiencing PMS and assessed its psychometric properties. They found significantly high test–retest correlations for all three subscales of the modified form and concluded that the WHYMPI, modified for PMS, remains a reliable instrument for assessing partner response to premenstrual symptoms.

Medical Management

Medical management of PMS symptoms can include nutritional intervention, psychotropic medication, ovulation suppression, estrogen therapy, and surgical therapy. Nutritionally, deficiencies of nutrients such as pyridoxine, calcium, magnesium, and vitamin E are thought to make a small contribution to PMS. Serotonin deficiency in the central nervous system seems to play a larger role than nutritional deficiencies through affecting carbohydrate cravings and mood disturbances (Brezezinski, Wurtman, & Wurtman, 1990). High-carbohydrate and low-fat, low-salt diets are recommended. Psychotropic medications, especially selective serotonin reuptake inhibitors, can also have a positive effect on mood (Steiner et al., 1995).

Oral contraceptives are widely used to treat severe PMS symptoms, with the goal of either ovulation suppression or estrogen supplementation. Oral contraceptives do decrease dysmenorrhea and PMS symptoms for the majority of women but also can aggravate symptoms in women with established, severe PMS. Other methods of estrogen therapy include the estroderm patch and subcutaneous estradial implants. For women who are psychologically and socially disabled due to PMS, surgical therapy, involving hysterectomy and bilateral salpingoophorectomy (surgical removal of one or both fallopian tubes and ovaries), has been used as a last resort.

Couples Intervention

The treatment plan for couples with PMS should be designed around the results of the assessment and can use as its focus cognitive–behavioral couples therapy (CBCT). The goals of the treatment are to address all aspects of the assessment deemed to be important contributing or maintenance variables to the PMS symptomatology. The treatment plan therefore will include the following elements: (a) a cognitive component to define and restructure any cognitive distortions contributing to depression symptoms, PMS illness behavior, or neuroticism; (b) a behavioral component to address any reinforcement for PMS symptomatology and role burden for the partner of the patient with PMS; and (c) an affective component to address both partners' feelings about PMS symptoms as well as general relationship issues.

The cognitive component of treatment often is an appropriate beginning point because cognitive distortions associated with depression are severe enough to interfere with both individual and couple functioning. CBCT has been used, with mixed results, for the treatment of depression among couples in which one partner is depressed. The details of these studies are beyond the scope of this chapter (see Baucom & Epstein, 1990, for a review). However, the techniques have been found to ameliorate cognitive distortions related to and separate from a diagnosis of depression. A cognitive approach with couples entails modifying thoughts that distort partners' experiences of their interactions, increase distress about their relationship, and induce destructive and stressful behavior. Collecting evidence to determine the validity or reasonableness of each person's cognitions about the relationship is central to the therapeutic process. Steps of this process include defining rigid and distorted cognitions, testing cognitions by examining their logic or illogic, and modifying cognitions through thinking of alternative, more accurate explanations for an event.

Next, a behavioral component can be introduced to intervene on behaviors that may be exacerbating PMS illness behaviors. For example, we, along with others (e.g., Kerns et al., 1991), have found that a solicitous response style by a partner may in fact increase illness behaviors. In addition, a distracting response style can decrease negative moods (Canar et al., 1998). Therefore, couples can be taught to problem solve around PMS symptomatology to decrease any negative effect of partner behaviors and increase any positive effect. For example, the partner without PMS symptoms will be taught how to not reinforce symptoms of PMS through solicitous behavior as well as not criticizing the partner. Problem-solving skills can be taught to help patients and partners cope with PMS-related symptoms, role strain, and decision making around PMS symptomatology. Problem-solving skills, as explained by Baucom and Epstein (1990), involve defining the problem or goal, generating possible solutions, and the choice and acceptance of a solution by both the patient and her partner.

Third, an affective component should be included in treatment to have each partner express their feelings about the symptomatology as well as to increase general intimacy between the woman and her partner. Research on couples' communication has provided evidence that unhappy couples engage in a higher frequency and intensity of hostile exchanges and a lower frequency of supportive or affectional emotional exchanges compared with happy couples (Rankin-Esquer, Miller, Myers, & Taylor, 1997). Emotional expressiveness training (EET) instructs couples to express their own emotions, listen to the emotions of their partner, and give praise or reinforcement for emotional expression. Many couples are unable to express their emotions in a productive manner (Baucom & Epstein, 1990). To assist in these communication difficulties, couples are taught the specific EET skills, including directions for expressing emotions as well as being an empathic responder. The content of discussions in this component should include response to symptoms by both partners and day-to-day issues of behavior change, as well as more global issues.

A Case Study: Maria and Arnoldo

Maria and Arnoldo have been together for 5 years, 4 of which have been a committed relationship. Maria is 32, and Arnoldo is 31. They have no children, and both work outside of the home. Maria works as a computer consultant for a large accounting firm, whereas Arnoldo is a district manager for a pharmaceutical company. They put a high value on joint activities but are extremely busy with their careers and have to consciously make an effort to spend time together. Walks, bike riding, museums, and church functions are a few of the things they enjoy. They attempt to attend church every Sunday together because both believe spirituality to be an important facet of their lives.

Recently, Arnoldo's job led to frequent travel, often with his spending at least 3 days per week away from home. Initially, Maria was supportive of this change in his position but then began to experience feelings of neglect and jealousy. Their conversations frequently led to arguments, concluding with Arnoldo's leaving the house and returning after Maria had gone to sleep. Although Maria had always experienced changes in mood just before the beginning of her period, she recently began to complain of severe pain, feelings of isolation, and a depressed mood. Arnoldo dismissed her complaints as "normal female problems," making Maria feel that her symptoms did not warrant a visit to a health care professional.

As her symptoms persisted, the relationship became increasingly strained. Maria had often sought the company of friends while Arnoldo was out of town, but as she and her husband became increasingly distant, she relied more heavily on her friends for emotional support. Maria's symptoms eventually became intolerable to her, and she made an appointment at her local health care clinic.

The problems faced by Maria and Arnoldo include her feelings of isolation and jealousy due to Arnoldo's absence and his seeming disregard for these feelings. His leaving in the middle of arguments suggests the couple may be characterized by a pursuer–distancer cycle of behavior, where Maria increasingly pushes for attention and reassurance while Arnoldo withdraws and minimizes the importance of complaints.

At Maria's medical visit, it was determined that her symptoms of pain, irritability, and depressed mood occur primarily during her luteal menstrual phase and are consistent with a diagnosis of PMS. Maria expressed that although both she and others could tell when she was about to get her period, she had never experienced problems of this severity until 3 months ago, leading the physician to ask about any life changes or stress beginning at that time. After some thought, Maria remembered that was about the time that Arnoldo began to travel frequently. The doctor decided to change the level of estrogen in her oral contraceptive prescription, to prescribe an antidepressant for her mood, and to refer her to the clinic's psychologist for an assessment.

As part of the psychological assessment, Maria was asked to prospectively rate her symptoms over the next 2 months to confirm a PMS diagnosis. Concerned about the stress that her relationship might be having on her physically, the psychologist suggested that she and Arnoldo attend couples therapy. Couples therapy would entail a formal assessment of their relationship, including a relationship history, communication strengths and weaknesses, cognitions concerning PMS and their relationship, and ability to solve problems effectively. Because of the negative behavioral pattern of pursuing–distancing, treatment could include EET and cognitive restructuring, to help the couple better express their thoughts and feelings. It was hoped that this training would ameliorate the severity and frequency of Maria's premenstrual symptoms by reducing relationship distress.

CONCLUSIONS AND FUTURE DIRECTIONS

Although the amount of research in this area of investigation is slim, the initial findings are exciting because they have used a biopsychosocial approach to understanding PMS. To recognize that psychological factors can be affected by physiological causes and vice versa is a major step in the understanding of relationship adjustment and satisfaction. It is our hope that future research will expand on what has been outlined in this chapter and that health professionals can benefit from these findings.

In summary, then, our review suggests the following findings: (a) There seems to be a reciprocal association between PMS symptom severity and relationship satisfaction, (b) stress created by PMS can have a negative impact on a relationship, and (c) relationship satisfaction can affect the decision to seek health care. With respect to treatment, a thorough assessment of PMS symptom severity; relationship satisfaction; and the behaviors, emotions, and thoughts that each partner has regarding PMS symptoms is necessary to determine the proper course of treatment. Medical management, including nutritional intervention, psychotropic medication, ovulation suppression, estrogen therapy, and surgical therapy, is appropriate when premenstrual symptoms are causing stress in day-to-day life and intimate relationships. Also, nonmedical treatments include physical activity, progressive muscle relaxation, and biofeedback and can be prescribed if medical intervention is judged as unnecessary or ineffective. Last, if relationship stress is caused by PMS symptoms, CBCT is extremely useful to help partners improve communication and problem solving and change negative, harmful thoughts concerning both PMS and the relationship.

Future research could benefit from improving on the methodology in future investigations. The continued use of prospective methods for data collection can portray an accurate and reliable report of PMS symptomatology. The data obtained from the use of psychometrically sound instruments should be the basis for a consensus definition of PMS.

As discussed earlier, a comprehensive definition of PMS should focus on conceptualizing PMS on a continuum and understanding that PMS is a product of multiple etiological factors. This conceptualization means considering the biological, psychological, and relationship factors related to PMS.

In particular, research that focuses on identifying sources of reinforcement or learned behavior for PMS could aid in the prediction of premenstrual symptoms and severity and therefore provide useful information for those working this population. The significant other may influence symptom reporting and severity, relationship satisfaction, and help-seeking behavior. Finally, research regarding cohabiting lesbian couples and the correlation of their PMS symptomatology could strengthen the understanding of the role of intimate relationships in this syndrome.

REFERENCES

Abraham, G. E., Elsner, C. W., & Lucas, L. A. (1978). Hormonal and behavioral changes during the menstrual cycle. *Senologia, 3,* 33–40.

American Psychiatric Association. (1994). *Diagnostic and statistical manual of mental disorders* (4th ed.). Washington, DC: Author.

Andersch, B., Wendestam, C., Hahn, L., & Ohman, R. (1986). Premenstrual complaints. I. Prevalence of premenstrual symptoms in a Swedish urban population. *Journal of Psychosomatic Obstetrics and Gynaecology, 5,* 39–49.

Backstrom, T., & Carstensen, H. (1974). Estrogen and progesterone in plasma in relation to premenstrual tension. *Journal of Steroid and Biochemistry, 5,* 257–260.

Backstrom, T., & Hammarback, S. (1991). Premenstrual syndrome—Psychiatric or gynaecological disorder. *Annals of Medicine, 23,* 625–633.

Bancroft, J., Rennie, D., & Warner, P. (1994). Vulnerability to perimenstrual mood change: The relevance of a past history of depressive disorder. *Psychosomatic Medicine, 56,* 225–231.

Baucom, D. H., & Epstein, N. (1990). *Cognitive–behavioral marital therapy.* New York: Brunner/Mazel.

Beck, A. T., Ward, C. H., Mendelson, M., Mock, J., & Erbaugh, J. (1961). An inventory for measuring depression. *Archives of General Psychiatry, 4,* 561–571.

Brezezinski, A., Wurtman, J., & Wurtman, R. (1990). D-Fenfluramine suppresses the increased calorie and carbohydrate intakes and improves the mood of women with premenstrual depression. *Obstetrics and Gynecology, 76,* 296.

Brown, M. A., & Zimmer, P. A. (1985). *Couples' experience of premenstrual symptomatology: A family impact study.* Paper presented at the Sixth Conference of the Society for Menstrual Cycle Research, Galveston, TX.

Canar, W. J., DeMarco, G., Sher, T. G., & Young, M. A. (1998). *A test–retest reliability analysis of the WHYMPII modified for the study of partner response toward symptoms of PMS.* Poster presented at the 18th Annual Convention of the Society of Behavioral Medicine, San Francisco, CA.

Chisholm, G., Jung, S. O., Cumming, C. E., & Fox, E. E. (1990). Premenstrual anxiety and depression: Comparison of objective psychological tests with a retrospective questionnaire. *Acta Psychiatrica Scandinavica, 81,* 52–57.

Clare, A. W. (1985). Invited review: Hormones, behavior and the menstrual cycle. *Journal of Psychosomatic Research, 29,* 225–233.

Coppen, A., & Kessel, N. (1963). Menstruation and personality. *British Journal of Psychiatry, 109,* 711–725.

Costa, P. T., & McCrae, R. R. (1987). Neuroticism, somatic complaints, and disease: Is the bark worse than the bite? *Journal of Personality, 55,* 299–316.

Coughlin, P. C. (1990). Premenstrual syndrome: How marital satisfaction and role choice affect symptom severity. *Social Work, 35,* 351–355.

DeJong, R., Rubinow, D. R., Roy-Byrne, P. P., Hoban, M. C., Grover, G. N., & Post, R. M. (1985). Premenstrual mood disorder and psychiatric illness. *American Journal of Psychiatry, 142,* 1359–1361.

Endicott, J., Halbreich, U., Schacht, S., & Nee, J. (1981). Premenstrual changes and affective disorders. *Psychosomatic Medicine, 6,* 519–529.

Eysenck, S. B. G., & Eysenck, H. J. (1964). An improved short questionnaire for the measurement of extraversion and neuroticism. *Life Sciences, 3,* 1103–1109.

Frank, R. T. (1931). The hormonal causes of premenstrual tension. *Archives of Neurology and Psychiatry, 26,* 1053–1057.

Futterman, L. A., Jones, J. E., Miccio-Fonseca, L. C., & Quigley, M. E. T. (1988). Assessing premenstrual syndrome using the premenstrual experience assessment. *Psychological Reports, 63,* 19–34.

Gath, D., Osborn, M., Bungay, G., Iles, S., Day, A., Bond, A., & Passingham, C. (1987). Psychiatric disorder and gynaecological symptoms in middle aged women: A community survey. *British Journal of Medicine, 294,* 213–218.

Gottman, J. M. (1979). *Marital interaction.* New York: Academic Press.

Halbreich, U., & Endicott, J. (1985). Relationship of dysphoric premenstrual changes to depressive disorders. *Acta Psychiatrica Scandinavica, 71,* 331–338.

Hallman, J. (1986). The premenstrual syndrome—An equivalent of depression? *Acta Psychiatrica Scandinavica, 73*, 403–411.

Hargrove, J. T., & Abraham, G. E. (1982). The incidence of premenstrual tension in a gynecologic clinic. *Journal of Reproductive Medicine, 27*, 721–724.

Harrison, W. M., Endicott, J., Nee, J., Glick, H., & Rabkin, J. G. (1989). Characteristics of women seeking treatment for premenstrual syndrome. *Psychosomatics, 30*, 405–411.

Hart, W. G., & Russell, J. W. (1986). A prospective comparison study of premenstrual symptoms. *The Medical Journal of Australia, 144*, 466–468.

Helgeson, V. S. (1993). The onset of chronic illness: Its effect on the patient–spouse relationship. *Journal of Social and Clinical Psychology, 12*, 406–428.

House, J. S., Robbins, C., & Metzner, H. L. (1982). The association of social relationships and activities with mortality: Prospective evidence from the Tecumseh Community Health Study. *American Journal of Epidemiology, 116*, 123–140.

Hurt, S. W., Schnurr, P. P., Severino, S. K., Freeman, E. W., Gise, L. H., Rivera-Tovar, A., & Steege, J. F. (1992). Late luteal phase dysphoric disorder in 670 women evaluated for premenstrual complaints. *American Journal of Psychiatry, 149*, 525–530.

Jorgenson, J., Rossignol, A. M., & Bonnlander, H. (1993). Evidence against multiple premenstrual syndromes: Results of a multivariate profile analysis of premenstrual symptomatology. *Journal of Psychosomatic Research, 37*, 257–263.

Kashiwagi, T., McClure, J. H., & Wetzel, R. D. (1981). Premenstrual effective syndrome and psychiatric disorder. *Diseases of the Nervous System, 37*, 116–119.

Kerns, R. D., Southwick, S., Giller, E. L., Haythornthwaite, J. A., Jacob, M. C., & Rosenberg, R. (1991). The relationship between reports of pain-related social interactions and expressions of pain and affective distress. *Behavior Therapy, 22*, 101–111.

Kerns, R. D., Turk, D. C., & Rudy, T. E. (1985). The West Haven–Yale Multidimensional Pain Inventory (WHYMPI). *Pain, 23*, 345–356.

Keye, W. R. (Ed.). (1988). *The premenstrual syndrome.* Philadelphia: W.B. Saunders.

Kiecolt-Glaser, J. K., Kennedy, S., Malkoff, S., Fisher, L., Speicher, C. E., & Glaser, R. (1988). Marital discord and immunity in males. *Psychosomatic Medicine, 50*, 213–229.

Levitt, E. E., & Lubin, B. (1967). Some personality factors associated with menstrual attitude. *Journal of Psychosomatic Research, 11*, 267–270.

Logue, C. M., & Moos, R. H. (1986). Perimenstrual symptoms prevalence and risk factors. *Psychosomatic Medicine, 48*, 388–414.

Mackenzie, T. B., Wilcox, K., & Baron, H. (1986). Lifetime prevalence of psychiatric disorders in women with premenstrual difficulties. *Journal of Affective Disorders, 10*, 15–19.

McDaniels, S. (1988). The interpersonal politics of premenstrual syndrome. *Family Systems Medicine, 6*, 134–149.

Mechanic, D. (1978). Sex, illness, illness behavior, and the use of health services. *Social Science and Medicine, 12*, 207–214.

Merikangas, K. R., Foeldenyi, M., & Angst, J. (1993). Patterns of menstrual disturbance in the community: Results of the Zurich cohort study. *European Archives of Psychiatry and Clinical Neuroscience, 243*, 23–32.

Monday, M. R., Brush, M. U., & Taylor, R. W. (1981). Correlation between progesterone, estradiol, and aldosterone levels in premenstrual syndrome. *Clinical Endocrinology, 14*, 1–9.

Moos, R. H. (1969). Typology of menstrual cycle symptoms. *American Journal of Obstetrics and Gynecology, 103*, 390–402.

Morse, C. A., Dennerstein, L., Varnavides, K., & Burrows, G. D. (1988). Menstrual cycle symptoms: Comparison of a non-clinical sample with a patient group. *Journal of Affective Disorders, 14*, 41–50.

Mortola, J. F. (1992). Issues in the diagnosis and research of premenstrual syndrome. *Clinical Obstetrics and Gynecology, 35*, 587–598.

Muse, K. N., Cetel, N. S., Futterman, L. A., & Yen, S. S. C. (1984). The premenstrual syndrome: Effects of "medical oophorectomy." *New England Journal of Medicine, 311*, 1345–1349.

Parker, P. D. (1994). Premenstrual syndrome. *American Family Physician, 50*, 1309–1317.

Parlee, M. B. (1973). The premenstrual syndrome. *Psychological Bulletin, 80*, 454.

Pretzer, J. L., Epstein, N., & Fleming, B. (1991). Marital Attitude Survey: A measure of dysfunctional attributions and expectancies. *Journal of Cognitive Psychotherapy: An International Quarterly, 5*, 131–148.

Radloff, L. S. (1977). A self-report depression scale for research in the general population. *Applied Psychological Measurement, 1*, 385–401.

Rankin-Esquer, L. A., Miller, N. H., Myers, D., & Taylor, C. B. (1997). Marital status and outcome in patients with coronary heart disease. *Journal of Clinical Psychology in Medical Settings, 4*, 417–435.

Rapkin, A. J., Chang, L. H., & Reading, A. E. (1987). Premenstrual syndrome: A double blind placebo controlled study of treatment with progesterone vaginal suppositories. *Journal of Obstetrics and Gynecology, 7*, 217–225.

Reading, A. E. (1992). Cognitive model of premenstrual syndrome. *Clinical Obstetrics and Gynecology, 35*, 693–700.

Reis, H. T., Wheeler, L., Kernis, M. H., Spiegel, N., & Nezlek, J. (1985). On specificity in the impact of social participation on physical and psychological health. *Journal of Personality and Social Psychology, 48*, 456–471.

Rivera-Tovar, A. D., & Frank, E. (1990). Late luteal phase dysphoric disorder in young women. *American Journal of Psychiatry, 147*, 1634–1636.

Rothman, K. J. (1976). Causes. *American Journal of Epidemiology, 104*, 587–592.

Rubinow, D. R. (1992). Premenstrual syndrome: New views. *The Journal of the American Medical Association, 268*, 1908–1912.

Rubinow, D. R., & Roy-Byrne, P. P. (1984). Premenstrual syndrome: Overview from a methodological perspective. *American Journal of Psychiatry, 141*, 163–172.

Ryser, R., & Feinauer, L. L. (1992). Premenstrual syndrome and the marital relationship. *American Journal of Family Therapy, 20*, 179–190.

Sampson, G. A., & Jenner, F. A. (1977). Studies of daily recordings from the Moos Menstrual Distress Questionnaire. *British Journal of Psychiatry, 130,* 263–271.

Sanders, D., Warner, P., Backstrom, T., & Bancroft, J. (1983). Mood, sexuality, hormones and the menstrual cycle. *Psychosomatic Medicine, 45,* 487–501.

Scambler, A., & Scambler, G. (1985). Menstrual symptoms, attitudes and consulting behavior. *Social Science and Medicine, 20,* 1065–1068.

Schagen van Leeuwen, J. H., teVelde, E. R., Kop, W. J., van der Ploeg, H. M., & Haspels, A. A. (1993). A simple strategy to detect significant premenstrual changes. *Journal of Psychosomatic Obstetrics and Gynaecology, 14,* 211–222.

Schmaling, K. B., & Sher, T. G. (1997). Physical health and relationships. In W. K. Halford & H. J. Markman (Eds.), *Clinical handbook of marriage and couples interventions* (pp. 323–345). New York: Wiley.

Siegel, J. (1986). Marital dynamics of women with premenstrual tension syndrome. *Family Systems Medicine, 4,* 358–366.

Simon, H. (1978). *Mind and madness in ancient Greece.* New York: Cornell University Press.

Smith, S., & Schiff, I. (Eds.). (1993). *Modern management of premenstrual syndrome.* New York: Norton.

Spanier, G. B. (1976). Measuring dyadic adjustment: New scales for assessing the quality of marriage and similar dyads. *Journal of Marriage and the Family, 38,* 15–28.

Steege, J. F., Stout, A. L., & Rupp, S. L. (1988). Clinical features. In W. R. Keye (Ed.), *The premenstrual syndrome* (pp. 113–127). Philadelphia: W.B. Saunders.

Steiner, M., Steinberg, S., Stewart, D., Carter, D., Berger, C., Reid, R., Grover, D., & Streiner, D. (1995). Fluoxetine in the treatment of premenstrual dysphoria. *New England Journal of Medicine, 332,* 1529–1534.

Stout, A. L., & Steege, J. F. (1985). Psychological assessment of women seeking treatment for premenstrual syndrome. *Journal of Psychosomatic Research, 29,* 621–629.

Sveinsdottir, H., & Marteinsdottir, G. (1991). Retrospective assessment of premenstrual changes in Icelandic women. *Health Care for Women International, 12,* 303–315.

Thompson, D. R., & Cordle, C. J. (1988). Support of wives of myocardial infarction patients. *Journal of Advanced Nursing, 13,* 223–228.

Van den Akker, O., & Steptoe, A. (1985). The pattern and prevalence of symptoms during the menstrual cycle. *British Journal of Psychiatry, 147,* 164–169.

Whitehead, W. E., Morrison, A., Crowell, M. D., Heller, B. R., Courtland Robinson, J., Benjamin, C., & Horn, S. (1992). Development of a scale to measure childhood learning of illness behavior. *Western Journal of Nursing Research, 14,* 170–185.

Widholm, O., & Kantero, R. L. (1971). A statistical analysis of the menstrual patterns of 8,000 Finnish girls and their mothers. *Acta Obstetricia et Gynecologica Scandinavica, 14,* 3–36.

Woods, N. F. (1992). A commentary by Woods [to Whitehead]. *Western Journal of Nursing Research, 14,* 183–184.

World Health Organization. (1981). A cross-cultural study of menstruation: Implications for contraceptive development and use. *Studies in Family Planning, 12,* 3–16.

Yonkers, K., & White, K. (1992). Premenstrual exacerbation of depression: One process or two? *Journal of Clinical Psychiatry, 53,* 289–292.

9

COUPLES FACING FERTILITY PROBLEMS

LAURI A. PASCH AND ANDREW CHRISTENSEN

Consider the following interactions, in which two couples discuss what next steps to take regarding treatment for their fertility problem, specifically, how each partner feels about adopting a child.

INTERACTION 1: LORENZO AND MARIA

Maria: You said at one point that you would agree that we would adopt.

Lorenzo: I said we would talk about it.

Maria: No, you *agreed* that we would adopt. I'm not willing not to have a child in my life. I told you that before. If in a year, we're still going through this . . .

Lorenzo: A year? There are people who try for 3 years, and after a year you're going to throw in the towel and say let's adopt? That's ridiculous.

Maria: Why is that ridiculous? I'm almost 40.

Lorenzo: That doesn't mean anything in this day and age.

241

Maria: To me, it means something.

Lorenzo: Well, how about how I feel?

INTERACTION 2: MICHAEL AND ARLENE

Michael: Well, it seems like you feel more comfortable with the idea of adopting. For you it's more a matter of when, not like tomorrow, but I think you are more emotionally ready.

Arlene: I think you're right, but it's pretty obvious we both would prefer having a child who is biologically ours.

Michael: I just don't know if I will feel the same about an adopted child as I would about our child. I mean, I think I would, but I guess I worry about how others would feel. It's just such a shame. . . .

Arlene: I know. . . . But I know we are going to be great parents, whatever happens. I mean I don't want us to lose sight of that.

This chapter concerns the complex issues that couples with fertility problems face and how partners work together in responding to them. Consider the two interactions presented above, which we observed in one of our studies of couples with fertility problems (see Pasch, 1994; Pasch, Dunkel-Schetter, & Christensen, 1995). These brief interactions provide a hint of the complexity of the issues that couples face. Considering whether to pursue adoption is just one of a myriad of treatment-related decisions couples must make, and these decisions may be revisited many times over the course of several years. These interactions also illustrate how fertility problems affect the couple as a unit. Partners need each other's cooperation to achieve their goals, and this can cause a major problem when their goals or preferred strategies for reaching them differ dramatically, as in the case of Maria and Lorenzo. Finally, the quality of the interactions gives us a sense of the variability between couples in their ability to communicate with each other. Arlene and Michael seemed to be able to explore feelings with each other and share intimacy regarding their joint problem, whereas Lorenzo and Maria quickly fell into accusations and defensiveness. Whereas Arlene and Michael's relationship will probably grow closer and more intimate as a result of sharing this problem with each other, Lorenzo and Maria may grow further apart.

In this chapter, we present an introduction to the psychology of couples and infertility. The chapter is divided into four sections. In the first section, we present background information on infertility and introduce the complexity of the issues couples and health professionals working with them may face. The second section provides a review of the relatively small empirical research literature pertaining to the broad question of how fertility problems affect couples. Several excellent sources have recently appeared on the topic (e.g., Leiblum, 1997; Zoldbrod, 1993). However, these sources tend to be clinically based, and there remains a clear absence of well-designed empirical studies. The third section concerns assessment and treatment. For the medical professional, we provide suggestions regarding provision of couple-friendly care. For the mental health professional, we provide guidance regarding working with couples who experience significant relationship distress associated with having a fertility problem. Although there is no research to support the use of any particular approach, we present one based on recent work with distressed couples in general (see Christensen, Jacobson, & Babcock, 1995; Jacobson & Christensen, 1996) and incorporate examples from our work with infertile couples. In the fourth section, we delineate some of the key challenges to be faced in future work, from a conceptual, methodological, and applied perspective.

BACKGROUND

Infertility is medically defined as the inability of a couple to conceive after 12 months of regular intercourse without contraception (Office of Technology Assessment [OTA], 1988). There are few reliable sources of demographic information about infertility in the United States. The 1995 National Survey of Family Growth found that 8% of married couples with wives age 15 to 44 experience infertility, which translates into approximately 2.4 million married couples; an unknown number of potential parents among unmarried couples and singles also are infertile (Abma, Chandra, Mosher, Peterson, & Piccinino, 1997).

The definition of *infertility* is used to screen couples for fertility treatment and is not intended to measure sterility, which is considered a more permanent condition. Therefore, a woman may be fertile at one point in her life but infertile later, due to increasing age, tubal damage resulting from pelvic inflammatory disease, and many other causes. Similarly, an individual may have no difficulty having children with one partner but may be infertile with another. In our experience, couples prefer to be referred to as *experiencing fertility problems*, because of a finality commonly associated with the term *infertile*. Indeed, estimates suggest that as many as half of couples who have met the medical definition of *infertile* are eventually successful in bearing a child, either through medical intervention or simply with the passage of time (OTA, 1988).

The past two decades have seen major advances in medical technology aimed at diagnosing and treating fertility problems. The year 1998 signaled the 20th anniversary of the first "test-tube baby," that is, the first child born by means of in vitro fertilization (IVF). IVF is a technique in which drugs are used to stimulate the maturation of a number of oocytes, mature oocytes are removed from the ovary using ultrasound-guided aspiration, fertilization is attempted in the laboratory using the man's sperm, and the resulting embryos are transferred into the uterus. IVF and similar, more recently developed techniques, including gamete intrafallopian transfer (GIFT) and zygote intrafallopian transfer (ZIFT), are collectively termed *assisted reproductive technologies* (ARTs). According to data from 1996, the success rate (defined as live births) for a given ART treatment cycle (i.e., stimulation, retrieval, fertilization, and transfer) was about 22% (Centers for Disease Control and Prevention, 1999). Thus, despite advances in their success, the vast majority of ART attempts still do not lead to the valued goal of a baby. Many couples make multiple attempts and are still not successful. Although ARTs and other advances now offer the possibility of pregnancy for couples who would otherwise not have been able to have a child, there is little doubt that they are associated with significant stress and have the potential for negative psychological consequences, particularly when they fail. The decision not to try an ART also may be associated with distress, as couples may find themselves regretting the decision not to try everything possible. New advances in technology can intensify this problem, as couples may feel obligated to revisit their decision as hopes for success are renewed.

Couples considering the use of ARTs and other fertility treatments face an enormous constellation of complex decisions and challenges. For example, one important issue facing those who use IVF is the number of embryos to transfer into the uterus. Because of the high cost of each cycle, many couples want to maximize their chance of success in a given cycle by transferring several embryos, with the hope that at least one of them will implant and lead to the much wanted baby. However, this practice carries the risk of multiple gestations. Because of the high-risk nature of multiple-gestation pregnancies, couples may have to decide whether to use a procedure called *selective reduction* to reduce the number of fetuses, with the goal of increasing the chance of any surviving (see Laruelle & Englert, 1996). To avoid these problems, couples can choose to have fewer embryos transferred but then face the costs associated with a greater number of treatment attempts.

Another complex issue couples may face is whether to use donor gametes when either oocyte or sperm quality is not satisfactory. The use of donor gametes offers these couples the opportunity to experience pregnancy and to have a child who is genetically related to one of the parents. The use of donor oocytes has increased dramatically in recent years, as a result of the finding that the most significant barrier to conception with advanced maternal age is deterioration of the older woman's oocytes (Sauer, Paulson, & Lobo, 1992). Oocytes from a younger donor are stimulated by means of drugs, retrieved from her ovary, fertilized in the laboratory with the recipient's partner's sperm, and then transferred to the recipient's uterus. When using donor gametes (oocytes or sperm), couples must consider what type of donor to use (i.e., known or anonymous), characteristics to look for in a donor, how they will feel about having a child that is genetically related to one parent and not the other, what they will tell the child and other people regarding the child's genetic heritage, and so forth (see Braverman, 1993).

These are just a few of the many issues couples face, all of which have significant psychological, financial, and social ramifications. It is also important to realize that these decisions are made under conditions of extreme stress and vulnerability. Couples usually consider these techniques after years of trying other, less invasive approaches. Greenfeld and Haseltine (1986) have reported that ART patients in their study had, on average, spent 6.4 years trying to get pregnant and had been through 2 years of evaluation and treatment for their fertility problem. When many couples face these decisions, they feel they have no time to waste, because the chances of success fall with each passing year of the woman's life. They also occur within the broader context of the couple's life, which may involve securing jobs, reaching educational goals, changing careers, managing work stress, relocating, dealing with family problems, dealing with other medical problems, and so forth. Fertility problems can create barriers in this broader context. For example, individuals may put off changing jobs or going back to school to maintain their medical insurance, or couples may wait to relocate or buy a home until the children are born.

A unique aspect of the experience of infertility is that it is truly a couples' issue, whether it is examined from an epidemiological, medical, psychological, or sociocultural perspective. As a result, it is different from other medical problems, including those described in this volume, which, although clearly affecting both partners, actually characterize only the afflicted partner. Epidemiologically, couples meet the criteria for infertility, not individuals, and individuals can change categories depending on partner characteristics. Medically, the diagnosis and treatment of infertility require active participation of both members of the couple. Although in the past, infertility was considered to be mainly a woman's problem, estimates now suggest that the biological problem is equally likely to be male as female and even more likely to involve both partners (OTA, 1988). With regard to treatment, a partner with no reproductive abnormalities may find himself or herself undergoing extensive medical procedures to circumvent a problem in the partner. For example, IVF is now frequently used with couples with male factor infertility. Also, no type of medical treatment invades private aspects of couple relationships (i.e., the timing and performance of sexual intercourse) as does infertility treatment. Psychologically, regardless of which partner has the etiological factors, both partners find themselves unable to have a child. Although the experience may be somewhat different for the afflicted partner and the nonafflicted partner, both face the loss of their own parenting potential and experience the distress and life alteration associated with that loss. Furthermore, from a sociocultural perspective, bearing children is often considered necessary to fulfill one's marital roles (Nachtigall, Becker, & Wozny, 1992). Couples who are unable to fulfill their childbearing goals can experience difficulty feeling a part of the social fabric of society (see Becker & Nachtigall, 1994).

Because infertility affects the couple as a unit, it presents unique challenges for the couple relationship. Below, we review the research that has been conducted to date relevant to the association between fertility problems and the couple relationship.

ASSOCIATION OF ILLNESS AND COUPLE FACTORS

Do Fertility Problems Lead to Relationship and Sexual Problems?

The clinical–anecdotal literature suggests a number of negative effects of the experience of infertility on the couple relationship, including anger, hostility, blaming of each other, dissatisfaction with a lack of partner support, anxiety about the status of the relationship (particularly by the partner with the biological problem), isolation from each other, and a high likelihood of separation (e.g., Cook, 1987; Mahlstedt, 1985; see Dunkel-Schetter & Lobel, 1991, for a review). The descriptive literature does suggest some positive effects as well, including increased closeness and feelings of support (e.g., Mazor, 1984). The descriptive literature on effects on the sexual relationship is uniformly negative, reporting diminished desire and arousal, ejaculatory problems, lack of orgasm, lower frequency of sexual relations, and sexual dissatisfaction (e.g., Woollett, 1985; see Dunkel-Schetter & Lobel, 1991, for a review). These problems are thought to result from both fears of inadequacy and the deleterious impact of infertility treatment, which involves having sexual intercourse by the calendar, loss of privacy, and the reduction of the act of sexual intercourse to a clinical act of reproduction (see Leiblum, 1994).

However, Dunkel-Schetter and Lobel (1991) and Stanton and Danoff-Burg (1995) reviewed the well-designed quantitative research that used control groups or standardized measures and adequate sampling methods and size. They concluded that the evidence consistently revealed no impairment in relationship or sexual functioning as a result of infertility (see also Leiblum, 1994). In fact, two controlled studies of couples seeking treatment for fertility problems found that relationship satisfaction was higher in infertile couples than in controls who had no fertility problem (Callan & Hennessey, 1989; Downey & McKinney, 1992). Most controlled studies of sexual functioning found that infertile individuals were within the normal range of sexual satisfaction and functioning (i.e., Daniluk, 1988).

It might be that significant relationship and sexual problems are most likely to develop after extended periods of failure to conceive, but very few well-designed studies have followed couples long enough to address this question. However, Leiblum, Kemmann, and Lane (1987) studied 59 couples before and after a failed cycle of IVF. Although both women and men reported symptoms of depression, they continued to report high levels of relationship satisfaction compared with norms. The study also found that over 50% of couples reported improved communication, increased sensitivity to their partner's feelings, and increased sense of closeness as a result of infertility. Only 2%–4 % reported decreases in these aspects of relationship quality, and the remainder reported no changes. Additionally, 20% of wives reported that their infertility difficulties had improved the frequency of sexual relations and increased sexual satisfaction, 14% of both husbands and wives reported lower frequency, and the remainder reported no changes. Further research is needed to fully examine the long-term effects of failure, as well as the effects of success, on the couple relationship.

It is also important to view the experience of infertility within the broader context of couples' lives and to consider how infertility compares with pregnancy and parenthood. This is of particular interest given the well-known, small, but reliable reduction in relationship satisfaction after the birth of a first child (see Belsky, 1990). One of the few longitudinal studies of infertility revealed that previously infertile couples who had a child over the 2-year course of the study ($n = 73$) on average reported more positive life quality but lower relationship satisfaction than couples who remained childless ($n = 101$; but note that nonstandardized measures were used; Abbey, Andrews, & Halman, 1994). Thus, it did not appear that the continued experience of failure to conceive resulted in significant relationship problems, and in fact, any negative effect was less than that associated with becoming parents.

What accounts for the discrepancy between clinical–anecdotal reports, which suggest significant problems, and quantitative research, which does not? A number of explanations have been offered, including (a) lack of sensitivity of the global measures used in quantitative research, (b) desire on the part of research participants to appear more healthy, so that they will be considered good candidates for infertility treatment, and (c) overgeneralization of the problems experienced by a small number of patients who seek mental health treatment to the infertility population in general (Dunkel-Schetter & Lobel, 1991). There is probably some truth to each of these explanations. However, as Dunkel-Schetter and Lobel have concluded, perhaps the most compelling reason for the discrepancy is that there is substantial variability between infertile couples in how they are affected. Some couples experience serious relationship problems, whereas others emerge closer and more satisfied with their relationship than before. Therefore, it is not surprising that the quantitative research has not found that infertile couples, on average, are more distressed in their relationships or have more sexual problems than do other couples.

In our view, a more interesting question than whether infertile couples experience more or less relationship distress and sexual problems than other couples is what leads to the variability between couples. Why do some couples report significant relationship problems and others report a strengthening of their relationship as a result of "going through this together"? Both clinical–anecdotal reports and quantitative research have recently begun to suggest that one explanation for this variability involves the match between partners in their response to infertility. It has been suggested that relationship problems may develop to the extent that couples have incompatible ways of responding to the fertility problem. This hypothesis is addressed in detail below.

The Association Between Couple Factors and Relationship Distress

Consider Michele and Gerald, whom we interviewed in a study of couples with fertility problems (Pasch, 1994). Michele and Gerald were both very distressed about the difficulty they were having in getting pregnant. They had tried using IVF, but Gerald's sperm did not fertilize any oocytes. Most likely, their only chance for Michele to become pregnant was to use donor sperm. Gerald was the type of person who liked to consider all avenues before he made a decision, particularly when emotional issues were involved. Michele preferred to make decisions quickly and not to dwell on problems. Before they encountered a fertility problem, this difference had not caused much of a problem, because they had not been faced with any difficult decisions that they had to make together. In response to the fertility problem, Gerald constantly wanted to talk with Michele about what they should do. Michele felt the problem was too hard to talk about and tried not to think about it too much. When Gerald tried to talk to Michele, she became quiet and somewhat withdrawn, and she could not stand to listen to Gerald's incessant calculations about probabilities and costs and so forth. Gerald found her withdrawal intolerable and asserted that Michele's lack of responsiveness was a sign of hostility toward him for having a low sperm count. He complained that Michele's refusal to work with him in making a decision was ruining their chances of ever having a child. This problem communicating began to trickle into other aspects of their relationship, including their sexual relationship. Gerald began to wonder if Michele was really the right woman for him, because she would not open up to him when it really mattered.

This is an example of the dynamics that can result when partners differ in their appraisal or coping with the fertility problem. There are many similar examples in the descriptive literature on infertile couples (i.e., Epstein & Rosenberg, 1997; Mahlstedt, 1985; Salzer, 1991). For example, on the basis of her clinical experience working with couples with fertility problems, Mahlstedt (1985) made the following observations:

> Men often cope with their pain by keeping it to themselves or focusing on their wives. Women often cope by talking continually with their

husbands, who feeling powerless to take away the pain, sometimes stop listening. In order to get him involved, she escalates her complaints and he, in response, retreats even farther and may even cease participating in the treatment process. In these cases, the woman feels abandoned when she needs her husband most, and he feels overwhelmed because she seems to need him so much. They begin to resent each other and become depressed not only by their failure to conceive but also by their loss of closeness and ability to understand each other. (p. 337)

In keeping with Mahlstedt's (1985) observations, there is strong evidence from a number of studies for differences between men and women in their response to fertility problems. For example, there is evidence that (a) having children is more important to women than to men (Berg, Wilson, & Weingartner, 1991); (b) women's self-esteem is more affected by having fertility problems (Pasch, 1994); (c) women experience more distress associated with infertility and are at greater risk for depression after failed treatment efforts (see Stanton & Danoff-Burg, 1995); and (d) women are more involved and invested in fertility treatment (Pasch, 1994). Regarding coping strategies, women are more likely to use escape–avoidance, seeking support, and emotional expression, whereas men are more likely to use distancing and self-control in response to infertility (Abbey, Andrews, & Halman, 1991; Pasch et al., 1995; Stanton, 1991; Stanton, Tennen, Affleck, & Mendola, 1992). These differences may well be the source of many of the relationship problems couples experience. However, although there are differences between men and women in general, within a particular couple, differences do not necessarily fall along gendered lines. In our own work, we have occasionally encountered couples in which the man was more invested in having children than the woman and couples in which the man was more interested in talking and sharing feelings than the woman (as in the case of Michele and Gerald).

A few recent studies have begun to address the question of whether differences between partners in appraisal and coping are associated with relationship problems. Levin, Sher, and Theodos (1997) studied 46 couples undergoing treatment for fertility problems. They found that for wives, relationship satisfaction was relatively low when the wife used emotion-oriented coping infrequently but the husband used it frequently. However, they also found that relationship satisfaction was relatively low when both partners rarely used of task-oriented strategies. Perhaps in this case, both partners become frustrated and blame each other for not focusing on strategies aimed at solving the fertility problem.

In our own research, we studied 48 couples seeking treatment for fertility problems (Pasch, 1994). We were interested in examining how each partner's response to infertility (i.e., her or his appraisal of the meaning of the problem, involvement in treatment, and coping strategies) was related to the couple's ability to communicate effectively regarding their fertility problem. To measure communication, we asked each couple to participate in an interaction task in which they discussed a difficult issue related to their fertility problem with each other for 15 minutes. The resulting interactions were audiotaped and coded by trained raters on a number of different communication dimensions. Common topics for the discussions were making decisions about treatments, making decisions about whether to consider adoption or to use donor gametes, commitment to having children, emotional reactions to the fertility problem, how much to talk about the fertility problem, the effect of the fertility problem on other life plans, and telling others about the fertility problem. Overall, more destructive communication was associated with (a) one partner (usually the woman) being relatively more invested in having children than the other; (b) husbands being relatively low in involvement in treatment, regardless of wives' involvement; (c) one partner (usually the woman) being relatively high in the use of seeking support when her partner was relatively low; and (d) one partner (usually the man) being relatively high in the use of distancing when his partner was relatively low. Relatively high levels of destructive communication during the interaction task were associated with lower global relationship satisfaction and a more negative perceived impact of the fertility problem on the relationship.

The Association Between Couple Factors and Individual Distress

There is substantial variability in the impact of infertility on individual functioning (see Stanton & Dunkel-Schetter, 1991). In recent years, there has been a shift in research away from studying whether infertile individuals are more distressed than other people and toward examining the risk or protective factors associated with enhancing or hindering psychological adjustment (e.g., Litt, Tennen, Affleck, & Klock, 1992; Stanton, 1991; Tennen, Affleck, & Mendola, 1991).

The quality of the couple relationship may be particularly important for infertile couples as a protective factor, given that the stigma associated with infertility leads some individuals to retreat from their broader social networks to avoid embarrassment and receiving unhelpful advice (Abbey et al., 1991). There is some evidence for a concurrent association between relationship satisfaction and individual distress, although studies suffer from the lack of standardized measures. McEwan, Costello, and Taylor (1987) studied 62 women in infertile couples and found that those who reported having a confiding relationship with their partner experienced more positive psychological adjustment to infertility (see also Abbey et al., 1991). However, no studies have examined relationship quality before infertility, so the direction of the effect remains unclear. Only one study with an adequate size has examined whether a strong couple relationship is protective against distress after ART failure. Newton, Hearn, and Yuzpe (1990) found that pre-IVF measures of relationship cohesion, expressiveness, and conflict were not significant predictors of depression or anxiety after IVF failure ($n = 151$ women and 122 men).

Because infertility affects couples as a unit, there also has been interest in how the appraisal, coping, and adjustment of one partner may be related to the psychological adjustment of the other. Only a few preliminary studies have addressed this question. Stanton et al. (1992) studied 72 couples who were seeking treatment for infertility and found that the only variable of one partner that was related to the other's adjustment was coping through seeking support. As wives sought more support, their husbands reported less distress. Levin et al. (1997) found that husbands, but not wives, were more distressed to the extent that both partners were high in the use of emotional-oriented coping. Pasch et al. (1995) found that husbands were more distressed to the extent that they used escape–avoidance and to the extent that their wives exhibited more demanding behaviors during the laboratory communication task. Wives were more distressed to the extent that they or their partner used escape–avoidance and to the extent that they were more demanding and expressed more negative affect and less positive affect during the laboratory communication task.

Couple Decision Making Regarding Fertility Treatment

Another important topic of research on couples with fertility problems is the study of how couples make decisions regarding treatment. As described earlier, couples are faced with an increasingly complex set of issues with enormous ramifications for their future, encompassing the nature and origin of the family they build together. Research on unassisted reproductive decision making has shown that how couples decide if and when to have children is an extremely complex process, in part because of the fact that proceptive behavior (actions taken toward the goal of having children) requires the participation of both partners, who may have different desires and intentions (Miller, 1994). Couple decision making regarding assisted reproduction is even more complex because treatment involves intense commitment on the part of both partners.

A few studies have described differences between men and women in factors relevant to treatment decisions. It has been reported that women are more likely to take the initiative to seek treatment and are more likely to be responsible for making decisions about treatment (Greil, Leitko, & Porter, 1988; McGrade & Tolor, 1981). Pepe and Bryne (1991) studied 40 women who had experienced failed fertility treatment and had ended treatment. Participants were asked who was responsible for initiating and terminating fertility treatment. Regarding initiating treatment, 61% of the women felt it was a shared decision, 36% felt it was mostly or totally their own decision, and only 3% felt it was their husband's decision. Regarding terminating treatment, 61% felt it was a shared decision, 16% felt it was mostly or totally their decision, and 19% felt it was mostly or totally their husband's decision. These results suggest that whereas women play a larger role in initiating treatment than their partner, men become more involved in treatment decision making in regard to termination of treatment. This study also showed that women were less satisfied with their relationship (before, during, and after treatment, reported retrospectively) to the extent that the decision to initiate treatment was not shared, suggesting that relationship distress is associated with proceeding with treatment without the full support of the husband.

Related to the findings that women are more invested in having children than are men, they also appear to be more willing to try any treatment that might lead to success. Collins, Freeman, Boxer, and Tureck (1992) found that women were more likely than men to report that they would "do anything" to have a child ($N = 200$ couples). Frank (1990) had 40 men and 107 women rank the importance of various factors in decisions about treatment. Although men and women tended to give similar rankings, men ranked consideration of possible side effects and risks of treatment higher than women, whereas women were more concerned with whether the treatment would be successful.

There is evidence that women's perceptions of how treatment has impacted their relationship is a factor in their decision to continue treatment. Mao and Wood (1984) found that strain on the couple relationship was one of the major reasons for withdrawing from ART treatment; other reasons were financial costs, anxiety, depression, medical barriers, and disruption to lives and careers ($N = 121$). Daniluk, Pattinson, Zouvez, and Mitchell (1993) studied 41 men and 51 women who had previously tried ART, succeeded, and were now considering ART again to increase their family size. Individuals were more likely to intend to try ART again if they perceived a positive impact of infertility on their relationship and if they reported more dyadic affection after parenthood.

Callan, Kloske, Kashima, and Hennessey (1988) used a formal theoretical model (the theory of reasoned action) to examine how women make decisions regarding infertility treatment. They studied 53 women who had made at least one previous ART attempt and found that those who intended to try ART again were more likely than those who did not intend to try again to believe that using an ART would allow them to become a mother, have their own child, have a happier relationship, have more sense of purpose in life, be like other women, have the emotional benefits and costs of having children, reduce negative comments about their relationship, and experience an increased quality of life. Women who intended to undergo ART treatment were also more likely to think that their actions would be supported by other infertile women, their husband, and their physician. Those who did not intend to try ART again were more likely to believe that significant others would want them to stop. Although the use of a formal theoretical model represents a major advance in the literature, because Callan et al. did not study men, the factors that might affect each partner's ability to translate his or her intentions into actual proceptive behavior and how couples resolve differing intentions remain unclear.

ASSESSMENT AND INTERVENTION

As we and others have previously argued, attention to the potential negative psychological effects of the experience of infertility and its treatment and to ways to avoid negative effects should be central in the minds of all health care professionals who work with couples with fertility problems (Leiblum, 1997; Pasch & Dunkel-Schetter, 1997). Below, we offer our recommendations regarding working with infertile couples, from the points of view of both the medical professional and the mental health professional. In the absence of a more complete empirical base from which to guide intervention efforts, our recommendations are based on the limited research that is available, a compilation of the recommendations of others working in this field, and our own experience with couples in general.

Recommendations for Medical Professionals

Many suggestions have been offered to physicians and medical staff who work with infertile couples regarding how to manage psychological issues (see Daniluk, 1997; Pasch & Dunkel-Schetter, 1997). Here, we focus on the issues specific to the consideration of the couple as a unit. There appears to be agreement among those working in the field that due to the dyadic nature of infertility, diagnostic and treatment planning should include both members of the couple (Daniluk, 1997). Encouraging joint attendance and participation is thought to set the tone for the couple to see infertility as a joint problem regardless of which member has the biological problem. Failure to include both partners can lead to multiple problems, from one member of the couple participating in a treatment protocol that he or she finds objectionable to one member becoming a parent by a means with which she or he is not comfortable (e.g., donor sperm).

As described earlier, research has shown that men tend to be less likely to suggest seeking treatment, less involved in treatment, and less involved in making decisions about treatment options. In part, this is because most of the medical tests and interventions are focused on the woman, and the woman is naturally more attuned to the process of trying to become pregnant because she experiences the physical signs of ovulation, pregnancy, and failure. We found that couples' communication was more constructive and that both perceived the impact of the fertility problem as more positive if the husband was involved in treatment (Pasch et al., 1995). Involvement of the male partner included attending appointments, accessing resources about infertility, being present for medical procedures, and generally staying informed of the process.

One reason that the man may become uninvolved in treatment decision making is that the woman becomes the expert in dealing with treatment and the man, being relatively uninformed, feels he has little to offer. Sudore, Croughan-Minihane, Pasch, Neuhaus, and Camarano (1998) investigated the extent to which 29 men and 39 women knew the infertility diagnosis that was recorded in their medical charts by their physician. Although both partners' knowledge was often inaccurate and incomplete, knowledge by men was extremely low: 28% of wives and 46% of husbands could not report even one diagnosis that was recorded in the medical chart (there was an average of 2.5 diagnoses per couple). Attention by physicians to ensuring that the male partner is informed of the diagnosis may lead to less disengagement over time as the treatment process continues.

Unfortunately, eliciting the participation of the less involved partner is not always easy. Physicians and other medical staff can encourage the participation of a partner who seems less interested by making it clear that his or her opinion is important and valued and that his or her desires will be included in the decision-making process if he or she is willing to express them. This nonjudgmental approach is important because men may on the surface appear disinterested when actually they are feeling excluded or feel they have nothing to offer because most of the medical investigations involve the woman.

Because partners may disagree about what treatment approach to take, how far to proceed with treatment, whether to consider adoption, and so forth, physicians and medical staff should be prepared to work with both members of the couple to explore positives and negatives associated with the various options. It should be emphasized that differences between partners are normal and can be satisfactorily worked through. Normalizing differences can help partners develop a platform for considering their predicament: "our problem with what to do about using IVF," as opposed to "he will not agree to trying IVF." Suggestions for counseling couples who have reached a decision-making impasse are described in the next section.

Recommendations for Mental Health Professionals

As described earlier, there is little evidence that infertility leads to impairment in relationship functioning for most couples. Nevertheless, there is significant variability between couples, and some couples do experience significant relationship problems as a result of dealing with fertility problems and the associated stressors. Although many authors have advocated the provision of counseling, including couples counseling, as a component of infertility treatment programs, there is relatively little known regarding the types of interventions that are most useful. Cognitive–behavioral approaches have received some attention (see Zoldbrod, 1993) and are known to be effective approaches to couples treatment in general (see Baucom, Mueser, Shoham, Daiuto, & Stickle, 1998). No controlled research has evaluated the usefulness of couples treatment for couples with fertility problems.

In this section, we provide our suggestions for working with couples with fertility problems who experience significant relationship distress. The approach described is particularly appropriate for couples who have reached some kind of stalemate, for example, when one partner insists on continued medical treatment, and the other refuses. As described earlier, many couples experience significant distress associated with infertility but are able to use their resources to manage the distress before it leads to relationship problems per se. These couples may not need the kind of therapy we describe but may benefit from more general counseling approaches, including providing information, support, and help with decision making (Leiblum, 1997). Also, our approach is based on the assumption that both members of the couple are willing to participate in counseling. Soliciting the participation of a less invested partner is not always easy but can be attempted by nonjudgmentally inviting the less invested partner to participate, emphasizing that his or her opinions and desires are as important as those of his or her partner.

The approach we describe is based on the principles of integrative couples therapy (ICT), a couples therapy approach developed by Christensen et al. (1995) and Jacobson and Christensen (1996). ICT is based on behavioral principles and uses techniques such as communication and problem-solving-skills training, which partners can use to accommodate each other. What it adds is a focus on promoting intimacy through increasing partners' acceptance and understanding of each other. This focus on mutual understanding is particularly relevant to couples with fertility problems, or couples who are encountering any type of stressful circumstance, because stressful circumstances can lead to self-focus and an inability to see the other's point of view (Wood, Saltzberg, & Goldsamt, 1990). ICT helps couples explore their own and their partner's feelings and thoughts about central issues of concern to them. For a complete description, the reader should refer to Jacobson and Christensen (1996) or Christensen et al. (1995).

Step 1: Assessment—Development of the Formulation

The assessment phase of ICT has several goals, including determining the distress level of the couple, gauging the level of commitment to the relationship, and evaluating any violence in the couple. Achievement of these goals is often facilitated by the use of standardized measures such as the Dyadic Adjustment Scale (Spanier, 1976) and the Conflict Tactics Scale

(Straus, 1979). Perhaps the most important part of an ICT assessment is the development of a formulation, which will be the basis for the treatment. The formulation is an analysis of the couple's core conflict and is identified through targeted discussions with the couple. To develop a formulation, the therapist must first identify the theme of the couple's conflict, which is usually a difference between partners. Common sources of conflict for couples with fertility problems include differences in desire and commitment to having children, modes of emotional expression, desire for sharing feelings and talking about the fertility problem, preference for specific medical treatments, and length of time and amount of money to spend on fertility treatments. For example, consider Jackie and Roger, who had been trying to have a child for 4 years. Jackie saw having a child as the most important thing in her life. She felt that her life would not be complete until they succeeded. She wanted to try every treatment possible, even if the chances of it working were very remote. When they first started trying, Roger wanted very much to have children but thought it would not be detrimental to him if they did not. After they were unsuccessful for a while, he came to the conclusion that they were just not meant to have children. He wanted their lives to go on and for there to be an end point to the constant focus on getting pregnant. He felt he was at his wit's end with medical treatments and was very distressed about the financial burden. So the theme of their conflict was differences in commitment to having a child.

Once a theme has been identified, the therapist identifies the pattern of interaction that develops between the couple around this theme. In Jackie and Roger's case, Jackie was constantly making demands on Roger to participate more and to agree to spending more and more money on expensive treatments. She castigated him for his lack of commitment. Roger withdrew from her, unable to deal with her insistent tone, accusations, and mood swings. When they had first started having fertility problems, Roger had tried to be understanding when Jackie was upset, but later, when Jackie got upset after she got her period, he outright refused to talk to her.

Having identified the pattern of interaction, the therapist tries to understand what the emotional outcome of this conflict is for each partner. Often, partners each feel trapped, unable to get the other to do what they want. In Jackie and Roger's case, Roger felt he did not know Jackie anymore, she did not seem like herself because she was so obsessed with getting pregnant, and he could not find a way to persuade her to "get over it." Jackie could not believe her husband was so insensitive, and she could not find a way to get him to be responsive to her needs. Both felt alone and misunderstood.

After the assessment phase, the ICT therapist gives couples feedback about their assessment. The therapist shares the formulation with the couple, inviting them to add or detract as they see fit. Because the formulation is a nonblaming analysis of the couple's conflict, the goal is for the couple to adopt it as their own view of their problem.

Step 2: Treatment—Acceptance-Building Strategies

After the assessment and feedback sessions, the work of therapy involves (a) identifying incidents in the couple's daily life that are manifestations of the theme and patterns of interaction (e.g., an upcoming event that may trigger the problem or a recent negative or positive event relating to the problem) and (b) using a set of techniques to help the couple increase intimacy through acceptance and understanding of each other. Several of these techniques, as applied to couples with fertility problems, are described below. Throughout this section, we emphasize acceptance-building strategies involved in ICT because they are not well known. Traditional change-oriented strategies such as communication skills building and behavior exchange do play an important, albeit adjunctive role; however, they are described extensively elsewhere (e.g., Jacobson & Christensen, 1996; Jacobson & Margolin, 1979).

Empathic joining around the problem. When couples are facing incompatibilities of the magnitude of Roger and Jackie's, they are usually unable to see anything but the negative aspects of each other's behavior. The first strategy in ICT is feedback about the therapist's formulation of the problem. Because the formulation focuses on the pain that each partner is experiencing and the efforts each has already made, however misguided, to accommodate the other, it is a first step toward their becoming more sympathetic with each other's position. During the initial feedback session, the therapist might say the following to Roger and Jackie:

> A major problem I see the two of you as having comes from a difference in your commitment to having a child. You, Jackie, are extremely committed to having a child by whatever means necessary, whereas Roger, you originally wanted very much to have a child, but over time you have become much less committed, in response to all the medical problems the two of you have encountered. This is actually a common difference between people; in fact, many couples have one partner who is more invested in having children than the other. But when couples encounter difficulty getting pregnant, it can become a big problem because dealing with a fertility problem usually requires a lot of time, money, and energy from both partners, not just the one who really wants children. I think the stress of dealing with this situation has led each of you to become more extreme in your positions and has generated a painful sequence of communication between the two of you. Initially, you, Jackie, feeling distraught, would seek support from Roger, and he tried to offer comfort and reassurance. But when that did not work, he became frustrated and maybe even felt helpless, because there was nothing he could do to make you feel better. Over time, Jackie became increasingly demanding of you, Roger, because she wasn't getting the support she needed, and you started to withdraw from her. Now, as soon as Jackie brings up the fertility issue, Roger, you sense the pressure,

feel put upon, and do not want to touch the issue. So it is hardly surprising that Jackie is blaming Roger and always putting demands on him and Roger is retreating in an angry silence. And it is clear that both of you are feeling angry and misunderstood.

The formulation is the first step in promoting empathy between the pair but it is rarely sufficient on its own. Further work focuses on individual incidents that reflect the conflict between them. For example, therapy sessions might focus on what transpired the last time Jackie got her period, the feelings each had, and the pattern of interaction that occurred between them; or on what might happen when they get their next results of a diagnostic test. The clinical purpose for these discussions is to promote the idea that the problems arise from differences between partners and less so from inadequacies or malicious intent of either partner and to promote the non-blaming "language of acceptance," that is, to promote an empathic context for understanding each partner's behavior in the face of their differences.

Unified detachment. A second strategy used in ICT to increase emotional acceptance is to promote a descriptive, detached, externalized view of the problem. The therapist helps the couple to examine the sequence of their conflict, including the events and feelings that trigger it, in a detached way. The goal is for the couple to begin to talk about their problem as an "it" as opposed to a "you" or "me." This reduces the focus on blaming one partner or the other and provides the couple with a platform for thinking about the problem. For example, consider Maria and Lorenzo, whose interaction appeared at the beginning of this chapter. They had reached a total stalemate regarding treatment. Maria has blocked fallopian tubes. With the help of her doctor, she had come to the conclusion that her chances of success with IVF were very remote. She wanted to pursue adoption, but Lorenzo was dead set against it. They could not even talk about the problem anymore, because their discussions deteriorated to accusations and expressions of contempt. Maria called him "stubborn" and "cruel" for not allowing her to have a child in her life, and Lorenzo called her "foolish for wanting to raise the child of some drug-addicted mother." Through discussions about the problem and situations in which they are confronted with it, the therapist would try to encourage a detached view of this problem as "their problem with different views about adoption" as opposed to the fault of one or the other. The therapist might engage them in an analysis of the triggers that lead to their angry discussions or a comparison of discussions that go rather well with those that go poorly. The therapist might help them develop a humorous or metaphorical label for their struggle, such as the "child crusade." All these efforts could promote a more detached view of their difficulty and facilitate more acceptance of each other.

Tolerance building. Accepting one's partner is often difficult because of the pain associated with the partner's negative behaviors. For example,

Roger could have been more understanding of Jackie's desperate need for a child if she had not constantly criticized him for not being more committed to infertility treatment. Another strategy for increasing acceptance is building each partner's ability to tolerate the negative aspects of his or her partner's behavior. One way ICT therapists do this is to point out the positive, or less negative, aspects of the partner's negative behaviors, thus making them more tolerable. For example, the ICT therapist may help Roger to interpret Jackie's criticisms as a reflection of her feelings of helplessness at not having been able to get pregnant, and her view, albeit misguided, that badgering him will bring her closer to her goal. The therapist can then try to identify how Jackie's behavior fits into the bigger picture of their connection to each other. For example, perhaps Jackie's ability to stick to a goal, no matter what, was something that initially attracted Roger to her, because he tended to give up on his goals as soon as he ran into any obstacles. In using this technique, ICT therapists are careful not to deny that the negative behaviors of the partner may be painful, but instead to emphasize how the behaviors are part of a greater constellation of traits that make up their partner, some parts of which are easy to appreciate.

Greater self-care. Another avenue toward greater acceptance is to increase each partner's ability to protect and care for herself or himself in the face of negative behaviors of the other. This strategy is based on the idea that if partners have a set of skills for dealing with negative partner behaviors, they will be less upset when those negative behaviors occur, their interactions will be less likely to escalate, and they will be able to recover from negative interactions more quickly. Encouraging self-care is particularly important for couples faced with fertility problems, or other major stressful life events, because the stress and demands associated with these events can increase both partners' needs for support while simultaneously decreasing their ability to provide support to their partner (Christensen & Pasch, 1993).

Recall Michele and Gerald, who had different ways of coping with their fertility problem. Gerald wanted to talk incessantly with Michele about the various options facing them regarding donor sperm, whereas Michele wanted to just make a decision and go on. To help increase Gerald's ability to tolerate Michele's lack of responsiveness, the therapist might encourage Gerald to attend an informational seminar on male infertility or to find someone who has had a similar decision to make with whom he could share some of his concerns. This strategy would be consistent with Gottlieb and Wagner's (1991) work with couples with ill children. They reported that receiving emotional support from others was one successful way wives adapted to their husbands' lack of emotional expressiveness. Although powerful, these strategies must be used carefully because there is a potential for them to be seen as a way of absolving responsibility, that is, suggesting that Michele did not have to participate in the decision-making process. Specifically, it would be emphasized that Michele could not be expected to respond in just the way Gerald wanted her to all the time, so by having someone else to talk to, Gerald would not have to become furious when Michele was not as willing to listen as he would like.

An interesting outcome of many acceptance-building strategies is that they often do lead to behavior change, although they are not designed to do so. For example, knowing that Gerald had, at least in theory, taken some responsibility for managing his own obsessive need to consider all options might take some of the pressure off Michele and she might have actually been able to be more emotionally available to him. Similarly, if Maria and Lorenzo were able to see their difference of opinion about adoption as "their problem," they might have been be able to cease the use of self-defeating strategies to solve it and see a more straightforward solution (e.g., borrowing money to allow them to use a private adoption agency).

CONCLUSIONS AND FUTURE DIRECTIONS

Recent years have seen a number of advances in the understanding of the psychology of couples and infertility. The preponderance of studies suggests that global relationship and sexual functioning are not lower in infertile couples than in couples in general, although there is considerable variability. A small number of studies have begun to identify factors (i.e., coping) that might account for this variability. These advances notwithstanding, it is evident that the research literature contains more gaps than answers. In this section, we delineate some of the key challenges to be faced in three domains: conceptual frameworks, methodological considerations, and issues in clinical applications.

Conceptual Frameworks

Our current understanding of the psychology of couples and infertility is hampered by the atheoretical nature of much of the research. Most research has been purely descriptive, examining the level of adjustment of infertile couples. More recent work has used a stress and coping framework to identify the processes that determine the level of adjustment (see Stanton & Dunkel-Schetter, 1991). Although the use of this well-established theoretical model represents a major advance, the traditional stress and coping model is limited because it does not fully appreciate the dyadic context in which medical problems occur. Attention to the dyadic context is particularly important in consideration of infertility, which we have argued is even more of a couples issue than many other medical problems. A departure from the traditional stress and coping framework is evident in the few studies reviewed earlier that examine how the coping efforts of one partner may affect the adjustment of the other or how differences between partners may affect communication, the overall relationship, and each partner's adjustment (see Levin et al., 1997; Pasch et al., 1995; Stanton et al., 1992). We therefore encourage the development of more dyad-oriented theoretical frameworks, as have begun to be put forth in other research areas (see Revenson, 1994).

In addition, to date, most of the research on the psychology of infertility in the United States must be thought of as a psychology of White, relatively affluent couples who seek medical treatment for their difficulty conceiving. Most research has been conducted through medical settings that provide advanced infertility evaluation and treatment, services to which only a segment of the population has access. As a result, we know little about the experience of couples with fertility problems who do not seek treatment at all, either because of lack of financial resources or otherwise, or those who terminate treatment. Furthermore, there is a clear need to include individuals from ethnic minority groups and individuals from lower socioeconomic groups. This is particularly important in the light of evidence that some of these individuals are at high risk for experiencing fertility problems (OTA, 1988). Although there has been recent attention to the issues lesbian couples face when they experience fertility problems or choose to make use of reproductive technologies to have children (see Chan, Raboy, & Patterson, 1998; Jacob, 1997), they have also been largely neglected. It is clear that lesbian couples face additional barriers, because the sociopolitical system often questions their rights to make use of reproductive technologies and their suitability as parents (see Golombok & Tasker, 1994).

Methodological Considerations

Unfortunately, the literature on couples and infertility is not as strong methodologically as it should be to adequately address important questions about how infertility and reproductive technologies affect couples. The common methodological weaknesses include small sample sizes, poor sampling methods, use of nonstandardized measures, and the lack of adequate control groups. Also, the vast majority of studies have been conducted by investigators who were affiliated with the infertility treatment center in which the research was conducted. This may have several consequences. First, many studies have used data from routine initial assessments with patients. Ambiguity regarding the purpose of the assessments may lead patients to hide emotional or relationship problems, fearing that revealing problems might lead to rejection from the program. Therefore, the validity of their responses is questionable. Additionally, previous researchers have had substantial difficulties in studying patients who experienced ART failures, perhaps because they linked the researchers with the treatment facility that failed to help them achieve a pregnancy (Adler, Keyes, & Robertson, 1991). Patients who did participate in follow-up studies may be those who were most satisfied with the treatment they received.

Another critical weakness in the literature is that only a few studies are prospective and longitudinal (Downey & McKinney, 1990). In the absence of prospective, longitudinal research, we know little about the psychological consequences of the possible paths couples take as they struggle with infertility and of outcomes they encounter. Knowledge of the long-term outcomes of ARTs and other choices (including the decision not to pursue treatment) is important because these decisions have far-reaching implications for later family life. The few longitudinal studies that do exist suggest that it is critical to examine outcomes in the broader context of couples' lives (see Abbey et al., 1994). We also know little about risk factors for later poor adjustment, information that is critical to the design of research-based assessment and intervention programs.

Issues in Clinical Applications

How should research be translated into clinical applications that will promote the well-being of couples facing fertility problems? Considerably more research of the types identified above is necessary before this goal can be realized. Nevertheless, below, we identify several applications that would assist health professionals in guiding patients through the treatment process.

First, one of the critical roles mental health professionals play in infertility treatment is conducting pretreatment assessments with couples. There is considerable variability among practices in the purpose of these assessments, including providing information and support and identifying patients in need of special treatment (i.e., for depression), to avoid undue stress over the course of treatment, as well as identifying patients who are considered inappropriate for participation in the ART program. At present, the empirical grounds for making these decisions are weak. Therefore, the development of research-based assessment protocols is an important application of empirical research. Prospective, longitudinal research that identifies those couples at greatest risk for negative psychological outcomes will provide an empirical basis for making these decisions and will facilitate the targeting of psychological services to those patients at highest risk and thus prevent the development of serious negative outcomes.

Second, given the complexity and uncertainty of the new reproductive options, there is a need for the development of decision-making aids for couples faced with fertility-treatment decisions. These aids might be in the form of reading materials or videotapes that provide information regarding particular procedures and contain stories of couples who have chosen to undergo various treatments with various possible outcomes, as well as of couples who have elected not to use the procedure, have adopted a child, or have chosen to remain without children. These materials should be developed based on the elements of informed decision making as defined in behavioral decision theories (i.e., identification of the full range of child-related options, consideration of risks and benefits, and assessment of the likelihood and personal value associated with each risk and benefit; see Hodne, 1995). Additionally, because of the dyadic nature of infertility treatment, the decision-making aids should address the issue of resolving differences between partners.

REFERENCES

Abbey, A., Andrews, F. M., & Halman, L. J. (1991). The importance of social relationships for infertile couples' well-being. In A. L. Stanton & C. Dunkel-Schetter (Eds.), *Infertility: Perspectives from stress and coping research* (pp. 61–86). New York: Plenum.

Abbey, A., Andrews, F., & Halman, L. J. (1994). Infertility and parenthood: Does becoming a parent increase well-being? *Journal of Consulting and Clinical Psychology, 62*, 398–403.

Abma, J., Chandra, A., Mosher, W. D., Peterson, L. S., & Piccinino, L. J. (1997). Fertility, family planning, and women's health: New data from the 1995 National Survey of Family Growth. *Vital and Health Statistics: Series 23. Data from the National Survey of Family Growth, 19*, 1–114.

Adler, N. E., Keyes, S., & Robertson, P. (1991). Psychological issues in reproductive technologies: Pregnancy-inducing technology and diagnostic screening. In J. Rodin & A. Collins (Eds.), *Women and new reproductive technologies: Medical, psychosocial, legal, and ethical dilemmas* (pp. 111–133). Hillsdale, NJ: Erlbaum.

Baucom, D. H., Meuser, K. T., Shoham, V., Daiuto, A., & Stickle, T. R. (1998). Empirically supported couple and family interventions for marital distress and adult mental health problems. *Journal of Consulting and Clinical Psychology, 66*, 53–88.

Becker, G., & Nachtigall, R. D. (1994). "Born to be a mother": The cultural construction of risk in infertility treatment in the U.S. *Social Science Medicine, 39*, 507–518.

Belsky, J. (1990). Children and marriage. In F. D. Fincham & T. N. Bradbury (Eds.), *The psychology of marriage: Basic issues and applications* (pp. 172–200). New York: Guilford Press.

Berg, B. J., Wilson, J. F., & Weingartner, P. J. (1991). Psychological sequelae of infertility treatment: The role of gender and sex-role identification. *Social Science and Medicine, 33*, 1071–1080.

Braverman, A. M. (1993). Survey results on the current practice of ovum donation. *Fertility and Sterility, 59*, 1216–1220.

Callan, V. J., & Hennessey, J. F. (1989). Psychological adjustment to infertility: A unique comparison of two groups of infertile women, mothers, and women childless by choice. *Journal of Reproductive and Infant Psychology, 7*, 105–112.

Callan, V. J., Kloske, B., Kashima, Y., & Hennessey, J. F. (1988). Toward understanding women's decisions to continue or stop in vitro fertilization: The role of social, psychological, and background factors. *Journal of in Vitro Fertilization and Embryo Transfer, 5,* 363–369.

Centers for Disease Control and Prevention. (1999). *1996 assisted reproductive technology success rates: National summary and fertility clinic reports.* [On-line report]. Available: http://www.cdc.gov/nccdphp/drh/art.htm.

Chan, R. W., Raboy, B., & Patterson, C. J. (1998). Psychosocial adjustment among children conceived via donor insemination by lesbian and heterosexual mothers. *Child Development, 69,* 443–457.

Christensen, A., Jacobson, N. S., & Babcock, J. C. (1995). Integrative behavioral couple therapy. In N. S. Jacobson & A. S. Gurman (Eds.), *Clinical handbook of couple therapy* (pp. 31–64). New York: Guilford Press.

Christensen, A., & Pasch, L. (1993). The sequence of marital conflict: An analysis of seven phases of marital conflict in distressed and nondistressed couples. *Clinical Psychology Review, 13,* 3–14.

Collins, A., Freeman, E. W., Boxer, A. S., & Tureck, R. (1992). Perceptions of infertility and treatment stress in females as compared with males entering in vitro fertilization treatment. *Fertility and Sterility, 57,* 350–356.

Cook, E. P. (1987). Characteristics of the biopsychosocial crisis of infertility. *Journal of Counseling and Development, 65,* 465–470.

Daniluk, J. C. (1988). Infertility: Intrapersonal and interpersonal impact. *Fertility and Sterility, 49,* 982–990.

Daniluk, J. (1997). Helping patients cope with infertility. *Clinical Obstetrics and Gynecology, 40,* 661–672.

Daniluk, J., Pattinson, T., Zouvez, C., & Mitchell, J. (1993). Factors related to couples' decisions to attempt in vitro fertilization. *Journal of Assisted Reproduction and Genetics, 10,* 310–316.

Downey, J., & McKinney, M. (1990). Psychiatric research and the new reproductive technologies. In N. L. Stotland (Ed.), *Psychiatric aspects of reproductive technology* (pp. 155–168). Washington, DC: American Psychiatric Press.

Downey, J., & McKinney, M. (1992). The psychiatric status of women presenting for infertility evaluation. *American Journal of Orthopsychiatry, 62,* 196–205.

Dunkel-Schetter, C., & Lobel, M. (1991). Psychological reactions to infertility. In A. L. Stanton & C. Dunkel-Schetter (Eds.), *Infertility: Perspectives from stress and coping research* (pp. 29–60). New York: Plenum.

Epstein, Y. M., & Rosenberg, H. S. (1997). He does, she doesn't; she does, he doesn't: Couple conflicts about infertility. In S. R. Leiblum (Ed.), *Infertility: Psychological issues and counseling strategies* (pp. 129–148). New York: Wiley.

Frank, D. I. (1990). Gender differences in decision making about infertility treatment. *Applied Nursing Research, 3,* 56–62.

Golombok, S., & Tasker, F. (1994). Donor insemination for single heterosexual and lesbian women: Issues concerning the welfare of the child. *Human Reproduction, 9,* 1972–1976.

Gottlieb, B. H., & Wagner, F. (1991). Stress and support processes in close relationships. In J. Eckenrode (Ed.), *The social context of coping* (pp. 165–188). New York: Plenum.

Greenfeld, D., & Haseltine, F. (1986). Candidate selection and psychosocial considerations of in-vitro fertilization procedures. *Clinical Obstetrics and Gynecology, 29,* 119–126.

Greil, A. L., Leitko, T. A., & Porter, K. L. (1988). Infertility: His and hers. *Gender and Society, 2,* 172–199.

Hodne, C. J. (1995). Medical decision making. In M. O'Hara, R. C. Reiter, S. R. Johnson, A. Milburn, & J. Engeldinger (Eds.), *Psychological aspects of women's reproductive health* (pp. 267–290). Springer.

Jacob, M. C. (1997). Concerns of single women and lesbian couples considering conception through assisted reproduction. In S. R. Leiblum (Ed.), *Infertility: Psychological issues and counseling strategies* (pp. 189–206). New York: Wiley.

Jacobson, N. S., & Christensen, A. (1996). *Integrative couple therapy: Promoting acceptance and change.* New York: Norton.

Jacobson, N. S., & Margolin, G. (1979). *Marital therapy: Strategies based on social learning and behavior exchange principles.* New York: Brunner/Mazel.

Laruelle, C., & Englert, Y. (1996). Psychological study of in vitro fertilization–embryo transfer participants' attitudes toward the destiny of their supernumerary embryos. *Fertility and Sterility, 63,* 1047–1050.

Leiblum, S. R. (1994). The impact of infertility on sexual and marital satisfaction. *Annual Review of Sex Research, 4,* 99–120.

Leiblum, S. R. (1997). (Ed.) *Infertility: Psychological issues and counseling strategies.* New York: Wiley.

Leiblum, S. R., Kemmann, E., & Lane, M. K. (1987). The psychological concomitants of in vitro fertilization. *Journal of Psychosomatic Obstetrics and Gynecology, 6,* 165–178.

Levin, J. B., Sher, T., & Theodos, V. (1997). The effect of intracouple coping concordance on psychological and marital distress in infertility patients. *Journal of Clinical Psychology in Medical Settings, 4,* 361–372.

Litt, M. D., Tennen, H., Affleck, G., & Klock, S. (1992). Coping and cognitive factors in adaptation to in vitro fertilization failure. *Journal of Behavioral Medicine, 15,* 171–187.

Mahlstedt, P. P. (1985). The psychological component of infertility. *Fertility and Sterility, 43,* 335–346.

Mao, K, & Wood, C. (1984). Barriers to treatment of infertility by in vitro fertilization and embryo transfer. *The Medical Journal of Australia, 140,* 532–533.

Mazor, M. D. (1984). Emotional reactions to infertility. In M. D. Mazor & H. F. Simons (Eds.), *Infertility: Medical, emotional, and social considerations* (pp. 23–35). New York: Human Sciences Press.

McEwan, K. L., Costello, C. G., & Taylor, P. J. (1987). Adjustment to infertility. *Journal of Abnormal Psychology, 96,* 108–116.

McGrade, J. L., & Tolor, A. (1981). The reaction to infertility and the infertility investigation: A comparison of the responses of men and women. *Infertility, 4,* 7–27.

Miller, W. B. (1994). Childbearing motivations, desires, and intentions: A theoretical framework. *Genetic, Social, and General Psychology Monographs, 120,* 223–258.

Nachtigall, R. D., Becker, G., & Wozny, M. (1992). The effects of gender-specific diagnosis on men's and women's response to infertility. *Fertility and Sterility, 57,* 113–121.

Newton, C. R., Hearn, M. T., & Yuzpe, A. A. (1990). Psychological assessment and follow-up after in vitro fertilization: Assessing the impact of failure. *Fertility and Sterility, 54,* 879–886.

Office of Technology Assessment. (1988). *Infertility: Medical and social choices* (Publication No. OTA-BA-358). Washington, DC: U.S. Government Printing Office.

Pasch, L. A. (1994). *Fertility problems and marital relationships: The effects of appraisal and coping differences on communication.* Unpublished doctoral dissertation, University of California, Los Angeles.

Pasch, L. A., & Dunkel-Schetter, C. (1997). Fertility problems: Complex issues for women and couples. In S. J. Gallant, G. P. Keita, & R. Royak-Schaler (Eds.), *Health care for women: Psychological, social, and behavioral influences* (pp. 187–201). Washington, DC: American Psychological Association.

Pasch, L. A., Dunkel-Schetter, C., & Christensen, A. (1995, August). Communication in couples with fertility problems. In S. Manne (Chair), *Couples with severe medical problems.* Symposium conducted at the 103rd Annual Convention of the American Psychological Association, New York.

Pepe, M. V., & Byrne, T. J. (1991). Women's perceptions of immediate and long-term effects of failed infertility treatment on marital and sexual satisfaction. *Family Relations, 40,* 303–309.

Revenson, T. A. (1994). Social support and marital coping with chronic illness. *Annals of Behavioral Medicine, 16,* 122–130.

Salzer, L. P. (1991). *Surviving infertility.* New York: Harper Perennial.

Sauer, M. V., Paulson, R. J., & Lobo, R. A. (1992). Reversing the natural decline in human fertility. *Journal of the American Medical Association, 268,* 1275–1279.

Spanier, G. B. (1976). Measuring dyadic adjustment: New scales for assessing the quality of marriage and similar dyads. *Journal of Marriage and the Family, 38,* 15–28.

Stanton, A. L. (1991). Cognitive appraisals, coping processes, and adjustment to infertility. In A. L. Stanton & C. Dunkel-Schetter (Eds.), *Infertility: Perspectives from stress and coping research* (pp. 87–108). New York: Plenum.

Stanton, A. L., & Danoff-Burg, S. (1995). Selected issues in women's reproductive health: Psychological perspectives. In A. L. Stanton & S. J. Gallant (Eds.), *The psychology of women's health* (pp. 261–305). Washington, DC: American Psychological Association.

Stanton, A. L., & Dunkel-Schetter, C. (Eds.). (1991). *Infertility: Perspectives from stress and coping research*. New York: Plenum.

Stanton, A. L., Tennen, H., Affleck, G., & Mendola, R. (1992). Coping and adjustment to infertility. *Journal of Social and Clinical Psychology, 11*, 1–13.

Straus, M.A. (1979). Measuring intrafamily conflict and violence: The Conflict Tactics Scale. *Journal of Marriage and the Family, 41*, 75–86.

Sudore, R., Croughan-Minihane, M., Pasch, L., Neuhaus, J., & Camarano, L. (1998). *The validity of self-reported infertility diagnoses*. Manuscript submitted for publication.

Tennen, H., Affleck, G., & Mendola, R. (1991). Causal explanations for infertility: Their relation to control appraisals and psychological adjustment. In A. L. Stanton & C. Dunkel-Schetter (Eds.), *Infertility: Perspectives from stress and coping research* (pp. 109–131). New York: Plenum.

Wood, J. V., Saltzberg, J. A., & Goldsamt, L. A. (1990). Does affect induce self-focused attention? *Journal of Personality and Social Psychology, 58*, 899–908.

Woollett, A. (1985). Childlessness: Strategies for coping with infertility. *International Journal of Behavioral Development, 8*, 473–482.

Zoldbrod, A. P. (1993). *Men, women, and infertility: Intervention and treatment strategies*. New York: Lexington Books.

10

ALCOHOL PROBLEMS AND COUPLES: DRINKING IN AN INTIMATE RELATIONAL CONTEXT

LINDA J. ROBERTS AND KIRSTEN D. LINNEY

More than 90% of Americans will marry, and the majority will drink alcohol in the course of celebrating and cementing their nuptial bond. Drinking, at least on occasion, is currently the norm in our society. Americans are not alone: Alcohol is currently used in most societies in the world, and its use dates as far back in time as recorded history. In many societies, alcohol has played a functional if not beneficial role in medicine, food preservation, religious ceremonies, and celebrations. The medicinal and celebratory properties of alcohol, however, represent only part of the story of this popular substance. Alcohol use also has brought significant adverse effects to individuals, families, and communities throughout the world. In the United States, it is estimated that the adverse effects from alcohol abuse and dependence cost $148 billion annually in lost productivity, treatment, medical consequences, accidents, and crime (Harwood, Fountain, & Livermore, 1998).

Preparation of this chapter was supported by National Institute on Alcohol Abuse and Alcoholism Grant K21-AA00149 awarded to Linda J. Roberts.

269

Despite the fact that couples around the globe ritually "lift their glasses" to toast their marital bond, marriage appears to exert a protective effect with respect to drinking problems (for recent reviews, see Leonard & Rothbard, 1999; L. J. Roberts & Leonard, 1997). Compared with both the divorced and the never married, married individuals are likely to drink less and have fewer alcohol-related problems (Bachman, Wadsworth, O'Malley, Johnston, & Schulenberg, 1997; Clark & Hilton, 1991). Nonetheless, a majority of married individuals do drink, 73% of married men and 63% of married women (Hilton, 1988), and they are not immune to the adverse effects of alcohol consumption. Further, mixing marriage and drinking brings a new arena for problems: When alcohol problems arise in a marriage or other intimate partnership, adverse consequences affect not only the drinker but the partner (see McCrady & Hay, 1987).

How does drinking affect relationship processes? And how do close, intimate relationships affect drinking patterns? The answers to these questions are not simple, and unfortunately, the empirical data to address them are still limited. The alcohol field has been dominated by studies of the drinking behavior and drinking problems of men, using models focusing on individual-level variables. Only recently have women's drinking and the interpersonal context of drinking received attention. To complicate matters, drinking is interwoven within the fabric of an intimate relationship in diverse and complex ways. As we will argue, to fully understand the drinking behavior of intimate partners, it is imperative that we understand the relational context of their drinking. Conversely, to fully understand a couple's relationship dynamics, we need to appraise the role of alcohol in the relationship. The following vignette describes a young married couple who participated in one of our research studies and serves to illustrate some of the multicolored threads that interweave drinking and relationship processes:

Dawn and Randy met in a bar. An initial bond formed over drinks, and a more intense relationship soon followed. Before she met Randy, Dawn had enjoyed "getting drunk" with friends, but she had limited her drinking to weekends. This couple's courtship, however, revolved around frequent visits to bars. Dawn found herself drinking whenever she went out with Randy, and as her contact with him increased, her consumption increased. After they married, their bar visits decreased, but not their drinking. Randy drank every day after work, and Dawn often joined him; drinking together seemed to be a way to spend time together. On weekends, they still frequented bars. To both of them, having fun or "partying" was synonymous with drinking heavily. Alcohol also played a role in their sex life; drinking became an important prelude to sex.

Parenthood led to changes in their drinking patterns. Dawn needed to care for their young children, which meant she could no longer accompany Randy to the bars on weekends. She often drank at home alone. Randy started to go to the bars by himself on weeknights. Being left behind upset Dawn, and she had growing fears that Randy was "cheating on her." During her pregnancies, she felt particularly vulnerable to losing him to another woman, and she continued to drink and party with him despite the risk to her fetus. Randy, on the hand, began to go to bars on weeknights as a way to escape the demands of his wife. This only intensified Dawn's efforts to be with him and to drink with him. However, when Dawn accompanied him to the bars, the night would often end in shouting matches and, on occasion, physical aggression. The stress in their life increased. Randy's employment was inconsistent, their finances were strained, and their two young children demanded a lot of time and energy. Bickering and fights between them became frequent. Their relationship was becoming brittle, and drinking together was no longer helping them achieve a sense of closeness.

As this vignette suggests, Randy and Dawn's drinking cannot be fully understood in isolation from the context of their intimate relationship. Individual factors, such as each partner's developmental history, personality, and genetic vulnerability, do influence drinking behaviors, but relationship processes also contribute and interact with individual vulnerabilities in significant ways. For example, Dawn was influenced by Randy's heavier drinking habits; she found herself consuming more alcohol as they mutually structured their leisure time. Not drinking would have meant not being with her husband, and Dawn felt an overwhelming need for his presence. Their relationship dynamics in interaction with Dawn's personality led to an increase in her drinking. Randy, on the other hand, found that regular drinking at the bars provided an escape from family stress and Dawn's unrelenting demand for attention.

Randy and Dawn's developing relationship influenced their drinking behaviors, but their drinking also influenced their relationship: Directly and indirectly, drinking caused a host of serious relationship problems, including conflict, physical violence, jealousy, and ultimately estrangement. Despite the clearly negative role that alcohol played, it was used in an attempt to attain positive relationship goals. Early in their relationship, Randy and Dawn believed that drinking would help them avoid conflict, achieve closeness, enhance sexual relations, and provide shared fun times. Whether drinking ever helped them achieve these ends is unclear. What is clear is that as their drinking pattern became increasingly characterized by frequent and heavy consumption, their problems escalated and eventually the fabric of their marriage frayed and disintegrated. When we recontacted Dawn and Randy for a follow-up 3 years later, they were no longer married. Their story illustrates primary conclusions from our review of the empirical literature, and we return to them at various points to provide a real-life example of what research suggests about the reciprocal relationships between drinking and relationship dynamics.

BACKGROUND

Alcohol Problems

What does it mean to drink too much? The answer has varied across cultures and time—and often has been fraught with controversy. Despite tremendous strides in our understanding of the neurobiological, psychological, and social consequences of alcohol, the controversy continues. There is no scientifically consensual definition of what constitutes hazardous drinking, nor is there consensus on other basic terminology (M. B. Sobell & Sobell, 1993).[1]

Although discrepancies surround the precise definition and boundary conditions for *alcohol dependence*, there is consensus that it represents a pernicious condition requiring intervention. Dependent drinkers, or alcoholics, have been the primary focus of treatment efforts in the United States since the 1930s. However, in an influential report, the Institute of Medicine (IOM; 1990) recently called for a "broadening of the base for treatment" and the adoption of an *alcohol problems perspective*. The alcohol problems framework is purposely broad; it seeks to expand societal concern, and concomitantly the population targeted for prevention and intervention efforts, beyond alcoholism. The alcohol problems perspective explicitly recognizes the tremendous heterogeneity in the severity, duration, progression, etiology, consequences, and manifestations of alcohol problems. As shown in Figure 10.1, alcohol consumption and problems can be viewed on a continuum ranging from no alcohol problems following little consumption to severe problems often associated, although not exclusively, with heavy consumption. The nondependent problem drinker (see M. B. Sobell & Sobell, 1993) is someone who has or could experience serious negative consequences (or problems) as a result of drinking. Although Randy and Dawn's drinking patterns are quite different, they both could be described as problem drinkers. Drinking caused relationship problems for both of them, and Randy's drinking contributed to his periods of unemployment and was directly related to several arrests and physical injuries. While Dawn was pregnant, any heavy drinking on her part could be considered an alcohol problem because of the significant risk alcohol poses to the developing fetus.

---

[1] A large array of terms are currently used to describe alcohol-related problems (e.g., *alcohol abuse, alcohol misuse, alcoholism, alcohol problems, alcohol dependence, alcohol-related disabilities, dependent drinking, problem drinking, risky drinking,* or *excessive drinking*) but with little consensus on precise definitions or distinguishing characteristics.

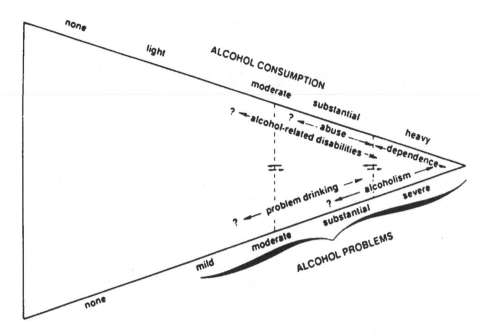

Figure 10.1. A terminological map of alcohol consumption and problems. The triangle represents the population of the United States. The alcohol consumption of the population ranges from none to heavy (along the upper side of the triangle), and the problems experienced in association with alcohol consumption range from none to severe (along the lower side of the triangle.) The two-way arrows and the dotted lines indicate that both from an individual and a population perspective, consumption levels and the degree of problems vary from time to time. The scope of terms that are often used refer to individuals and groups according to their consumption levels and the degree of their problems is illustrated; question marks indicate that the lower boundary for many of the terms is uncertain. From *Broadening the Base of Treatment for Alcohol Problems* (p. 30), by the Institute of Medicine, 1990, Washington, DC: National Academy Press. Copyright 1990 by the National Academy of Sciences. Reprinted with permission.

The nomenclature of the *Diagnostic and Statistical Manual of Mental Disorders* (4th ed.; *DSM–IV*; American Psychiatric Association, 1994) recognizes two alcohol use disorders: alcohol dependence and alcohol abuse. Alcohol dependence is based on the idea of an alcohol dependence syndrome (G. Edwards & Gross, 1976), consisting of multiple symptoms including tolerance, signs of withdrawal, and diminished control over drinking. Alcohol abuse, on the other hand, is defined as a maladaptive pattern of drinking leading to significant impairment or distress. A person diagnosed with alcohol abuse drinks despite alcohol-related physical, social, psychological, or occupational problems or drinks in situations that put him or her at substantial risk for adverse consequences.

In one of the few studies to date using *DSM–IV* criteria (Grant et al., 1994), 4.4% of adults age 18 years and older were classified as alcohol dependent, a somewhat lower but comparable rate to earlier studies; 7.4% of adults were identified as having an alcohol use disorder (alcohol dependence and abuse combined). This translates into a population estimate of nearly 14 million Americans. Epidemiological data also confirm the well-known discrepancy in rates of drinking problems for men and women. Men are two to three times more likely than women to have alcohol use disorders.

The population estimates for alcohol use disorders do not include the millions of other adults who engage in risky drinking patterns that could potentially lead to alcohol problems but do not meet *DSM–IV* diagnostic criteria. Cahalan (1970) conducted the first national survey specifically looking at alcohol problems. Results indicated that 43% of men and 21% of women reported experiencing one or more alcohol-related problem during the previous 3 years. According to the IOM (1990) report, the ratio of problem drinkers to alcohol-dependent individuals is approximately 4:1, making problem drinkers the largest number of persons adversely affected by alcohol use. Despite the evidence that problem drinking is more prevalent than alcohol dependence, detection, treatment, and prevention efforts for this group of drinkers are currently not given the same attention as dependency and other severe alcohol problems.

Although heavy drinking is not pathonomic of alcohol problems, it is clearly a risk factor (Midanik, Tam, Greenfield, & Caetano, 1996; Room, Bondy, & Ferris, 1995). That is, not all heavy drinkers have alcohol problems despite the markedly higher probability of problems among heavy drinkers. Percentages of respondents who drink heavily or at risky levels are much higher than the rates for alcohol use disorders (Kessler et al., 1994; Midanik & Clark, 1994). Like alcohol problems, consumption patterns again reflect markedly different rates for men and women; men drink larger amounts and more often than women.

The Effects of Alcohol on Health and Behavior

Drinking affects human physiology and behavior in varied and complex ways (for a comprehensive discussion, see the Ninth Special Report to the U.S. Congress on Alcohol and Health by the National Institute on Alcohol Abuse and Alcoholism; NIAAA, 1997). Chronic heavy alcohol use can produce changes in brain structure and size, as well as in personality, perceptions, learning, and memory (Evert & Oscar-Berman, 1995). Chronic use also is associated with liver disease, heart disease, cancers, pancreatitis, depressions in immune system functioning, and malnutrition (Segal & Sisson, 1985). Further, when pregnant women drink even moderately, adverse health effects can be inflicted on a developing fetus (see Abel & Sokol, 1986).

The consequences of acute alcohol consumption on the brain and body are dependent on many different factors, including dosage, metabolism, tolerance, body weight, and gender. Although complex, the acute pharmacological effects of alcohol ingestion are relatively straightforward compared with the psychological or *expectancy* effects of alcohol. In an early study, Marlatt and Rohsenow (1980) demonstrated that the expectancy of having received a drink had a stronger effect on cognitive processes than whether alcohol was actually consumed. Later studies have replicated this essential finding: In a number of domains, expectancies appear to be of critical importance in determining behavioral responses under drinking conditions (for meta-analysis, see Hull & Bond, 1986).

To add to this complexity, the effects of alcohol on social behavior and emotions are extremely varied irrespective of expectancies. Experimental research confirms a pattern of seemingly paradoxical effects: Alcohol can both enhance and compromise interpersonal functioning. For example, alcohol has been shown to facilitate self-disclosure (e.g., P. M. Miller, Ingham, Plant, & Miller, 1977) and helping behavior (e.g., Steele, Critchlow, & Liu, 1985) but also to increase aggression (e.g., Ito, Miller, & Pollock, 1996) and risk taking (e.g., MacDonald, Zanna, & Fong, 1995). Further, the variability in social effects cannot be explained by drinking expectancies and individual differences in reactivity to alcohol alone (Steele & Josephs, 1990). In their ethnographic account of drinking behavior, MacAndrew and Edgerton (1969; quoted in Steele and Josephs, 1990) put it this way:

> The same man in the same bar, drinking approximately the same amount of alcohol, may, on three nights running, be, say, surly and belligerent on the first evening, the spirit of amiability on the second, and morose and withdrawn on the third. How can the same substance make the same person feel like conquering the world one night and "crying in their beer" the next? (p. 922)

Steele and Josephs (1990) have suggested a model to answer this question. In their model, alcohol ingestion creates a single direct pharmacological effect: *impaired information processing*. This "alcohol myopia" interacts with the drinker's environmental and situational context to produce a diverse array of alcohol-affected social behaviors. Alcohol alters perception and thought so that the intoxicated person cannot effectively process multiple stimuli or cues. The alcohol-induced myopia, or shortsightedness, causes the drinker to attend to only the most proximal or salient cues and to disregard distal cues. Distal cues are often cues that would normally inhibit antisocial behaviors. For example, while intoxicated, Randy once became so enraged with Dawn that he hit her while they were in a bar, leading to his arrest. In this situation, the salient cue for Randy was that Dawn was angrily pressuring him to leave. Under sober conditions, social norms would inhibit his use of force, especially force displayed in public, but because of his intoxication, these distal cues were not as salient as his wife's pressure. According to the model, when an alcohol-impaired person is in an environment that contains salient provoking cues for the instigation of aggression, that person will be more disposed to not attend to internal and external cues that are relevant to the inhibition of aggression. The sober individual who is faced with the same salient instigating cues has the cognitive resources to be able to attend to, access, process, and respond to cues (e.g., situational dangers, norms, or internal moral prohibitions) that signal the importance of behavioral inhibition.

In summary, to understand the effects of alcohol and alcohol-related social problems, we must consider not only the pharmacological properties of alcohol but also a complex convergence of non-alcohol-specific factors, including the genetic makeup and personality of the individual, drinking motives and expectancies, the immediate social environment, and the broader social, cultural, and historical context of drinking. When we drink, what we are doing, where we are, and who we are with all work to influence how alcohol affects behavioral outcomes. Intimate partners can be an important force in this broad constellation of factors affecting and being affected by alcohol use.

The Etiology of Alcohol Problems

Although a unitary disease conceptualization of alcohol abuse and dependence has dominated the alcohol field for the past 50 years, a multifactorial etiological model has gradually challenged this traditional view. Scientists increasingly refer to *biopsychosocial* models of causation (Engel, 1977) to explain social behavioral disturbances. Among alcohol researchers, a growing consensus favors the idea that the etiology of alcohol problems is best conceptualized within such multifactorial frameworks (Fitzgerald, Davies, Zucker, & Klinger, 1994; IOM, 1990; Tarter & Vanyukov, 1994). The notion of a uniform etiological pathway has been eschewed in favor of a model with interacting biological, psychological, and social processes and a multiplicity of paths. For example, although sons of alcoholic fathers are at risk of developing alcohol problems, an inherited vulnerability may not cause a problem unless the environment also provides a risk factor, for example, social pressures to drink.

Within the multifactorial framework, the interactions between a drinker and an intimate partner are significant strands in the tangled web of etiological factors. Understanding a drinker's immediate social environment is necessary for understanding not only the etiology but also the maintenance of and remedies for alcohol problems. Before reviewing the literature on these empirical connections, we briefly review the history of the ways the drinker's intimate partner has been incorporated in models of the "alcohol-complicated marriage."

Models for Alcohol Problems in Marriage: A Historical Account

Until recently, the alcohol field focused almost exclusively on the individual alcoholic, particularly the male alcoholic, with little attention to the drinker's familial and relational context. Although some early theorists discussed partners of alcoholics, or more precisely wives of alcoholics, conceptualizations remained fundamentally individualistic in approach, stressing deficits or pathology in the psychological functioning of the partner rather than the relationship between the partners. Historically, the first model to incorporate a consideration of the partner was a codisease or, more broadly, a *codeficit* model. Early formulations and support for this model were based on impressions of psychodynamically oriented clinicians who observed that spouses of alcoholics evidenced a broad spectrum of neurotic symptoms (Jacob, 1987). For example, Whalen (1953) argued that women married to alcoholic partners chose their heavy-drinking partner to resolve their own psychodynamic conflicts.

Joan Jackson's work in the 1950s and 1960s heralded an alternative model of the relationship between a drinker and his partner, a model Orford (1990) has referred to as the *stress victim* model. In her classic paper, Jackson (1954) argued that an appropriate way to understand the behavior of a woman married to an alcoholic was to see her as attempting to cope with an acute stress or family crisis. The model acknowledges the presence of psychological difficulties for the woman but explains these as a consequence of the hardships associated with living with a heavy drinker. Jackson promoted the idea that the observed psychological problems of the wives of alcoholics decreased as their husband's drinking problems were resolved (Kogan & Jackson, 1965a, 1965b). The birth and growth of Al-Anon during this same time period institutionalized a recognition of the important ways an individual's drinking behavior influences close others.

Like the codeficit model, the stress victim model has been criticized on both conceptual and methodological grounds (for reviews and critiques of this early research, see P. Edwards, Harvey, & Whitehead, 1973; Jacob & Seilhamer, 1982; McCrady & Hay, 1987; Paolino & McCrady, 1977). The model fails to explain a variety of observations, including the high rate of assortative mating on drinking (Jacob & Bremer, 1986; McLeod, 1993); the marital difficulties encountered by two heavily drinking partners; and the existence of intimate partnerships in which conflict, distress, and poor psychological functioning predate heavy drinking. Although the model has spawned research that identifies and describes the coping behaviors of partners of problem drinkers (e.g., Orford et al., 1975; Rychtarik, 1990), it has not led to an understanding of the temporal, situational, and relationship contexts of these coping behaviors. Interpersonal interaction and relationship variables are absent from both the stress victim and the codeficit models. Moreover, although the stress victim model explicitly acknowledges the effects that a heavy drinker may have on her or his family, it is fundamentally a unidirectional model.

In the past 25 years, the *family systems* and *family interaction* perspectives have significantly advanced our understanding of the interface of alcohol and family relationships, most notably through the work of Ted Jacob (e.g., Jacob & Krahn, 1988; Jacob & Leonard, 1988) and Peter Steinglass (e.g., Steinglass, 1987). Although the family systems and family interaction traditions have somewhat different historical roots and emphases, the terms can be used interchangeably to characterize an influential conceptual model (Jacob, 1987). Unlike its predecessors, an *interaction–systems* model emphasizes both relational processes and bidirectional effects or mutual influence between relational and drinking variables:

> The data most important in exploring [relationships between the spouse and the etiology and maintenance of drinking] have been absent—the actual *patterns* of interaction between spouse and partner that potentiate or maintain the abusive drinking. . . . Empirically based *descriptions* of family interactions involving an alcoholic are the *necessary building blocks* for theoretical, treatment and prevention efforts to be forged in the years ahead. (Jacob, 1987, p. 164, italics in original)

The fundamental task for the researcher guided by an interaction–systems model is to describe interaction patterns between a drinker and his or her partner and to explain how these relational processes interact with other variables relevant to couple and individual outcomes. Whereas prior models have been predicated on the assumption that the drinker's partner was either a "victim or villain," the interactional–systems model acknowledges the possibility of adaptive functions for drinking within the family context (Jacob, 1987).

THE ASSOCIATION BETWEEN DRINKING AND COUPLE FACTORS

In this section, we critically review the literature relevant to the mixing of alcohol with couple relationships. Because extant studies are almost exclusively limited to married samples, we focus on marital relationships. Acknowledging the multifactorial nature of the development of alcohol problems leads us to examine not only the way couple factors interface with alcoholism and problem drinking but also the way couple factors interface with normative drinking. Thus, we examine not only the relationship between problem drinking and couple factors but also that between alcohol consumption and couple factors. We integrate research from diverse populations of drinkers, including treated alcoholics and community samples of both problem and nonproblem drinkers.

Although bidirectional effects between drinking and couple factors are now acknowledged explicitly in the dominant explanatory models in the field, existing research is nonetheless limited either to the analysis of simple associations between drinking variables and couple variables or to an examination of a unidirectional influence process. We review the evidence for an association between drinking variables and both marital dissolution and marital quality and examine the evidence available for three directional hypotheses: (a) Drinking leads to marital disruptions, (b) drinking leads to decrements in marital quality, and (c) marital distress leads to drinking.[2] Finally, we review literature that has looked directly at variables that may mediate the relationship between drinking and marital quality, including communication and interactional dynamics, sexual relations, and violence.

Marital Disruptions and Drinking

Establishing the Association

Partners often report that a drinking problem precipitated their divorce (e.g., Levinger, 1966). Such reports, however, may be subject to significant bias and distortion. Evidence for an association between drinking and relationship dissolution also is found in numerous studies demonstrating higher rates of heavy drinking and alcoholism among divorced samples than among married samples (for reviews, see Leonard & Rothbard, 1999; Paolino & McCrady, 1977). These cross-sectional studies, however, cannot illuminate the causal role of drinking problems in marital disruptions. The observed association may as easily reflect the effects of being divorced as the causal impact of alcohol problems; moreover, it is probable that in many cases both alcohol and marital problems arise from underlying common multifactorial sources (e.g., personality dispositions). Unfortunately, drinking behavior has consistently been overlooked as a predictor in large prospective studies of marital dissolution. As L. K. White (1990) has noted in her decade review of divorce studies, "respondents' accounts of their own divorces illuminate several factors that receive little attention in the empirical literature . . . [including] alcoholism" (p. 908).

Directional Influences

Three recent studies have attempted to establish a temporal relationship between drinking and marital disruptions (Amato & Rogers, 1997;

---

[2]The studies we review in the Directional Influences sections are not experimental and are not able to make strong claims about causality. However, they are differentiated from the studies we review in the Establishing the Association sections by virtue of their attention to the temporal ordering of the drinking and relationship variables and, usually, by use of a longitudinal design.

Kessler, Walters, & Forthofer, 1998; Leonard & Roberts, 1998b). Amato and Rogers (1997) examined the role of perceptions of marital problems, as reported by spouses, in divorce up to 12 years later. Results indicated that if either partner's drinking or drug use was a marital issue for the couple early in the study, the couple was more likely to divorce in the subsequent years. Although this study falls short of identifying problem drinking as a precursor to marital dissolution, it demonstrates that the perception of a difficulty or incompatibility with respect to drinking (or drug use) is a significant predictor of later divorce.

Using retrospective reports of the timing of the onset of alcohol use disorders and the termination of marriage, results from the National Comorbidity Survey demonstrated that problem drinking at one point in time increases the likelihood of a subsequent marital disruption (Kessler et al., 1998). A limitation of the study, however, was that the temporal locations of the onset of an alcohol problem and a marital disruption were based on respondents' recall rather than on a longitudinal design. Further, as the authors pointed out, unmeasured *third* variables, such as personality disorders, could have led both to an alcohol use disorder and to subsequent adverse marital outcomes.

In a third study, Leonard and Roberts (1998b) assessed both marital adjustment and drinking behavior in newlyweds at two points in time and controlled for a group of relevant third variables. Using data from the Buffalo Newlywed Study (BNS), they examined the relation of married couples' alcohol consumption and alcohol problems to the occurrence of marital disruptions. The BNS was a study of over 500 couples recruited as they applied for their marriage license and assessed premarriage, at their first anniversary, and at their third anniversary. Drinking variables at the time of marriage were used to predict subsequent marital disruptions, statistically controlling for sociodemographics, personality characteristics, and conflict behaviors. Husband's alcohol consumption and husband's problem drinking each were uniquely predictive of marital disruptions. However, the findings for wives were quite different. Neither the wife's alcohol consumption nor her alcohol-related problems accounted for unique varience in marital disruptions. Thus, early in the marriage, the husband's drinking, but not the wife's, uniquely predicted instability.

Marital Quality and Drinking

Establishing the Association

Problem drinking and marital quality. Alcohol problems are common in couples presenting for marital therapy (Halford & Osgarby, 1993), and marital problems are common in drinkers presenting for alcohol treatment (O'Farrell & Birchler, 1987). For example, among Australian couples seeking marital therapy, Halford and Osgarby (1993) found that more than four fifths of the couples reported marital disagreements about alcohol abuse at least frequently and one third of the men met criteria for alcoholism. In research comparing alcoholic and control samples, higher rates of marital distress are typically found in the alcoholic samples (e.g., Jacob, Dunn, & Leonard, 1983; O'Farrell & Birchler, 1987; Perodeau & Kohn, 1989). In addition, poor marital and family functioning has been found to be associated with relapse among treated alcoholics (Moos, Bromet, Tsu, & Moos, 1979; Moos & Moos, 1984).

Although research linking lower marital quality and drinking problems in the treatment literature is fairly consistent, the generalizability of research findings to the population of alcoholics or problem drinkers is uncertain. The association of marital quality and drinking behavior may be much different in couples in which the drinker is not seeking therapy, for example, the presence of marital disharmony may play a role in the instigation of treatment (Steinberg, Epstein, McCrady, & Hirsch, 1997). Further, extant research on relationship functioning among alcoholics has focused on a limited subsample of problem drinkers: married, middle-to-upper-middle-class, White men with no other psychopathology (McCrady & Epstein, 1995a). Community and general population studies are an important but neglected piece of the picture.

Despite considerable variability in methodology, participant characteristics, and assessment measures, in community-based data sets, problem drinking is associated with lower marital quality (Grzywacz & Marks, 1999; McLeod; 1993; Roberts, Leonard, & Senchak, 1994). In contrast to treatment-based studies, these community-based studies have used larger samples and have addressed both male and female problem drinking. For example, in McLeod's (1993) study, respondents who met criteria for current alcohol dependence evidenced significantly poorer marital quality. Roberts et al. (1994), in analyses of the BNS data set described earlier, found that both husband and wife problem drinking evidenced significant associations with marital adjustment even after controlling for the partner's drinking. Using a large data set that allowed tests for gender differences, Grzywacz and Marks (1999) found a negative association between problem drinking and marital quality that was not qualified by gender.

Consumption patterns and marital quality. Gender differences arise in studies examining consumption and marital outcomes. In a sample of young Finnish and Estonian couples, Holmila (1988) found that husbands' frequent drinking was associated with lower marital quality, but wives' frequent drinking was not. Holmila, however, examined only the frequency of drinking, not the amount consumed. In another study using the BNS data set (Roberts et al., 1994), two consumption variables, the frequency of drinking and the typical quantity consumed, were used to predict marital quality over and above the effects of problem drinking.[3] Consumption patterns evidenced significant, independent relationships with marital adjustment and marital intimacy. Specifically, if partners typically drank larger quantities of alcohol, their spouses reported lower marital adjustment. This suggests that even when alcohol consumption has not resulted in negative consequences or dependence symptoms, heavy drinking is related to poorer marital functioning. Frequent drinking did not have a negative impact on marriage. In fact, in the absence of problem drinking, frequent drinking, by either husbands or wives, predicted greater reported intimacy among wives.

Using a community sample of couples not limited to newlyweds, Roberts and Linney (1998) found significant relationships between both husbands' and wives' drinking and marital functioning. Husbands' heavy drinking and frequent drinking each independently contributed to the prediction of lower marital quality, together accounting for an additional 5% of the variance after the consideration of wives' drinking and sociodemographic variables. In contrast, wives' typical quantity was unrelated to marital quality, but wives' frequent drinking again was related to higher reported marital quality.

The positive association between wives' frequent drinking and marital quality that Roberts et al. (1994) and Roberts and Linney (1998) found deserves comment. Although unexpected, a positive association between drinking and marital intimacy should not be surprising given cultural beliefs about the effects of alcohol on behavior. Research has demonstrated that although individuals recognize the negative behavioral effects of drinking, they also identify a number of positive effects of drinking, including increases in affective expression and enhancements in both sexual and nonsexual intimacy (Beckman, 1979; Klassen & Wilsnack, 1986; S. C. Wilsnack, 1984). For example, most women drinkers report that drinking makes them more able to "open up" and feel closer to persons with whom they share a drink (R. W. Wilsnack, Wilsnack, & Klassen, 1987). These expectancies, rather than the pharmacologic action of the alcohol, may account for many of the positive effects of alcohol consumption (see Hull & Bond, 1986). Note that no positive associations were found for higher quantities of consumption and that in these community samples, the frequently drinking wives were typically light drinkers. Thus, the positive association of frequent drinking and marital quality does not suggest an effect related to alcohol impairment, as a significant finding for drinking larger quantities might. A finding related to drinking frequency may instead be interpreted as suggesting a drinking-context effect, that is, frequently drinking wives may more

_____

[3]Although the analytic strategy used precludes direct comparison with Holmila's (1988) results, examination of the zero-order correlations between the marital quality indexes and frequent drinking in the BNS data suggests comparability to Holmila's findings: A significant negative correlation with marital quality was found for husbands' but not wives' frequent drinking.

frequently be in relaxing, intimate, or fun contexts with their partner, which might explain the positive association with marital quality.

Another possible interpretation of the positive association is that given the fact that males generally drink more frequently than females, frequently drinking wives are effectively matching their husband's drinking level and this congruence accounts for the experience of marital intimacy. Support for the importance of the interaction between husband's and wife's drinking has been found in a number of studies (e.g., Holmila, 1988; Perodeau & Kohn, 1989; S. C. Wilsnack & Wilsnack, 1990); individual partners' consumption patterns may not be as important in affecting couple functioning as the relationship between husband's and wife's drinking patterns. For example, Roberts and Leonard (1998) used cluster analysis to create an empirical typology of "drinking partnerships" in early marriage and found that partnerships in which couples drank at similar levels and with one another were associated with higher marital functioning.

Directional Influences

Marital problems as a consequence of problem drinking. Research on samples of treated alcoholics has provided indirect evidence for the assertion that drinking problems contribute to the erosion of marital quality. During periods of abstinence, partners report more satisfying relationships (Nirenberg, Liepman, Begin, Doolittle, & Broffman, 1990; O'Farrell, Cutter, & Floyd, 1985), and when a drinking problem is resolved, marital functioning appears to improve (Moos, Finney, & Cronkite, 1990; Moos, Finney, & Gamble, 1982). Brennan, Moos, and Kelly (1994) have recently replicated this latter finding in a sample of late-life problem drinkers, demonstrating a positive effect of remission on marital quality even for couples in which problem drinking may have been a long-standing issue.

Two recent longitudinal studies suggest that drinking may predict decrements in marital quality over time. First, in a national study of women drinkers (S. C. Wilsnack & Wilsnack, 1990), wives' reports of their husband's heavier drinking in 1981 predicted decrements in the wives' marital quality in 1986. In the second study (Leonard & Roberts, 1998b), husband and wife alcohol consumption and alcohol problems at the time of marriage were used to predict the couple's marital quality 1 year later while controlling for baseline quality. Both husband and wife problem drinking and husband alcohol consumption predicted decrements in marital quality. However, in a more stringent test—the ability of the drinking variables to predict over and above a set of relevant sociodemographic, personality, and self-reported marital interaction variables—husbands' drinking did not provide a significant increment in predictability, but both of the wives' drinking variables did. Wives' alcohol problems were predictive of decrements in marital quality, but as in the cross-sectional analyses of the data set discussed earlier, wives' alcohol consumption was predictive of improved marital quality.

Adaptive consequences of drinking. The numerous studies documenting the negative effects of drinking notwithstanding, a number of research studies suggest that there may be positive, adaptive consequences of drinking for the family, even when the drinker is an alcoholic (Davis, Berenson, Steinglass, & Davis, 1974; Jacob et al., 1983). The work of Peter Steinglass and his colleagues (e.g., Steinglass, 1987) has been influential in this respect (for review of Steinglass's work see Jacob & Seilhamer, 1987). In one of the first studies using experimental drinking procedures with couples, Steinglass, Davis, and Berenson (1977) observed the daily interactions of 10 couples in which the husband, the wife, or both were in an inpatient treatment setting. A major focus of the research was the differentiation of interaction patterns in sober as compared with intoxicated states. In their thorough review of Steinglass's work, Jacob and Seilhamer (1987) have aptly summarized the results of these observations:

> Striking differences in patterns of interaction were observed between sober and intoxicated periods, differences that appeared to serve important "adaptive" functions for the couple. That is, the behavior that emerged during intoxicated periods appeared to potentiate or inhibit certain aspects of the relationship that, in effect, reduced tensions through the temporary solution to a conflictual or stressful process. In one case, for example, a sexually inhibited couple became more expressive and affectionate during intoxicated states, whereas another couple became assertive and effective when sobriety gave way to intoxication. For a third couple, previously suppressed anger, frustration and disappointment were more readily expressed during drinking than during nondrinking periods. (pp. 550–551)

Applying a systems theory perspective, Steinglass (1987) has argued that each partner's behavior during drinking periods can have adaptive consequences by restoring equilibrium in the marriage. These adaptive consequences for the couple's relationship then serve to reinforce and maintain a partner's abusive drinking. The alcoholic's drinking is seen as an organizing principle for the family; the drinking defines behavioral patterns for family members. The innovative work of Steinglass and his colleagues is largely responsible for the inauguration of "alcohol and the family" as an important research area and treatment focus. However, despite significant theoretical and methodological contributions to the field, Steinglass's empirical research program consists primarily of clinical observations on small samples without rigorous testing of major tenets and assumptions of the theory (see Jacob & Seilhamer, 1987, for a full critique of the research).

Jacob and his colleagues have undertaken a research program to assess the relationship between drinking and marital interaction in marriages complicated by alcoholism (see also Communication and International Dynamics section below). Two early studies in this research program (Dunn, Jacob, Hummon, & Seilhamer, 1987; Jacob et al., 1983) provide some initial support for the *adaptive maintenance* hypothesis proposed by Steinglass, but only for a subgroup of male alcoholics characterized by a steady as opposed to an episodic drinking pattern. Among steady drinkers, high levels of alcohol consumption in the prior month by the alcoholic were associated with high levels of marital satisfaction and low levels of psychiatric symptoms in the wife (Jacob et al., 1983). Similarly, in a study using time-series analyses to examine the temporal dependence between drinking and fluctuations in marital satisfaction, drinking by steady drinkers was followed by increases in the wives' marital satisfaction (Dunn et al., 1987). Unfortunately, small sample sizes compromised the generalizability of these results and, more important, the apparent positive consequences of the drinking suggested by these studies should not be interpreted in isolation of Jacob's (e.g., Haber & Jacob, 1997; Jacob & Krahn, 1988) consistent finding of observable negative consequences of drinking on the communicative behavior of couples.

Problem drinking as a consequence of marital problems. The notion that marital stress leads to drinking is often accepted uncritically as a logical extension of the widely accepted belief that individuals drink to cope with tension, stress, and disappointment. However, the tension-reduction hypothesis, which suggests that alcohol has tension-reducing properties that lead to its abuse, has not received consistent support (see Marlatt, 1976; Wilson, 1982, for reviews). Thus, the role of stress in drinking, along with the role of marital stress in particular, remains unsubstantiated. Although Steinglass suggests a path from marital problems to drinking, this as well as other tenets of the model has not been established empirically. However, in keeping with the notion of a causal link between marital stress and drinking, the literature on relapse among alcoholics suggests that marital problems and relationship stress are often precipitants of relapse (e.g., Cummings, Gordon, & Marlatt, 1980; Maisto, O'Farrell, Connors, McKay, & Pelcovits, 1988; O'Farrell, Hooley, Fals-Stewart, & Cutter, 1998).

We found only one longitudinal study examining marital strain and drinking in both husbands and wives (Romelsjo, Lazarus, Kaplan, & Cohen, 1991). This study was designed to examine stressful life situations as longitudinal predictors of alcohol outcomes in a general population sample over a 9-year period. Marital strain and other life stressors were only weak prospective predictors of changes in drinking. Marital problems evidenced stronger and more statistically significant associations with increases in men's drinking than women's drinking, in contrast to the clinical studies that suggest women more often than men report that their drinking was precipitated by marital stress (Dahlgren, 1979; Gorman & Peter, 1980). A second longitudinal study conducted only with women (Klassen, Wilsnack, Harris, & Wilsnack, 1991) found that a lack of intimacy in a woman's marriage predicted more problematic drinking 5 years later. This finding led the researchers to speculate that some women may drink in an attempt to achieve the intimacy they feel they are lacking in their marital relationship.

Relationship Processes and Drinking

In addition to examining evidence for an overall association between drinking and relationship quality and stability, we need to consider the role of relationship processes: the day-to-day dyadic interactions and relational events that may mediate or underlie the association of drinking behaviors and couple factors. Decrements in the quality of a couple's relationship may be a function of the extent to which drinking interferes with everyday relationship processes or causes stresses and hardships in family life (Dumka & Roosa, 1993; Zweben, 1986). Heavy drinking and dependent drinking have been hypothesized to alter marital and family functioning through a variety of processes, including depletion of economic resources, verbal and physical abuse, job problems, communication impairments, social isolation, neglect of household responsibilities, and sexual problems. As articulated in the interaction–systems model discussed earlier (Jacob, 1987), it is imperative that researchers attend to these relational processes to further our understanding of the alcohol–couple link. For example, many of these processes are evident to some degree in Randy and Dawn's relationship history. Only by examining the ways in which Randy's and Dawn's drinking was affected by and influenced their actual interactions can we understand the erosion of their marital satisfaction and their increase in drinking over time.

There is an impressive research literature on alcohol consumption and interpersonal processes, including conflict, aggression, self-disclosure, and risk taking. In contrast to the studies we have reviewed thus far, these investigations use observational methodologies, event-based analyses, and experimental paradigms, thus providing a more descriptive and dynamic understanding of the interplay of drinking and relational contexts. In this section, we examine the link between alcohol use and three relationship processes: communication and interactional dynamics, sexual relations, and violence.

Communication and Interactional Dynamics

Researchers have examined interactional characteristics that differentiate alcoholism-complicated relationships from other intimate relationships, as well as the impact of alcohol consumption on the interaction behaviors of both social- and problem-drinking couples. Because thorough reviews of this literature are available elsewhere (e.g., Jacob & Seilhamer, 1987; McCrady & Epstein, 1995a; Schaap, Schellekens, & Schippers, 1991), we provide only a selective review.

To capture the dynamic and reciprocal influence patterns that associate drinking and couple functioning, most research efforts have adopted the *con-*

flict paradigm that marital researchers (e.g. Gottman, 1979) have successfully used to differentiate distressed from nondistressed couples.[4] Using experimental drinking procedures with this paradigm enables researchers to examine the acute effects of alcohol consumption on naturalistic interactions between partners. Early attempts (e.g., Billings, Kessler, Gomberg, & Weiner, 1979; M. C. Roberts, Floyd, O'Farrell, & Cutter, 1985) suffered from a variety of methodological weaknesses including small sample size and a lack of appropriate control groups. To address these shortcomings, Jacob and his associates (e.g., Jacob & Krahn, 1988; Jacob & Leonard, 1988) have undertaken an impressive program of research on interaction behavior, to differentiate the marital and family interactions of couples with an alcoholic, depressed, or nondistressed husband. Couples with an alcoholic partner exhibit more negative and less positive behavior than nondistressed couples (e.g. Billings et al., 1979; Haber & Jacob, 1997; Jacob & Krahn, 1988). However, most studies (e.g., Billings et al., 1979; Jacob & Leonard, 1992; O'Farrell & Birchler, 1987) have not found differences between the interactions of couples with an alcoholic partner and nonalcoholic maritally distressed or psychiatric control couples, thus failing to support the contention that there are unique interactional dynamics in a drinking-complicated marriage as compared with a marriage with other stressful or dysfunctional conditions.

The work of Jacob and his colleagues is distinguished by an explicit recognition of the heterogeneity of alcohol-complicated relationships. As a first step in addressing this heterogeneity, their work has focused on the distinction between male alcoholics who are steady drinkers and those who have an episodic, or binge, pattern of drinking. When this typology was used to split their alcoholic group, interesting differences emerged (Jacob & Leonard, 1988). The interactions of couples containing an episodic drinker were more negative than those of both steady alcoholic couples and control couples. Further, comparing the interaction behavior of couples in drinking and nondrinking conditions revealed that couples in the episodic group were more negative and less task-focused on "drink night." Couples in the steady group, by contrast, exhibited higher rates of effective problem solving on drink night. Consistent with Steinglass's (1987) thesis of potential adaptive consequences of drinking, the behavior of steady alcoholics and their spouses demonstrates that at least under some conditions, positive interactional consequences may be associated with alcohol consumption.

A recent study (Haber & Jacob, 1997) further specifies characteristics that may moderate the relationship between drinking and couple interaction behavior. Haber and Jacob compared interaction behavior among couples

---

[4]In this paradigm, couples are asked to discuss and resolve a potential or actual conflict in their marriage while being videotaped in a naturalistic laboratory context. The videotapes are then systematically coded, and the couples' interactions can be described both in terms of the frequencies and the sequential structure of the codes.

with a male alcoholic, a female alcoholic, both partners alcoholic (concordant), and neither partner alcoholic (control) in both drink and no-drink conditions. Couples with a female alcoholic exhibited greater negativity and less positivity than couples with a male alcoholic and control couples, suggesting that an alcohol problem may play a different role in couples' relationships depending on the gender of the identified drinker.

In addition to an explicit focus on both male and female alcoholics, Haber and Jacob (1997) were the first to examine the *concordance between partners* with respect to alcohol abuse and its implications for interaction. Two alternate hypotheses were addressed: An *adaptive* hypothesis predicted that concordance would lead to team support and more adaptive interactive processes; on the other hand, a *maladaptive* hypothesis predicted that concordance would lead to a compounding of maladaptive features and greater interactive negativity. Although not significantly different from female alcoholic couples, concordant couples evidenced more negative and less positive behavior than male alcoholic couples and normal controls, supporting the *maladaptive* hypothesis. Further, female-alcoholic-only couples were found to have lower negativity in the drinking than nondrinking condition, whereas the opposite was true for female alcoholics with an alcoholic spouse (concordant couples). Haber and Jacob interpreted this as suggesting that drinking may be maladaptive for concordant couples but might serve some adaptive function for nonconcordant female alcoholics. The distinct patterns that emerged for the various couple subtypes underscore the importance of continued efforts to examine gender as well as the concordance in partners' drinking behaviors to understand the relationship between drinking and couple functioning.

Alcohol consumption does not appear to exert a uniformly detrimental impact on interpersonal interactions. Indeed, both social and problem drinkers maintain expectancies of enhanced interpersonal behavior as a result of alcohol consumption (Abrams & Wilson, 1979; Brown, Goldman, & Christiansen, 1985), and alcohol may indeed have positive effects on interpersonal behavior, at least for some individuals in some contexts (Frankenstein, Hay, & Nathan, 1985; Levenson, Sher, Grossman, Newman, & Newlin, 1980; Steele et al., 1985). For example, a number of studies have found that alcohol consumption increases affective expression for both the intoxicated and sober spouse (Frankenstein et al., 1985; Jacob & Krahn, 1988), suggesting a greater emotional openness between partners under drinking conditions. Future research efforts need to acknowledge both the positive and the negative interactional effects of alcohol consumption and to define the relational and situational conditions under which each is operative.

Sexual Relations

Shakespeare has epitomized the effects of alcohol on a person's sexuality: "It provokes the desire but it takes away the performance" (*Macbeth*, act

2, scene 3). Generally, empirical studies support Shakespeare's observation; individuals expect alcohol to be a "magic elixir" that increases sexual appetite, but physiologically, the substance may in fact impede arousal and sexual responsiveness (see Crowe & George, 1989, and S. C. Wilsnack, Plaud, Wilsnack, & Klassen, 1997, for reviews). Physiological evidence from laboratory studies indicates that alcohol consumption suppresses the sexual response for both men (e.g., Farkas & Rosen, 1976) and women (e.g., Wilson & Lawson, 1978). However, given the laboratory context of these studies, the findings may be of limited generalizability. Further, these conclusions refer only to arousal assessed with physiological markers. Inarguably, there is more to sexual responsiveness and arousal than mere bodily mechanics (Crowe & George, 1989; Goldman & Roehrich, 1991).[5] The role of alcohol in sexual responsiveness is complex. In their meta-analysis, Hull and Bond (1986) found the pharmacological effects of alcohol consumption on sexual arousal to be nonsignificant; however, the belief or expectancy that one had consumed alcohol exerted a strong positive effect on sexual arousal. Thus, alcohol expectancies appear to be the critical factor in any increases in sexual arousal associated with alcohol consumption.[6]

Studies using event-based methods to link specific occasions of drinking with specific instances of sexual relations have not found a particularly strong association between alcohol consumption and sexual activity (Harvey & Beckman, 1986; Leigh, 1993). Using a diary method, Leigh found that 40% of reported incidents of sexual intercourse were followed by drinking, but only 21% of drinking episodes were followed by sexual activity. In contrast, however, clinical and qualitative studies suggest that for some individuals, alcohol use may be motivated, in part, by desires to enhance sexual intimacy or, alternately, to avoid emotional intimacy while still engaging in sexual relations (Lammers, Schippers, & van der Staak, 1995; S. C. Wilsnack, 1991). In the Wilsnacks' longitudinal study of female drinkers, sexual dysfunction was related to drinking and predicted continuation of

---

[5]When participants in these laboratory studies were asked about their subjective arousal, an interesting gender difference emerged. Although men reported that their subjective arousal decreased as blood alcohol content increased (Farkas & Rosen, 1976; Malatesta, Pollack, Wilbanks, & Adams, 1979), women reported the opposite: Self-reported arousal increased as blood alcohol content increased (Malatesta, Pollack, Crotty, Peacock, 1982; Wilson & Lawson, 1978). Thus, women's subjective experience of arousal was not consistent with the physiological indicators, although for men, the subjective and objective measures were consistent. Shakespeare, perhaps having more insight into male than female sexuality, may have described the relationship between sexuality and alcohol more accurately for males than for females.

[6]Important gender differences in the relationship between alcohol and sexual arousal may be overlooked by the aggregation of studies for this meta-analysis. Alcohol administration studies involving women are scarce, but the few that exist suggest the effect of expectancy on arousal may be different for women than men. For example, Wilson and Lawson (1978) found that for women, believing they had consumed alcohol (expectancy set) was not enough to increase physical arousal. Yet for men, expectancy alone did increase sexual arousal (e.g., Briddell et al., 1978). Although the evidence is too sparse to make definitive conclusions about a gender difference, future efforts should explore the moderating effects of gender on the relationship between alcohol expectancies and sexuality-related issues.

drinking problems over time (S. C. Wilsnack, 1991). Further, women with alcohol problems more often reported that they and their partners drank before or during sexual activity, and women who reported both alcohol problems and sexual dysfunction in 1981 and subsequently divorced were less likely to continue to have alcohol problems in 1986. The latter finding led S. C. Wilsnack (1991) to speculate that some women may use alcohol to "treat" sexual problems. In a similar vein, a qualitative study (Lammers et al., 1995) identified a subgroup of alcohol-dependent women who were drinking in response to their problematic intimate relationships and who reported using alcohol to suppress their negative feelings toward their partner and to tolerate sexual relations. Despite these clinical observations and the familiar cultural assumptions about the facilitative role of alcohol in sexual relations, the simple association between drinking and sexual frequency has rarely been tested, much less the temporal or causal connection between drinking and sexual activity.

Violence

One of the clearest demonstrations of alcohol use negatively impacting the couple is the widely documented association between alcohol use and interpersonal violence (for a review, see L. J. Roberts, Roberts & Leonard, 1999). Several systematic studies have found that alcohol use, particularly heavy or problem drinking, is related to the likelihood of engaging in violent or aggressive acts toward one's spouse (e.g., Heyman, O'Leary, & Jouriles, 1995; Kantor & Straus, 1987; Leonard & Senchak, 1996). Coleman and Straus (1979), for example, reported a 1-year prevalence of severe marital violence of 30% among men who became intoxicated very often but of only 5% among men who occasionally became intoxicated and of 2% among those who never became intoxicated. In a national sample of male U.S. Army personnel, Pan, Neidig, and O'Leary (1994) found that having an alcohol problem significantly increased the likelihood of both mild and severe forms of husband-to-wife aggression. Further, in a number of these recent studies, the predictive relationship was found to hold even after controlling for sociodemographic and personality variables that could have produced a spurious relationship. In analyses of the BNS data set, husband's premarital drinking was a strong prospective predictor of husband-to-wife physical aggression 1 year later after controlling for premarital aggression, marital conflict styles, perceived power, husband's history of violence in family of origin, and husband personality characteristics, including hostility (Leonard & Senchak, 1996).

Furthermore, experimental evidence suggests a causal relationship between alcohol impairment and aggressive responding in a variety of interpersonal contexts. Two meta-analyses (Bushman & Cooper, 1990; Ito et al., 1996) of experimental studies assessing the causal relationship between alcohol, expectation of alcohol, and aggression concluded that alcohol has a robust main effect on human aggression across diverse controlled conditions. Heavy alcohol consumption may lead to or exacerbate marital aggression either because of a cognitive impairment or because of the presence of intoxication as an excuse for aggression (Leonard, 1993). Event-based studies of the proximal predictors of marital aggression and experimental studies designed to assess the acute effects of alcohol on aggressive men are critical to further document the relationship between intoxication and violence and to help specify the underlying causative mechanisms (see Leonard & Roberts, 1998a).

ASSESSMENT AND INTERVENTION

The evidence for an association between couple functioning and drinking suggests that practitioners should attend to the possibility of concurrent problems in these areas. Individuals or couples presenting with relationship problems should routinely be screened for the presence of alcohol problems (see also Halford & Osgarby, 1993), and issues of couple and family functioning should be routinely assessed in individuals presenting with alcohol problems (IOM, 1990). A variety of spouse- or partner-involved alcohol treatment programs are available that should be considered as treatment options when alcohol and marital problems coexist. In this section, we describe these couple-based treatment options, present evidence for their efficacy, and outline current approaches to assessment and screening of alcohol problems.

Assessment of Alcohol Problems

In keeping with dominant models of the etiology and maintenance of alcohol use disorders, assessment related to an alcohol use disorder is multifactorial, covering multiple areas of functioning (IOM, 1990; Maisto & Connors, 1990). The primary goals of assessment are to evaluate the severity of the alcohol problem, identify antecedents to drinking as well as consequences that reinforce or maintain the drinking, and identify cognitive, affective, and motivational aspects of the drinking behavior (McCrady & Epstein, 1995b). In treatment with couples, assessment also addresses the strengths and weaknesses of the couple's relationship, including how the partner responds to the drinking of the identified problem drinker (McCrady & Epstein, 1995b). Below we provide a brief introduction to four critical components of the assessment of alcohol problems, highlighting exemplary instruments (see NIAAA, 1995, for a comprehensive description and review of available instruments).[7]

---

[7]This NIAAA publication, "Assessing Alcohol Problems: A Guide for Clinicians and Researchers," describes and reviews available instruments for use in screening, diagnosis, treatment planning, treatment process assessment, and outcome evaluation. For easy access, portions of this guide appear at the NIAAA web site (www.niaaa.org).

Level and Pattern of Alcohol Use

Self-reports of the frequency and quantity of recent alcohol use are the most common indicators of alcohol use behavior. For assessing typical consumption during a given period of time, standard quantity–frequency questions provide typical frequency (e.g., number of days drinking), typical quantity (amount consumed), and, derived from these, a quantity–frequency index representing the average amount of ethanol consumed in a given time period. An alternative to quantity–frequency questions is the timeline follow-back procedure (L. C. Sobell & Sobell, 1992), a structured interview that assesses the number of days drinking and average amount consumed, as well as any patterns in drinking (e.g., binge drinking on weekends). Self-monitoring or diary records represent a third methodology for assessing consumption behavior. A major strength of diary reporting is that it may be used to simultaneously assess contextual information related to the respondent's drinking occasions (e.g., time, place, with whom one is drinking), which can be useful in treatment planning.

Dependence Symptoms and Severity of Problem

To assess signs and symptoms of an alcohol disorder, instruments range from interview-based measures such as the Psychiatric Research Interview for Substance and Mental Disorders (Hasin et al., 1996, formerly known as the Structured Clinical Interview for *DSM–III–R*; Spitzer, Williams, Gibbon, & First, 1990) or the Substance Use Disorder Diagnosis Schedule (Harrison & Hoffman, 1989) to self-report measures such as the Alcohol Dependence Scale (Skinner & Horn, 1984).

Consequences of Alcohol Use

Drinking consequences are distinct from dependence symptoms and should be measured separately (W. R. Miller, Westerberg, & Waldron, 1995). Negative drinking consequences commonly assessed include missing work, difficulties with marital or other family relationships, legal problems, and physical problems. The Drinker Inventory of Consequences (W. R. Miller, Tonigan, & Longabaugh, 1995) or the Drinking Problems Index (Finney, Moos, & Brennan, 1991) are examples of standardized instruments.

Motivational, Affective, Cognitive, and Interpersonal Factors

Understanding the motivational and contextual factors surrounding drinking behavior can aid in treatment planning. The University of Rhode Island Change Assessment (McConnaughy, Prochaska, & Velicer, 1983) and the Stages of Change Readiness and Treatment Eagerness Scale (W. R. Miller & Tonigan, 1996) assess motivation to change and can be useful in determining an appropriate intervention approach. The Alcohol Expectancy Questionnaire (Brown, Goldman, Inn, & Anderson, 1980) and numerous variations of this original instrument assess expectancies related to alcohol use, which have also been related to the motivation to drink. Note that alcohol and relationship assessments must be broadened to include other areas of psychological and interpersonal functioning (see IOM, 1990, for a comprehensive framework for guiding assessment, or Maisto & Connors, 1990, and W. R. Miller, Westerberg, & Waldron, 1995, for reviews).

Interventions for Severe Alcohol Problems

Numerous approaches are currently available for the treatment of severe alcohol problems. Although many treatments appear to be effective for at least some dependent drinkers, no one type is uniformly effective (IOM, 1990). Available treatments include pharmacological, behavioral, twelve-step (e.g., Alcoholics Anonymous), motivational enhancement, and marital and family approaches (see W. R. Miller & Hester, 1995, for a comprehensive volume on treatment approaches). Treatment of the dependent drinker generally includes management of alcohol withdrawal, management of alcohol-dependence issues, and relapse prevention.

Couples-Based Interventions

Involving the spouse or partner in treatment efforts is consistent with a variety of theoretical perspectives on the etiology and treatment of individual problem behaviors, including alcohol problems. Whether based in systems perspectives (Steinglass, 1987), social or family interaction models (Jacob, 1987), ecological models (Bronfenbrenner, 1977), or behavioral models (e.g., Bandura, 1977), successful individual change often is dependent on the behaviors of close others. Behavior therapists, for example, have cogently argued that when change is initiated by others in a client's interpersonal network at the same time that the client makes changes, outcomes are more likely to be maintained (Bandura, 1977). Although marital and family therapy approaches based on a family systems or a family disease conceptualization are widely practiced, there has been little or no research on their effectiveness; conversely, although a range of family- or partner-involved behavioral treatment approaches have received empirical support, these approaches have not been widely used by the alcohol-treatment community (O'Farrell, 1993; Rotunda & O'Farrell, 1997).

With severe problem drinkers, family- or partner-involved behavioral interventions have been successfully used at each of three basic stages of change: the initial commitment to change, the change itself, and posttreatment maintenance of change (see O'Farrell, 1993). Although a variety of couples behavioral approaches exist, most share the following goals: to educate the partners about alcohol, to teach the drinker's partner to terminate reinforcement contingencies that promote drinking and increase behaviors that support abstinence, and to ameliorate the partner's own distress. Sisson and Azrin (1986), for example, taught family members of problem drinkers community reinforcement skills that resulted in more treatment seeking and more drinking reduction than resulted with controls. Behavioral marital therapy (BMT) also has been used with problem drinkers and their spouses. The goal of BMT is to improve marital functioning by increasing positive marital and family activities, decreasing conflict, and teaching problem solving and communication skills (descriptions of the therapeutic process and case examples are provided in McCrady & Epstein, 1995b, and O'Farrell & Rotunda, 1997). A series of well-controlled outcome studies have been undertaken by McCrady and colleagues and O'Farrell and colleagues using BMT with problem drinkers and their partners (e.g., McCrady, Stout, Noel, Abrams, & Nelson, 1991; O'Farrell, Cutter, Choquette, Floyd, & Bayog, 1992). Treatment outcomes with spouse involvement were superior to individually oriented treatment modalities (see Baucom, Shoham, Mueser, Daiuto, & Stickle, 1998, and O'Farrell, 1992, 1994, for reviews; see M. E. Edwards & Steinglass, 1995, for meta-analysis). Although differences between BMT and other treatment groups tend to decrease over time, relapse-prevention sessions have been shown to help maintain the effectiveness of BMT (O'Farrell, Choquette & Cutter, 1998; O'Farrell, Choquette, Cutter, Brown, & McCourt, 1993).

Screening and Brief Intervention

To complement traditional intervention approaches for individuals with severe alcohol problems, there is a growing recognition of the importance of screening and brief intervention to reach the large numbers of individuals manifesting mild or moderate alcohol problems (IOM, 1990). As the IOM (1990) report has proposed, the target population for alcohol treatment needs to be "broadened"; the overall goal of treatment should be "to reduce or eliminate the use of alcohol as a contributing factor to physical, psychological, and social dysfunction and to arrest, retard, or reverse the progress of associated problems" (p. 46). Casting this wider net, Randy and Dawn both represent individuals that might appropriately be targeted for an alcohol-related intervention. Although Randy may be considered to have a severe drinking problem, Dawn does not appear to, and we do not have any evidence that either Randy or Dawn has symptoms of alcohol dependence. Nonetheless, each of the partners may benefit from an alcohol-related intervention to arrest, retard, or reverse the problems they experience associated with his or her alcohol use.

Recurrent physical, psychological, or relationship problems may often be secondary to alcohol problems. Screening for alcohol problems in settings where these problems are typically identified is especially important. Randy and Dawn's relationship history suggests a number of points at which this couple's drinking problems may have come to the attention of community practitioners and resulted in brief intervention or referral. For example, Randy's physical abuse of his wife came to the attention of law enforcement after he hit Dawn in a bar; Dawn's drinking during pregnancy presumably could have come to the attention of her doctor. Indeed, the identification and treatment of problem drinkers in health care settings have been identified as an important national health care priority (U.S. Public Health Service, 1991). A number of methods have been proposed to address this priority, including the use of physician-delivered brief intervention methods, brief behaviorally oriented treatment programs conducted by therapists, and computer-assisted counseling programs.

Brief interventions are time-limited, secondary prevention strategies that focus on reducing alcohol use in the nondependent drinker and thereby minimizing risks associated with drinking. Brief intervention procedures include assessment and direct feedback, contracting and goal setting, and self-help directed bibliotherapy. Brief behavioral treatment programs often additionally involve skill training in drinking moderation strategies, self-monitoring, and functional analysis of drinking. Several well-controlled outcome studies have substantiated the effectiveness of both brief intervention and behaviorally oriented drinking moderation programs (for meta-analysis, see Bien, Miller, & Tonigan, 1993). For example, Fleming, Barry, Manwell, Johnson, and London (1997) screened almost 20,000 patients for problem drinking and then randomized identified problem drinkers into a physician-administered brief intervention group or a control group. At the 12-month follow-up, the intervention group evidenced a significant reduction in 7-day alcohol use, binge-drinking episodes, frequency of excessive drinking, and, for men, length of hospital stays.

In contrast to intervention approaches with the dependent drinker, there have been very few systematic attempts to involve partners in interventions for drinkers with mild or moderate alcohol problems and no published, controlled studies examining the efficacy of doing so. However, given the evidence we have reviewed for an association between drinking and couple factors and the success of couple interventions for more severe problems, it may be advantageous to involve married or cohabiting partners in interventions with nondependent problem drinkers (see also IOM, 1990; Zweben & Barrett, 1993). Moreover, in addition to the evidence we have reviewed for the important role a partner may play in the maintenance and recovery from a severe alcohol problem, evidence also suggests a more fundamental connection between intimate partners' drinking behaviors. First, a substantial body of evidence supports the notion that spouses' drinking behaviors are positively associated (e.g., Corbett, Mora, & Ames, 1991; Hall, Hesselbrock, & Stabenau, 1983; McLeod, 1993). Although this may reflect an assortative mating process, a process of *interpersonal influence* also may be operative. It is commonly suggested that the direction of influence in drinking habits is from husband to wife (e.g., Cahalan, 1970; Jacob & Seilhamer, 1991; H. R. White, Bates, & Johnson, 1991), but wife-to-husband influence also has been documented. For example, Cronkite and Moos (1984) found that wives' alcohol consumption was a significant predictor of husbands' alcohol consumption 1 year later, controlling for baseline levels.

Thus, the drinking pattern of a person who is married (or in a similar intimate, cohabitant relationship) is not independent of the partner. An ongoing relationship like marriage necessitates what we have called a *drinking partnership*, a tacit agreement between partners with respect to drinking norms and behaviors (L. J. Roberts & Leonard, 1998). Either explicitly or implicitly, partners negotiate norms for alcohol use in their household (e.g., whether alcohol is served with meals or offered to guests, whether the refrigerator or liquor cabinet is "stocked"). Further, each partner becomes a salient feature of the other's drinking context, through direct modeling as well as the explicit or subtle communication of attitudes and values about drinking, including attempts to control or change the partner's drinking. We use the term *drinking partnership* to refer not only to the match or lack thereof between the husband's and wife's drinking levels but also to the patterning and contexts of their drinking. The drinking partnerships that couples mutually structure may take varied forms and have different relationships to both alcohol and marital problems (L. J. Roberts & Leonard, 1998).

Interventions designed for individuals with mild-to-moderate alcohol problems may benefit from involving the partner and directly addressing issues related to the drinking partnership. Returning again to Randy and Dawn, it would have been difficult for either partner to moderate his or her drinking without the cooperation and support of the other. Dawn, for example, was at least minimally aware of the potential risks her drinking posed to her developing fetus, but her husband's continued drinking and her desire to connect with him made it difficult for her to heed warnings. A couples-based intervention might have increased the likelihood that Dawn would moderate her drinking during pregnancy and after. Further, we would argue that an intervention that directly addressed the relationship dynamics that contributed to Dawn's and Randy's drinking behaviors (e.g., issues of intimacy and independence) would have had the greatest chance of making a difference in this couple's relationship trajectory.

CONCLUSIONS AND FUTURE DIRECTIONS

Achieving a precise understanding of the impact of alcohol problems on couple functioning and the influence of relationship factors on alcohol problems presents a formidable challenge to researchers, clinicians, and policymakers. On the basis of the research reviewed here, we can conclude that there is strong evidence for an association between the quality of a couple's relationship and drinking problems. However, beyond this simple assertion, extant findings are not easy to summarize. Undertaking research on the relationship between couple factors and alcohol use is complicated by the tremendous variability in individual drinking patterns and drinking contexts. Studies with differing samples, methodologies, control groups, and measures have found inconsistent results, attesting to this complexity. Further, empirical understandings of causal processes are still in an embryonic stage, and firm conclusions about the underlying reasons for the observed associations are not yet possible. As Halford and Osgarby (1993) have intimated, a "true" causal direction is likely to elude researchers, because alcohol and relationship problems may be reciprocally related or "exacerbate each other rather than invariably cause each other" (p. 245). Advances in our understanding of the interface of alcohol and couple factors will require inclusion of multiple levels of influence and acknowledgment and assessment of bidirectional effects. We recommend four directions for future research on drinking and couples.

Embrace Heterogenity and Broaden the Base

Echoing the theme of the IOM (1990) report, it is critical that we broaden the base of treatment for alcohol problems. Rather than focusing intervention efforts on the apex of the triangle depicted in Figure 10.1, we also need empirically grounded intervention efforts targeted at mild and moderate alcohol problems. Concomitantly, both in treatment and research efforts, we need to acknowledge and embrace the extreme heterogeneity in the manifestations and etiological trajectories of alcohol problems. Current research on couples and alcohol has not yet recruited samples that represent and model the heterogeneity of alcohol problems (McCrady & Epstein, 1995a). Research on female drinkers, minorities, same-sex couples, or individuals with comorbid drug problems or psychopathology, for example, is virtually absent. To advance our understanding of alcohol-related problems, we must study the considerable heterogeneity of alcohol problems even within existing subgroups (e.g., dependent drinkers) and search for homogeneous subgroups for study at the same time that the target population is substantially broadened.

Move Beyond Individual Drinking to Drinking Partnership

The drinking partnership, a conceptualization that includes the typical dosage of alcohol, as well as the drinking context and match (or lack thereof) between the husband's and the wife's drinking, may be a useful approach to the complexities inherent in the relationship between drinking and couple factors. Further, the partnership aspects of drinking need to be fully acknowledged in treatment efforts. The effectiveness of partner-involved interventions with severe problem drinkers, coupled with the evidence for reciprocal influence processes characterizing partner drinking in the intimate relational context, suggests that couple interventions may be a powerful tool for behavioral change among individuals manifesting mild-to-moderate alcohol problems. Expanding spouse- or partner-involved interventions from the province of alcoholism to the full spectrum of alcohol problems should be a priority in the years ahead.

Attend to Mediating and Moderating Variables

Future research needs to move beyond the examination of the overall association between drinking and couple factors to directly examine the role of both mediating and moderating factors in the relationship. For example, the connection between drinking and relational outcomes may be different at different stages in the development of a close relationship. Alcohol may play a different role early in a marriage, when a couple is still developing intimacy and a sexual bond, than later in a marriage, when there is less passion and more companionship. The presence of children may increase stress in the home, and the demands of parenting may radically alter the ways in which alcohol is used by the couple; further, the use of alcohol may take on a different meaning for couples with adolescents in the home as they consider what messages their drinking may send to an impressionable teenager. Many existing studies focus only on couples in one relationship stage (e.g., early marriage) or do not analyze for the potential moderating role of family development variables.

Another important moderating variable is gender of the drinker, but even this fundamental variable has not received sufficient attention in the literature (L. J. Roberts & Leonard, 1997). Although alcohol problems in both women and men result from a complex interplay of biological, psychological, and sociocultural factors, women's drinking may be particularly affected by interpersonal and relational factors (Olenick & Chalmers, 1991; S. C. Wilsnack, 1995). Attention to these factors will be critical in expanding our understanding of the processes that promote, maintain, or discourage alcohol use in women and, ultimately, in providing the basis for the development of effective intervention and prevention programs for women.

Further attention to the processes that mediate any observed relationship between drinking and couple factors also is essential. Examination of specific relationship processes will hasten our understanding of the association between drinking and relationship outcomes, as well as between relationship processes and drinking outcomes. Empirically based descriptions of the ways in which couples interact and influence each other over time are the necessary building blocks for theoretical understanding of the alcohol–couple link (Jacob, 1987). Studies that use qualitative interviewing, daily diary records, or direct observation of couple interactions are needed to increase understanding of drinking-related behaviors in the day-to-day lives of couples. A similar attention to process and mediating variables is needed in the treatment literature; little is known about the underlying processes or the "effective ingredients" of couple-based drinking interventions.

Examine Positive and Adaptive Functions of Alcohol Use

The association of alcohol problems with decrements in marital and family functioning is solidly rooted in the clinical and treatment literature, as well as in our public consciousness. However, coexisting with these negative expectancies are a host of positive expectancies about alcohol use, many of which are clearly linked to relational functioning. Although research is beginning to examine the impact of alcohol consumption on social behaviors relevant to relationship conflict and violence, a concomitant focus on the relational processes that drinkers believe alcohol positively affects would serve to advance the field. Particularly important in this respect are behaviors related to a couple's ability to establish and maintain intimacy. Like Randy and Dawn, many couples believe that alcohol facilitates intimate relating. Consider this passage from Carolyn Knapp's (1996) best-selling memoir of her struggle with alcoholism, in which she described the role alcohol played in her frequent meetings with a friend:

> When we drank together, my sense of time would shift. Sam would get there, and there'd be a slightly self-conscious twenty minutes or half hour until we'd eased our way into the drinks and conversation, and the next thing you knew, it would be two or three hours later and we'd be in the middle of some deep talk about family, or therapy, or work, and I'd feel *right there* genuinely united, as though we'd really spoken to and heard one another. . . . Drinking was the best way I knew, the fastest and simplest, to let my feelings out and to connect, just sit there and connect with another human being. (p. 68; italics in original)

Knapp directly related her alcohol use to a search for intimate, interpersonal connection, but only during recovery did she fully realize the ways in which alcohol served to sever and impede real connection with others. By attempting to identify positive relationship benefits that couples experience in their alcohol-affected interactions, we may be able to develop treatment and prevention efforts that help couples attain the same benefits, but without the use of alcohol.

REFERENCES

Abel, E. L., & Sokol, R. J. (1986). Fetal alcohol syndrome is now leading cause of mental retardation. *Lancet, 2,* 1222.

Abrams, D. B., & Wilson, G. T. (1979). Effects of alcohol on social anxiety in women: Cognitive versus physiological processes. *Journal of Abnormal Psychology, 88*, 161–173.

Amato, P. R., & Rogers, S. J. (1997). A longitudinal study of marital problems and subsequent divorce. *Journal of Marriage and the Family, 59*, 612–624.

American Psychiatric Association. (1994). *Diagnostic and statistical manual of mental disorders* (4th ed.). Washington, DC: Author.

Bachman, J. G., Wadsworth, K. N., O'Malley, P. M., Johnston, L. D. & Schulenberg, J. (1997). *Smoking, drinking and drug use in young adulthood: The impacts of new freedoms and new responsibilities.* Mahwah, NJ: Erlbaum.

Bandura, A. (1977). *Social learning theory.* Englewood Cliffs, NJ: Prentice Hall.

Baucom, D. H., Shoham, V., Mueser, K. T., Daiuto, A. D., & Stickle, T. R. (1998). Empirically supported couple and family interventions for marital distress and adult mental health problems. *Journal of Consulting and Clinical Psychology, 66*, 53–88.

Beckman, L J. (1979). *Journal of Studies on Alcohol, 40*, 272–282.

Bien, T. H., Miller, W. R., & Tonigan, J. S. (1993). Brief interventions for alcohol problems: A review. *Addiction, 88*, 315–336.

Billings, A., Kessler, M., Gomberg, C., & Weiner S. (1979). Marital conflict resolution of alcoholic and nonalcoholic couples during drinking and nondrinking sessions. *Journal of Studies on Alcohol, 3*, 183–195.

Brennan, P. L., Moos, R. H., & Kelly, K. M. (1994). Spouses of late-life problem drinkers: Functioning, coping responses, and family contexts. *Journal of Family Psychology, 8*, 447–457.

Briddell, D. W., Rimm, D. C., Caddy, G. R., Krawitz, G., Sholis, D. & Wunderlin, R. J. (1978). Effects of alcohol and cognitive set on sexual arousal to deviant stimuli. *Journal of Abnormal Psychology, 87*, 418–430.

Bronfenbrenner, U. (1977). Toward an experimental ecology of human development. *American Psychologist, 32*, 513–530.

Brown, S. A., Goldman, M. S., & Christiansen, B. A. (1985). Do alcohol expectancies mediate drinking patterns of adults? *Journal of Consulting and Clinical Psychology, 53*, 512–519.

Brown, S. A., Goldman, M. S., Inn, A., & Anderson, L. R. (1980). Expectations of reinforcement from alcohol: Their domain and relation to drinking patterns. *Journal of Consulting and Clinical Psychology, 48*, 419–426.

Bushman, B. J., & Cooper, H. M. (1990). Effects of alcohol on human aggression: An integrative research review. *Psychological Bulletin, 107*, 341–354.

Cahalan, D. (1970). *Problem drinkers: A national survey.* San Francisco: Jossey-Bass.

Clark, W. B., & Hilton, M. E. (1991). *Alcohol in America: Drinking practices and problems.* Albany: State University of New York Press.

Coleman, D. J., & Straus, M. A. (1979, August). *Alcohol abuse and family violence.* Paper presented at the annual meeting of the American Sociological Association, Boston.

Corbett, K., Mora, J. & Ames, G. (1991). Drinking patterns and drinking-related problems in Mexican-American husbands and wives. *Journal of Studies on Alcohol, 52*, 215–223.

Cronkite, R. C., & Moos, R. H. (1984). Sex and marital status in relation to the treatment and outcome of alcoholic patients. *Sex Roles, 11*, 93–112.

Crowe, L. C., & George, W. H. (1989). Alcohol and human sexuality: Review and integration. *Psychological Bulletin, 105*, 374–386.

Cummings, C., Gordon, J. R., & Marlatt, G. A. (1980). Relapse: Strategies of prevention and prediction. In W. R. Miller (Ed.), *Addictive behaviors: Treatment of alcoholism* (pp. 291–321). New York: Pergamon Press.

Dahlgren, L. (1979). Female alcoholics: IV. Marital situation and husbands. *Acta Psychiatrica Scandinavica, 59*, 59–69.

Davis, D. I., Berenson, D., Steinglass, P., & Davis, S. (1974). The adaptive consequences of drinking. *Psychiatry, 37*, 209–215.

Dumka, L. E., & Roosa, M. W. (1993). Factors mediating problem drinking and mothers' personal adjustment. *Journal of Family Psychology, 7*, 333–343.

Dunn, N. J., Jacob, T., Hummon, N., & Seilhamer, R. A. (1987). Marital stability in alcoholic-spouse relationships as a function of drinking pattern and location. *Journal of Abnormal Psychology, 96*, 99–107.

Edwards, G., & Gross, M. M. (1976). Alcohol dependence: Provisional description of a clinical syndrome. *British Medical Journal, 1*, 1058–1061.

Edwards, M. E., & Steinglass, P. (1995). Family therapy treatment outcomes for alcoholism. *Journal of Marital and Family Therapy, 21*, 475–509.

Edwards, P., Harvey, C., & Whitehead, P. C. (1973). Wives of alcoholics: A critical review and analysis. *Quarterly Journal of Studies on Alcohol, 34*(1, Pt. A), 112–132.

Engel, G. (1977). The need for a new medical model: A challenge for biomedicine. *Science, 196*, 129–136.

Evert, D. L., & Oscar-Berman, M. (1995). Alcohol related cognitive impairments: An overview of how alcoholism may affect the workings of the brain. *Alcohol Health and Research World, 19*, 89–96.

Farkas, G., & Rosen, R. C. (1976). The effects of ethanol on male sexual arousal. *Journal of Studies on Alcohol, 37*, 265–272.

Finney, W. J., Moos, R. H., & Brennan, P. L. (1991). The Drinking Problems Index: A measure to assess alcohol-related problems among older adults. *Journal of Substance Abuse, 3*, 395–404.

Fitzgerald, H. E., Davies, W. H., Zucker, R. A., & Klinger, M. (1994). Developmental systems theory and substance abuse. In L. L'Abate (Ed.), *Handbook of developmental family psychology and psychopathology* (pp. 350–372). New York: Wiley.

Fleming, M., Barry, K., Manwell, L., Johnson, K., & London, M. (1997). Brief physician advice for problem alcohol drinkers: A randomized control trial in community based primary care practices. *Journal of the American Medical Association, 277*, 1039–1045.

Frankenstein, W., Hay, W. M., & Nathan P. E. (1985). Effects of intoxication on alcoholics' marital communication and problem solving. *Journal of Studies on Alcohol, 46,* 1–6.

Goldman, M. S., & Roehrich, L. (1991). Alcohol expectancies and sexuality. *Alcohol Health and Research World, 15,* 126–132.

Gorman, D. M., & Peter, T. J. (1980). Types of life events and the onset of alcohol dependence. *British Journal of Addiction, 75,* 71–79.

Gottman, J. M. (1979). *Marital interaction: Experimental investigations.* New York: Academic Press.

Grant, B. F., Harford, T. C., Dawson, D. A., Chou, P., Dufour, M., & Pickering, R. (1994). Prevalence of *DSM–IV* alcohol abuse and dependence: United States, 1992. *Alcohol Health and Research World, 18,* 243–248.

Grzywacz, J. G., & Marks, N. F. (1999). Family solidarity and health behaviors: Evidence from the National Survey of Midlife Development in the United States (MIDUS). *Journal of Family Issues, 20,* 243–268.

Haber, J. R., & Jacob, T. (1997). Marital interactions of male versus female alcoholics. *Family Process, 36,* 385–402.

Halford, W. K., & Osgarby, S. M. (1993). Alcohol abuse in clients presenting with marital problems. *Journal of Family Psychology, 6,* 245–254.

Hall, R. L., Hesselbrock, V. M., & Stabenau, J. R. (1983). Familial distribution of alcohol use: II. Assortative mating of alcoholic probands. *Behavior Genetics, 13,* 373–382.

Harrison, P. A., & Hoffman, N. G. (1989). *SUDDS, Substance Use Disorder Diagnosis Schedule manual.* St. Paul, MN: New Standards.

Harvey, S. M., & Beckman, L. J. (1986). Alcohol consumption, female sexual behavior, and contraceptive use. *Journal of Studies on Alcohol, 47,* 327–332.

Harwood, H., Fountain, D., & Livermore, G. (1998). *Economic costs of alcohol and drug abuse in the United States, 1992.* Rockville, MD: National Institute on Drug Abuse.

Hasin, D. S., Trautman, K. D., Miele, G. M. Samat, S., Smith, M., & Endicott, J. (1996) Psychiatric research interview for substance and mental disorders (PRISM): Reliability for substance abusers. *American Journal of Psychiatry, 153,* 1153–1201.

Heyman, R. E., O'Leary, K. D., & Jouriles, E. N. (1995). Alcohol and aggressive personality styles: Potentiators of serious physical aggression against wives? *Journal of Family Psychology, 9,* 44–57.

Hilton, M. (1988). The demographic distribution of drinking patterns in 1984. *Drug and Alcohol Dependence, 22,* 37–47.

Holmila, M. (1988). *Wives, husbands, and alcohol: A study of informal drinking control within the family.* Helsinki, Finland: Finnish Foundation for Alcohol Studies.

Hull, J. G., & Bond, C. F. (1986). Social and behavioral consequences of alcohol consumption and expectancy. *Psychological Bulletin, 99,* 347–360.

Institute of Medicine. (1990). *Broadening the base of treatment for alcohol problems.* Washington, DC: National Academy Press.

Ito, T. A., Miller, N., & Pollock, V. E. (1996). Alcohol and aggression: A meta-analysis on the moderating effects of inhibitory cues, triggering events, and self-focused attention. *Psychological Bulletin, 120*, 60–82.

Jackson, J. (1954) The adjustment of the family to the crisis of alcoholism. *Quarterly Journal of Studies on Alcohol, 15*, 562–586.

Jacob, T. (1987). Alcoholism: A family interaction perspective. In P. C. Rivers (Ed.), *Nebraska Symposium on Motivation: Vol. 34. Alcohol and Addictive Behavior* (pp. 159–206). Lincoln: University of Nebraska Press.

Jacob, T., & Bremer, D. A. (1986). Assortative mating among men and women alcoholics. *Journal of Studies on Alcohol, 47*, 219–222.

Jacob, T., Dunn, N. J., & Leonard, K. E. (1983). Patterns of alcohol abuse and family stability. *Alcoholism: Clinical and Experimental Research, 7*, 382–385.

Jacob, T., & Krahn, G. L. (1988). Marital interactions of alcoholic couples: Comparison with depressed and nondistressed couples. *Journal of Consulting and Clinical Psychology, 56*, 73–79.

Jacob, T., & Leonard, K. E. (1988). Alcoholic–spouse interaction as a function of alcoholism subtype and alcohol consumption interaction. *Journal of Abnormal Psychology, 97*, 231–237.

Jacob, T., & Leonard, K. E. (1992). A sequential analysis of marital interactions involving male alcoholic, depressed and nondistressed males. *Journal of Abnormal Psychology, 101*, 647–656.

Jacob, T., & Seilhamer, R. A. (1982). The impact on spouses and how they cope. In J. Orford & J. Harwin (Eds.), *Alcohol and the family* (pp. 114–126). London: Crown Helm.

Jacob, T., & Seilhamer, R. A. (1987). Alcoholism and family interaction. In T. Jacob (Ed.), *Family interaction and psychopathology: Theories, methods, and findings* (p. 535–580). New York: Plenum.

Jacob, T., & Seilhamer, R. A. (1991). Alcoholism and the family. In D. J. Pittman & H. R. White (Eds.), Alcohol, culture, and social control monograph series: Society, culture, and drinking patterns reexamined (pp. 613–630). New Brunswick, NJ: Rutgers Center of Alcohol Studies.

Kantor, G. K., & Straus, M. A. (1987). The drunken bum theory of wife beating. *Social Problems, 34*, 213–230.

Kessler, R. C., Walters, E. E., & Forthofer, M. S. (1998). The social consequences of psychiatric disorders: III. Probability of marital stability. *The American Journal of Psychiatry, 155*, 1092–1096.

Kessler, R. C., McGonagle, K. A., Zhao, S. Nelson, C. H., Hughes, M., Eshleman, S., Wittchen, H. W., & Kendler, K. S. (1994). Lifetime and 12-month prevalence of *DSM–III–R* psychiatric disorders in the United States. *Archives of General Psychiatry, 51*, 8–19.

Klassen, A. D., & Wilsnack, S. C. (1986). Sexual experiences and drinking among women in a U.S. national survey. *Archives of Sexual Behavior, 15*, 363–392.

Klassen, A. D., Wilsnack, S. C., Harris, T. R., & Wilsnack, R. W. (1991, March). Partnership dissolution and remission of problem drinking in women: Findings from a U.S. longitudinal survey. In *Alcohol, family, and significant others*. Symposium sponsored by the Social Research Institute of Alcohol Studies and the Nordic Council for Alcohol and Drug Research, Helsinki, Finland.

Knapp, C. (1996). *Drinking: A love story*. New York: Dell.

Kogan, K. L., & Jackson, J. K. (1965a). Alcoholism: The fable of the noxious wife. *Mental Hygiene, 49*, 428–437.

Kogan, K. L., & Jackson, J. K. (1965b). Stress, personality and emotional disturbance in wives of alcohlics. *Quarterly Journal of Studies on Alcohol, 26*, 486–495.

Lammers, S. M. M., Schippers, G. M., & van der Staak, C. P. F. (1995). Submission and rebellion: Excessive drinking of women in problematic heterosexual partner relationships. *International Journal of Addictions, 30*, 901–917.

Leigh, B. C. (1993). Alcohol consumption and sexual activity as reported with a diary technique. *Journal of Abnormal Psychology, 102*, 490–493.

Leonard, K. E. (1993). Drinking patterns and intoxication in marital violence: Review, critique, and future directions for research. In S. E. Martin (Ed.), *Alcohol and interpersonal violence: Fostering multidisciplinary perspectives* (pp. 253–280). Rockville, MD: NIAAA.

Leonard, K. E., & Roberts, L. J. (1998a). The effects of alcohol on the marital interactions of aggressive and nonaggressive husbands and their wives. *Journal of Abnormal Psychology, 107*, 602–615.

Leonard, K. E., & Roberts, L. J. (1998b). Marital aggression, quality, and stability in the first year of marriage: Findings from the Buffalo Newlywed Study. T. N. Bradbury (Ed.), *The developmental course of marital dysfunction* (pp. 44–73). New York: Cambridge University Press.

Leonard, K. E., & Rothbard, J. C. (1999). Alcohol and the marriage effect. *Journal of Studies on Alcohol, 13*, 139–146.

Leonard, K. E., & Senchak, M. (1996). Prospective prediction of husband marital aggression within newlywed couples. *Journal of Abnormal Psychology, 105*, 369–380.

Levenson, R. W., Sher, K. J., Grossman, L. M., Newman, J., & Newlin, D. B. (1980). Alcohol and stress response dampening: Pharmacological effects, expectancy and tension reduction. *Journal of Abnormal Psychology, 89*, 528–538.

Levinger, G. (1966). Sources of marital dissatisfaction among applicants for divorce. *American Journal of Othopsychiatry, 32*, 803–807.

MacDonald, T. K., Zanna, M. P., & Fong, G. T. (1995). Decision making in altered states: Effects of alcohol on attitudes toward drinking and driving. *Journal of Personality and Social Psychology, 68*, 973–985.

Maisto, S. A., & Connors, G. J. (1990). Clinical diagnostic techniques and assessment tools in alcoholism research. *Alcohol Health and Research World, 14*, 232–238.

Maisto, S. A., O'Farrell, T. J., Connors, G. J., McKay, J., & Pelcovits, M. A. (1988). Alcoholics' attributions of factors affecting their relapse to drinking and reasons for terminating relapse events. *Addictive Behaviors, 13*, 79–82.

Malatesta, V. J., Pollack, R. H., Crotty, T. D., & Peacock, L. J. (1982). Acute alcohol intoxication and female orgasmic response. *Journal of Sex Research, 18,* 1–17.

Malatesta, V. J., Pollack, R. H., Wilbanks, W. A., & Adams, H. E. (1979). Alcohol effects on the orgasmic–ejaculatory response in human males. *Journal of Sex Research, 15,* 101–107.

Marlatt, G. A. (1976). Alcohol, stress, and cognitive control. In C. D. Spielberger & I. G. Sarason (Eds.), *Stress and anxiety* (Vol 3, pp. 271–296). New York: Hemisphere.

Marlatt, G. A., & Rohsenow, D. (1980). Cognitive processes in alcohol use: Expectancy and the balanced placebo design. N. K. Mello (Ed.), *Advances in substance abuse: Behavioral and biological research* (pp. 159–199). Greenwich, CT: JAI Press.

McConnaughy, E. A., Prochaska, J. O., & Velicer, W. F. (1983). Stages of change in psychotherapy: Measurement and sample profiles. *Psychotherapy Theory and Research Practice, 20,* 368–375.

McCrady, B. S., & Epstein, E. E. (1995a). Directions for research on alcoholic relationships: Marital- and individual-based models of heterogeneity. *Psychology of Addictive Behaviors, 9,* 157–166.

McCrady, B. S., & Epstein, E. E. (1995b). Marital therapy in the treatment of alcohol problems. In N. S. Jacobson & A. S. Gurman (Eds.), *Clinical handbook of couple therapy* (pp. 369–393). New York: Guilford Press.

McCrady, B. S., & Hay, W. (1987). Coping with problem drinking in the family. In J. Orford (Ed.), *Coping with disorder in the family* (pp. 86–116). London: Croom & Helm.

McCrady, B. S., Stout, R., Noel, N., Abrams, D., & Nelson, H. F. (1991). Effectiveness of three types of spouse-involved behavioral alcoholism treatment. *British Journal of Addiction, 86,* 1415–1424.

McLeod, J. D. (1993). Spouse concordance for alcohol dependence and heavy drinking: Evidence from a community sample. *Alcoholism Clinical and Experimental Research, 17,* 1146–1155.

Midanik, L. T., & Clark, W. B. (1994). Demographic distribution of U.S. drinking patterns in 1990: Description and trends from 1984. *American Journal of Public Health, 84,* 1218–1222.

Midanik, L. T., Tam, T. W., Greenfield, T., & Caetano, R. (1996). Risk functions for alcohol-related problems in a 1988 U.S. national sample. *Addictions, 91,* 1427–1437.

Miller, P. M., Ingham, J. G., Plant, M. A., & Miller, T. (1977). Alcohol consumption and self-disclosure. *British Journal of Addiction, 72,* 296–300.

Miller, W. R., & Hester, R. (1995). *Handbook of alcoholism treatment approaches: Effective alternatives.* New York: Allyn & Bacon.

Miller, W. R., & Tonigan, J. S. (1996). Assessing drinkers' motivations for change: The Stages of Change Readiness and Treatment Eagerness Scale (SOCRATES). *Psychology of Addictive Behaviors, 10,* 81–89.

Miller, W. R., Tonigan, J. S., & Longabaugh, R. (1995). *The Drinker Inventory of Consequences (DrInC): An instrument for assessing adverse consequences of alcohol abuse* (NIAAA Project MATCH Monograph Series, Vol 4). Bethesda, MD: U.S. Department of Health and Human Services.

Miller, W. R., Westerberg, V. S., & Waldron, H. B. (1995). Evaluating alcohol problems in adults and adolescents. In W. R. Miller & R. Hester (Eds.), *Handbook of alcoholism treatment approaches: Effective alternatives* (pp. 61–88). New York: Allyn & Bacon.

Moos, R. H., Bromet, E., Tsu, V., & Moos, B. (1979). Family characteristics and the outcome of treatment for alcoholism. *Journal of Studies on Alcohol, 40,* 78–88.

Moos, R. H., Finney, J. W., & Cronkite, R. C. (1990). *Alcoholism treatment: Context, process, and outcome.* New York: Oxford University Press.

Moos, R. H., Finney, J. W., & Gamble, W. (1982). The process of recovery from alcoholism: II. Comparing spouses of alcoholic patients and matched community controls. *Journal of Studies on Alcohol, 42,* 888–909.

Moos, R. H., & Moos, B. S. (1984). The process of recovery from alcoholism: 3. Comparing functioning in families of alcoholics and matched control families. *Journal of Studies on Alcohol, 45,* 111–118.

National Institute on Alcohol Abuse and Alcoholism. (1995). Assessing alcohol problems: A guide for clinicians and researchers. *NIAAA treatment handbook* (Series 4) Bethesda, MD: U.S. Department of Health and Human Services.

National Institute on Alcohol Abuse and Alcoholism. (1997). *Ninth special report to the U.S. Congress on Alcohol and Health.* Washington, DC: U. S. Government Printing Office.

Nirenberg, T. D., Liepman, M. R., Begin, A. M., Doolittle, R. H., & Broffman, T. E. (1990). The sexual relationship of male alcoholics and their female partners during periods of drinking and abstinence. *Journal of Studies on Alcohol, 51,* 565–568.

O'Farrell, T. J. (1992). Families and alcohol problems: An overview of treatment research. *Journal of Family Psychology, 5,* 339–359.

O'Farrell, T. J. (Ed.). (1993). *Treating alcohol problems: Marital and family interventions.* New York: Guilford Press.

O'Farrell, T. J. (1994). Marital therapy and spouse-involved treatment with alcoholic patients. *Behavior Therapy, 25,* 391–406.

O'Farrell, T. J., & Birchler, G. R. (1987). Marital relationships of alcoholic, conflicted, and nonconflicted couples. *Journal of Marital and Family Therapy, 13,* 259–274.

O'Farrell, T. J., Choquette, K. A., & Cutter, H. (1998). Couples relapse prevention sessions after behavioral marital therapy for male alcoholics: Outcomes during the three years after starting treatment. *Journal of Studies on Alcohol, 59,* 357–370.

O'Farrell, T. J., Choquette, K. A., Cutter, H., Brown, E., & McCourt, W. (1993). Behavioral marital therapy with and without additional relapse prevention sessions for alcoholics and their wives. *Journal of Studies on Alcohol, 54,* 652–666.

O'Farrell, T. J., Cutter, H. S. G., Choquette, K. A., Floyd, F. J., & Bayog, R. D. (1992). Behavioral marital therapy for male alcoholics: Marital and drinking adjustment during the two years after treatment. *Behavior Therapy, 23*, 529–549.

O'Farrell, T. J., Cutter, H. S. G., & Floyd, F. J. (1985). Evaluating behavioral marital therapy for male alcoholics: Effects on marital adjustment and communication from before to after treatment. *Behavior Therapy, 16*, 147–167.

O'Farrell, T. J., Hooley, J, Fals-Stewart, W. & Cutter, H. G. (1998). Expressed emotion and relaspe in alcoholic patients. *Journal of Consulting and Clinical Psychology, 66*, 744–752.

O'Farrell, T. J., & Rotunda, R. J. (1997). Couples interventions and alcohol abuse. In W. K. Halford & H. J. Markman (Eds.), *Clinical handbook of marriage and couples interventions* (pp. 555–588). Chichester, England: John Wiley and Sons.

Olenick, N. L., & Chalmers, D. K. (1991). Gender specific drinking styles in alcoholics and nonalcoholics. *Journal of Studies on Alcohol, 52*, 325–330.

Orford, J. (1990). Alcohol and the family. In L. T. Kozlowski, H. M. Annis, H. D. Cappell, F. B. Glaser, M. S. Goodstadt, Y. Israel, H. Kalant, E. M. Sellers, & E. R. Vingilis (Eds.), *Research advances in alcohol and drug problems* (Vol. 10, pp. 81–155). New York: Plenum.

Orford, J., Guthrie, S., Nicholls, P., Oppenheimer, E., Egert, S., & Hensman, C. (1975). Self-reported coping behavior of wives of alcoholics and its association with drinking outcome. *Journal of Studies on Alcohol, 36*, 1254–1267.

Pan, H. D., Neidig, P. H., & O'Leary, K. D. (1994). Predicting mild and severe husband-to-wife physical aggression. *Journal of Consulting and Clinical Psychology, 62*, 975–981.

Paolino, T. J., & McCrady, B. S. (1977). *The alcoholic marriage: Alternative perspectives.* New York: Grune & Stratton.

Perodeau, G. M., & Kohn, P. M. (1989). Sex differences in the martial functioning of treated alcoholics. *Drug and Alcohol Dependence, 23*, 1–11.

Roberts, L. J., & Leonard, K. E. (1997). Gender differences and similarities in the alcohol and marriage relationship. In S. Wilsnack & R. Wilsnack (Eds.), *Gender and alcohol: Individual and social perspectives* (pp. 289–311). New Brunswick, NJ: Rutgers Center of Alcohol Studies.

Roberts, L. J., & Leonard, K. E. (1998). An empirical typology of drinking partnerships and their relationship to marital functioning and drinking consequences. *Journal of Marriage and the Family, 60*, 515–526.

Roberts, L. J., Leonard, K. E., & Senchak, M. (1994, June). *Alcohol use, intimacy, and marital adjustment in early marriage.* Paper presented at the Annual Meeting for the Research Society on Alcoholism, Maui, HI.

Roberts, L. J., & Linney, K. D. (1998, November). *Alcohol use, marital functioning and the family life cycle.* Paper presented at the Annual Meeting of the National Council on Family Relations, Milwaukee, WI.

Roberts, L. J., Roberts, C. F., & Leonard, K. E. (1999). Alcohol, drugs, and interpersonal violence. In V. B. Van Hasselt & M. Hersen (Eds.), *Handbook of psychological approaches with violent criminal offenders: Contemporary strategies and issues* (pp. 493–519). New York: Plenum.

Roberts, M. C., Floyd, F. J., O'Farrell, T. J., & Cutter, H. S. (1985). Marital interactions and the duration of alcoholic husbands' sobriety. *American Journal of Drug and Alcohol Abuse, 11*, 303–313.

Romelsjo, A., Lazarus, N. B., Kaplan, G. A., & Cohen, R. D. (1991). The relationship between stressful life situations and changes in alcohol consumption in a general population sample. *British Journal of Addictions, 86*, 157–169.

Room, R., Bondy, S. J., & Ferris, J. (1995). The risk of harm to oneself from drinking. *Addiction, 90*, 499–513.

Rotunda, R. J., & O'Farrell, T. J. (1997). Marital and family therapy of alcohol use disorders: Bridging the gap between research and practice. *Professional Psychology: Research and Practice, 28*, 246–252.

Rychtarik, R. G. (1990). Alcohol-related coping skills in spouses of alcoholics: Assessment and implications for treatment. In R. L. Collins, K. E. Leonard, & J. S. Searles (Eds.), *Alcohol and the family* (pp. 356–379). New York: Guilford Press.

Schaap, C. P. D. R., Schellekens, I., & Schippers, G. M. (1991). Alcohol and marital interaction: The relationship between male alcoholism, interaction characteristics and marital therapy. In G. M. Schippers, S. M. M. Lammers, & C. P. D. R. Schapp (Eds.), *Contribution to the psychology of addiction* (pp. 65–86). Berwyn, PA: Swets & Zeitlinger.

Segal, R., & Sisson, B. V. (1985). Medical complications associated with alcohol use and the assessment of risk of physical damage. In T. E. Bratter & G. G. Forrest (Eds.), *Alcoholism and substance abuse* (pp. 137–175). New York: Free Press.

Sisson, R. W., & Azrin, N. H. (1986). Family-member involvement to initiate and promote treatment of problem drinkers. *Journal of Behavior Therapy and Experimental Psychiatry, 17*, 15–21.

Skinner, H. A., & Horn, J. L. (1984). *Alcohol Dependence Scale (ADS) user's guide.* Toronto, Ontario, Canada: Addiction Research Foundation.

Sobell, L. C., & Sobell, M. B. (1992). Timeline follow-back: A technique for assessing self-reported alcohol consumption. In R. Z. Litten & J. P. Allen (Eds.), *Measuring alcohol consumption: Psychosocial and biochemical methods* (pp. 41–72). Totowa, NJ: Humana Press.

Sobell, M. B., & Sobell, L. C. (1993). *Problem drinkers: Guided self-change treatment.* New York: Guilford Press.

Spitzer, R. L., Williams, J. B. W., Gibbon, M., & First, M. B. (1990). User's guide for the structured clinical interview for *DSM–III–R*: SCID. Washington, DC: American Psychiatric Press.

Steele, C. M., Critchlow, B., & Liu, T. J. (1985). Alcohol and social behavior: II. The helpful drunkard. *Journal of Personality and Social Psychology, 48*, 35–46.

Steele, C. M., & Josephs, R. A. (1990). Alcohol myopia: Its prized and dangerous effects. *American Psychologist, 45*, 921–933.

Steinberg, M. L., Epstein, E. E., McCrady, B. S., & Hirsch, L. S. (1997). Sources of motivation in a couples outpatient alcoholism treatment program. *American Journal of Drug and Alcohol Abuse, 23*(2), 191–205.

Steinglass, P. (with Bennett, L. A., Wolin, S. J., & Reiss, D.). (1987). *The alcoholic family*. New York: Basic Books.

Steinglass, P., Davis, D., & Berenson, D. (1977). Observations of conjointly hospitalized alcoholic couples during sobriety and intoxication: Implications for theory and therapy. *Family Process, 16,* 1–16.

Tarter, R. E., & Vanyukov, M. (1994). Alcoholism: A developmental disorder. *Journal of Consulting and Clinical Psychology, 62,* 1096–1107.

U.S. Public Health Service. (1991). *Healthy People 2000: National health promotion and disease prevention objectives* (DHHS Publication No. PHS 91-50212). Washington, DC: U.S. Department of Health and Human Services.

Whalen, T. (1953). Wives of alcoholics: Four types observed in a family service agency. *Quarterly Journal of Studies on Alcohol, 14,* 632–641.

White, H. R., Bates, M. E., & Johnson, V. (1991). Social reinforcement and alcohol consumption. In W. M. Cox (Ed.), *Why people drink: Parameters of alcohol as a social reinforcer* (pp. 233–261). New York: Gardner Press.

White, L. K. (1990). Determinants of divorce: A review of research in the eighties. *Journal of Marriage and the Family, 52,* 904–912.

Wilsnack, R. W., & Wilsnack, S. C. (1990, June). *Husbands and wives as drinking partners.* Paper presented at the 16th Annual Alcohol Epidemiology Symposium of the Kettil Brun Society for Social and Epidemiological Research on Alcohol, Budapest, Hungary.

Wilsnack, R. W., Wilsnack, S. C., & Klassen, A. D. (1987). Antecedents and consequences of drinking and drinking problems in women: Patterns from a U.S. national survey. In P. C. Rivers (Ed.), *Nebraska Symposium on Motivation: Vol. 34. Alcohol and addictive behavior* (pp. 85–158). Lincoln: University of Nebraska Press.

Wilsnack, S. C. (1984). Drinking, sexuality and sexual dysfunction in women. In S. C. Wilsnack & L. J. Beckman (Eds.), *Alcohol problems in women: Antecedents consequences, and intervention* (pp. 189–227). New York: Guilford Press.

Wilsnack, S. C. (1991). Sexuality and women's drinking: Findings from a U.S. national study. *Alcohol Health and Research World, 15,* 147–150.

Wilsnack, S. C. (1995). Alcohol use and alcohol problems in women. In A. L. Stanton & S. J. Gallant (Eds.), *The psychology of women's health: Progress and challenges in research and application* (pp. 381–443). Washington, DC: American Psychological Association.

Wilsnack, S. C., Plaud, J. J., Wilsnack, R. W., & Klassen, A. D. (1997). Sexuality, gender and alcohol use. In R. W. Wilsnack & S. C. Wilsnack (Eds.), *Gender and alcohol: Individual and social perspectives* (pp. 250–288). New Brunswick, NJ: Rutgers Center of Alcohol Research.

Wilsnack, S. C., & Wilsnack, R. W. (1990, June). *Marital drinking and the quality of marital relationships: Patterns from a U.S. longitudinal study.* Paper presented at the 35th International Institute on the Prevention and Treatment of Alcoholism, International Council on Alcohol and Addictions, Berlin, Germany.

Wilson, G. T. (1982). Alcohol and anxiety: Recent evidence on the tension reduction theory of alcohol use and abuse. In K. R. Blankstein & J. Polixy (Eds.), *Self-control and self-modification of emotional behavior* (pp. 117–142). New York: Plenum.

Wilson, G. T., & Lawson, D. M. (1978). Expectancies, alcohol, and sexual arousal in women. *Journal of Abnormal Psychology, 87*, 358–367.

Zweben, A. (1986). Problem drinking and marital adjustment. *Journal of Studies on Alcohol, 47*, 167–172.

Zweben, A., & Barrett, D. (1993). Brief couples treatment for alcohol problems. In T. J. O'Farrell (Ed.), *Treating alcohol problems: Marital and family interventions* (pp. 353–380). New York: Guilford Press.

11

COUPLE APPROACHES TO SMOKING CESSATION

CARLETON A. PALMER, DONALD H. BAUCOM, AND
COLLEEN M. MCBRIDE

In the mid-1980s, researchers in the area of smoking cessation began to include social support as part of a multifaceted approach to helping people stop smoking (e.g., Lichtenstein, Glasgow, & Abrams, 1986). As a result, a number of studies were conducted to examine (a) the effects of a person's social environment (including the smoker's partner and relationship characteristics) on his or her smoking behavior and (b) the impact of partner assistance and conjoint cessation on individual success. Research consistently demonstrated the importance of environmental barriers and social support in smoking cessation; in particular, having a partner who smoked was predictive of continued smoking. Unfortunately, interventions designed to increase support and conjoint cessation that included the partner in intervention consistently failed to demonstrate improved intervention outcomes relative to interventions that targeted only the individual. The consistent failure of these approaches led many researchers to conclude that partner-assisted approaches were, at best, ineffective and, at worst, detrimental, in cases when encouraging conjoint cessation undermined both partners' success. Since that time, little systematic research has examined the role of partners in smoking and smoking cessation.

Despite the prior lack of success of partner-assisted smoking-cessation interventions, we believe a couple approach to smoking cessation warrants further consideration. In the past 10 years, advances in conceptual models for involving the couple in one partner's attempts at behavior change indicate that previous interventions might not have used partners in an optimal fashion. In this chapter, we review the literature outlining the impact of a partner on a person's smoking behavior, and we propose a new framework for using a couple approach to smoking cessation that capitalizes on recent advances in the psychology of couples and illness.

INDIVIDUAL PERSPECTIVES ON SMOKING

The harmful effects of smoking are well documented. In particular, smoking is a major risk factor for cardiovascular disease and cancer, the two major causes of death in the United States. Smoking is causally linked to more than 400,000 deaths in the United States and 2.5 million deaths worldwide each year (Shopland & Burns, 1993). In addition, smoking has been estimated to cost society $100 billion annually due to medical care, accidents, and productivity losses associated with early mortality (Warner, 1993). Thus, smoking has dramatic individual and public health consequences. Despite these consequences, about 25% of the U.S. population continues to smoke, with the highest rates of smoking, up to 30%, observed among those with low education and income (Centers for Disease Control, 1992).

Over the past decade, self-help strategies have become an increasingly common modality for smoking-cessation interventions (Curry, 1993). Typically, these programs involve a variety of behavior-change strategies, including information about risks, self-monitoring (e.g., number of cigarettes and smoking circumstances), stimulus control (e.g., avoiding exposure to smoking cues), and the development of smoking substitutes (e.g., drinking water, deep breathing, increasing exercise; Lichtenstein, 1982). In addition, individuals might be assisted in the use of relaxation and more general stress-management strategies. Cessation programs also can include nicotine-replacement methods such as patches and gums (Jarvik & Henningfield, 1993). Such individual cessation approaches have had limited success, with 1-year quit rates approaching 10% for self-help programs (Curry, 1993) and 25% for more intensive group programs (Lando, 1993).

The majority of these programs have focused on the individual despite consistent indications that targeting the smoker's social context might be beneficial. For example, Kottke, Battista, DeFriese, and Brekke's (1988) meta-analysis of smoking-cessation interventions indicated that successful interventions provided personalized support and assistance over the longest possible time period. Correspondingly, they concluded that smoking is a social habit, and that changes in smoking behavior may be "best achieved through change in the social environment" (Kottke et al., 1988, p. 2889). Intimate relationships enable this type of ongoing assistance for behavior change. Such a conclusion is consistent with current approaches to other addictive behaviors, such as abuse of alcohol, where a person's intimate relationship is commonly taken into account (e.g., McCrady & Epstein, 1995).

ASSOCIATIONS BETWEEN SMOKING AND RELATIONSHIP FACTORS

Smoking Concordance in Relationships

Perhaps one of the most compelling reasons for approaching smoking cessation from a couple perspective is that smokers tend to have close relationships with other smokers. Previous studies have indicated significant concordance for smoking within relationships, both before marriage (Sutton, 1980) and during marriage (Venters, Jacobs, Luepker, Maiman, & Gillium, 1984). In a sample of pregnant women, McBride et al. (1998) observed that 52% of smokers were in a relationship with another smoker. The concordance for smoking among couples who are not married suggests that smoking status is a selection factor in these relationships. That is, smokers appear to choose other smokers when entering a relationship. In fact, among married couples, smoking concordance has been found to be higher than the concordance for level of physical activity, alcohol consumption, and dietary beliefs (Venters et al., 1984). In addition, partners who smoke appear to demonstrate convergence in their smoking habits. Venters et al. observed that in addition to smoking status, partners were similar in the amount they smoked and the timing of any decisions to quit. Thus, individuals who smoke may enter into relationships with other smokers and become more similar to their partners in their smoking habits.

Concordance for smoking within relationships compounds two primary issues related to smoking. First, the harmful effects of smoking are magnified when both individuals in a relationship smoke. For instance, smokers in a relationship are likely to regularly expose one another to passive smoke, which has documented health risks (Surgeon General, 1986). Smoking in the context of a relationship also introduces health risks to children, other family members, and friends who are exposed to their smoking. Particularly troublesome is the high rate of smoking among women during pregnancy (e.g., Floyd, Rimer, Giovino, Mullen, & Sullivan, 1993) and postpartum (e.g., Fingerhut, Kleinman, & Kendrick, 1990; McBride, Pirie, & Curry,

1992), which increases the risk for health problems in infants and children (Burchfiel et al., 1986; Environmental Protection Agency, 1992; Martinez, Cline, & Burrows, 1992; Wright et al., 1994).

Cessation is also complicated by concordance of smoking habits. Statistical models of partners' smoking over time indicate that partners who are concordant for smoking have highly stable smoking habits and do not tend to change their habits independently (Price, Chen, Cavalli-Sforza, & Feldman, 1981). In addition, research has indicated consistently that living with another smoker significantly increases the likelihood that a person who has quit smoking will relapse (Coppotelli & Orleans, 1985; Garvey, Bliss, Hitchcock, Hienhold, & Rosner, 1992; Graham & Gibson, 1971; Murray, Johnston, Dolce, Lee, & O'Hara, 1995). In fact, at least one study demonstrated that her or his partner's smoking had a greater impact on a person's maintenance of cessation than did smoking by other family members, friends, or coworkers (West, Graham, Swanson, & Wilkinson, 1977). The implication of these findings is that a sizable group of individuals who smoke will not be able to quit successfully unless their partner's smoking is addressed.

Although the finding that a partner's smoking negatively affects a person's attempts to quit is robust, the mechanisms by which this influence operates have not been systematically examined. Nevertheless, we can offer several possible ways that a partner's smoking might influence a person's cessation. One possibility is that smokers are unable to give their partner the support needed for quitting (cf. Mermelstein, Cohen, Lichtenstein, Baer, & Kamarck, 1986). In particular, because the partner is continuing to smoke, she or he may not be able to genuinely express support for the person's decision to quit. In addition, the partner may have difficulty helping the individual come up with strategies for avoiding smoking. In essence, it may be difficult for smoking partners to support thinking and behavior that are contrary to their own practices. Such an explanation is consistent with McBride et al.'s (1998) observation that women who lived with a partner who smoked perceived receiving significantly less support for cessation than women who lived with a nonsmoker. As we discuss later in this chapter, absence of support for quitting has important implications for a person's cessation.

Another possibility is that a smoking partner will continue to expose the individual to cues associated with smoking over the course of her or his cessation efforts (cf. Mermelstein et al., 1986). Clinical observations suggest that when husbands continue to smoke, it is difficult for them to completely hide their smoking from their partner who is attempting to quit smoking. Even when husbands attempt to conceal their smoking, their wives tend to experience regular exposures to the smells and tastes associated with smoking, and they often encounter packs of cigarettes around the house. These experiences may undermine the stimulus-control efforts of their partner. Over time, exposure to smoking-related cues may increase the difficulty of a person's attempts to quit smoking.

A third possible explanation for the link between partner smoking and cessation involves the relationship patterns that can develop around smoking. Doherty and Whitehead (1986) used a family systems perspective to suggest that smoking becomes ingrained into the interactions that smokers have with their significant others. In particular, they observed that smoking behavior can come to play an integral role in partner interactions around issues of inclusion and control (Whitehead & Doherty, 1989). The issue of inclusion can be particularly relevant when both partners smoke. In this instance, smoking may contribute to a couple's need for togetherness by giving them a habit and a time to share (e.g., sitting on the deck and smoking a cigarette together). The implication of such a perspective is that smoking patterns may be difficult to modify without restructuring more general interaction patterns in the relationship, particularly when both partners smoke. In essence, one partner's decision to quit smoking may disrupt a couple's routines related to spending time together. To the degree that such changes produce conflict or discomfort, it is reasonable to posit that individuals will avoid making the changes.

In summary, one of the more compelling reasons for approaching smoking cessation from a couple perspective is that often both people in a relationship are smokers. In such relationships, the individual and family health risks related to smoking are increased, and the likelihood that either person will quit independently from the other is decreased. Although the specific mechanisms through which partner smoking affects an individual's cessation require further investigation, interventions that address the smoking of both partners in a relationship are expected to make valuable contributions to traditional self-help approaches.

Partner Support

Another compelling reason for taking a couple approach to smoking cessation is the consistent finding that social support from a partner significantly predicts a person's attempts to quit. This finding has provided the rationale for cessation interventions that involve partners of smokers. The evidence along these lines suggests that smoking-specific support (i.e., support that is focal to smoking behavior) affects cessation. In addition, some studies have indicated that more general support, support intended to aid the general functioning of an individual, also affects cessation.

To assess smoking-specific support, Mermelstein, Lichtenstein, and McIntyre (1983) developed the Partner Interaction Questionnaire (PIQ). This self-report measure assesses the frequency and helpfulness of positive (e.g., rewarding, praising, helping a partner cope with urges to smoke) and negative (e.g., nagging, criticizing, monitoring smoking) behaviors from a partner in relation to smoking. The PIQ has been used in a number of studies to examine the impact of smoking-related support on individuals' attempts at cessation. In the earliest study, Mermelstein et al. (1983) observed that over a 6-month period, partners of successful quitters demonstrated more reinforcement and cooperative participation in relation to the smoker's efforts than did partners of individuals who never quit or who relapsed. Such partners also were rated as more helpful than partners of unsuccessful abstainers. In addition, negative partner behaviors, such as nagging and monitoring, were negatively correlated with individuals' success in abstaining from smoking. Thus, Mermelstein et al. (1983) demonstrated that positive, helpful behaviors from a partner correlate with the likelihood that a person will abstain from smoking, whereas negative, unhelpful partner behaviors are related to unsuccessful cessation efforts.

The influence of smoking-specific partner support has been observed with the PIQ across a number of studies, indicating that this effect is somewhat robust (Cohen & Lichtenstein, 1990; Mermelstein et al., 1986; Orleans et al., 1991; Roski, Schmid, & Lando, 1996). However, the pattern of results concerning smoking-specific support has varied across studies. Whereas some studies have demonstrated that positive support significantly predicted cessation (Coppotelli & Orleans, 1985; Mermelstein et al., 1983), findings have more consistently indicated that the lack of negative behaviors is most correlated with cessation (Glasgow, Klesges, & O'Neill, 1986; Gruder et al., 1993; Lichtenstein et al., 1986; Roski et al., 1996). The importance of negative behaviors may be a reflection of the more general finding in couples research that negative interactions are more predictive of individual and relationship functioning than are positive interactions.

In addressing this varying pattern of results, Cohen and Lichtenstein (1990) examined the ratio of positive to negative partner behaviors as a predictor of cessation. They observed that the ratio of positive to negative partner behaviors was a more consistent predictor of cessation over a 12-month period than was either index alone. Cohen and Lichtenstein concluded from these findings that individuals experience a general sense of support from their partners based on the relative frequency of positive and negative behaviors. Again, this conclusion corroborates the general pattern of findings observed in research on relationship quality, demonstrating that the ratio of positive to negative behaviors is related to an overall impression of the partner and the relationship. In a further refinement, Ginsberg, Hall, and Rosinsky (1991) observed that positive support that encourages the mastery and autonomy of the smoker may be particularly effective. In summary, it appears that increases in positive support from a partner (e.g., rewarding, encouraging, helping with plans and strategies) and decreases in negative behaviors (e.g., nagging, shunning, checking, or policing) are predictive of individuals' success at cessation.

A few studies have examined the impact of more general social support from a partner on a person's attempts at cessation. These studies have been conducted both in general populations of smokers and in relation to pregnant or postpartum women, in which a partner's general support is relevant to both smoking behavior and health outcomes for the woman and child, surrounding the pregnancy and birth (e.g., Collins, Dunkel-Schetter, Lobel, & Scrimshaw, 1993). In general, studies of general social support and cessation have followed from the supposition that smoking can serve to regulate negative affect in response to stress (Ockene, Nuttal, Benfari, Hurwitz, & Ockene, 1981). Thus, as Mermelstein et al. (1986) have suggested, general support may influence cessation by "helping to create a more manageable and calm interpersonal environment or by helping to alleviate daily hassles, stress, or negative emotions" (p. 447).

Although conceptualizations of general support have varied in the smoking-cessation literature, they typically have included an emotional component (e.g., listening, showing concern, comforting) and an instrumental component (e.g., helping with chores and tasks, providing practical advice). One exception is a study conducted by Ockene, Benfari, Nuttal, Hurwitz, and Ockene (1982), which used partner attendance at an individual's cessation classes as an indicator of social support. This study demonstrated that individuals with partners who were willing to become involved in the treatment were more likely to quit smoking than individuals without such partners. Using more typical measures of general support, Coppotelli and Orleans (1985) observed that women with partners who helped with responsibilities and problem solving and expressed empathy, concern, and understanding were more likely to maintain abstinence from smoking over an 8-week period compared with women without such partners. Similarly, Mermelstein et al. (1986) observed that perceived availability of general support predicted individuals' attempts at cessation and maintenance of cessation over 3 months. In particular, individuals' beliefs that they had someone with whom they could discuss their problems was a consistently significant predictor of cessation. Pollak and Mullen (1997) observed similar results in a sample of pregnant women who spontaneously quit smoking. They found that emotional and instrumental support from a partner predicted women's abstinence over a 6-week period.

Thus, both smoking-specific and general support predict cessation. These findings suggest that training a partner to be supportive in relation to smoking and life demands and to avoid negative behaviors related to smoking might benefit a person's attempts at cessation.

Interactions Between Partner Smoking Status and Support

Although smoking-specific and general support appear to benefit cessation on average, there is some evidence suggesting that the effectiveness of such support can be influenced by a partner's smoking status. For instance, Pollak and Mullen's (1997) findings suggest that general social support from a partner benefits cessation when the partner is a nonsmoker, but not when the partner is a smoker. In their study, women who received general support from a smoking partner were approximately five times more likely to return to smoking than women who received general support from a nonsmoking partner. At least one interpretation of these data is that a partner's continued smoking will override the effects of any social support that the partner provides. Such an effect may indicate that partner smoking status is a more powerful predictor of an individual's cessation than is social support. The interaction between partner smoking and partner support also might indicate that a partner's smoking decreases the amount of support that the individual perceives, as has been observed by other investigators (Aaronson, 1989; McBride et al., 1998). Thus, in cases in which the partner smokes, it may be as important or more important to help the partner stop smoking as it is to help the partner be supportive.

However, support from nonsmoking partners also can be problematic. Typically nonsmoking partners are interested in an individual's quitting, and they may even be willing to help the individual quit. However, studies have observed that nonsmokers tend to display more negative behaviors toward their partners' smoking than partners who smoke (McBride et al., 1998; Orleans et al., 1991). That is, they tend to use more coercive and negative strategies when "supporting" their partner's quitting. The reasons why nonsmoking partners tend to be more negative have not been investigated. However, it is likely that such behavior results at least in part from a lack of empathy or understanding related to the process of quitting smoking. Given that negative behaviors are an impediment to cessation, it is important that nonsmoking partners understand the quitting process and learn to avoid negative behaviors if not replace them with more genuinely supportive behaviors.

In summary then, it is important to take a partner's smoking status into account when examining the effects of support on cessation. Individuals with a smoking partner may not benefit from support if the partner continues to smoke. Individuals with a nonsmoking partner may experience more negative support than positive support, which can serve as an impediment to cessation. Such an interaction between smoking status and support has important implications for intervening with a couple around smoking cessation.

Partner Smoking, Support, and the Cessation Process

In addition to the interactions between partner smoking and partner support, some evidence suggests that these variables may influence a person's smoking behavior somewhat differently over the course of cessation efforts. In particular, findings indicate that partner support tends to predict cessation or maintenance of cessation over a short-term follow-up (e.g., Coppotelli & Orleans, 1985; Pollak & Mullen, 1997). By contrast, examinations of partner smoking status demonstrate that a partner's smoking has a consistent, negative impact on a person's long-term maintenance of cessation (e.g., Murray et al., 1995; Stevens, Greene, & Primavera, 1982; West et al., 1977); however, partner smoking status may not influence initial attempts at quitting (e.g., Gunn, 1983).

Such a pattern of results was observed by Mermelstein et al. (1986), in their 12-month follow-up of individuals participating in formal smoking-cessation programs. They observed significant effects of smoking-specific and general support on initial cessation attempts and short-term maintenance (3 months). At 12-month follow-up, the effects of support were no longer significant; however, the negative impact of having other smokers in the participants' social network had emerged as significant. In the context of these results, Mermelstein et al. (1986) proposed that smoking may consist of several distinct phases: initial cessation, short-term maintenance, and long-term maintenance. They suggested that support may help provide motivation and stress buffering as a person contemplates and begins a difficult behavior change. However, over the long term, individuals' abstinence may be more influenced by smoking in their environment than by general or smoking-specific support.

The decreasing influence of partner support during the cessation process raises important implications concerning the nature of social support. As Mermelstein et al. (1986) noted, support is a dynamic process that may change over time. In particular, partners may become less supportive as time passes and they perceive that smoking is no longer an issue for the individual. Partners also might become less supportive over time as they are frustrated by "slips" occurring in the individual's smoking. Thus, it may be important to provide support for the supporter, to ensure that a partner remains helpful during the quitting process.

Summary

In summarizing the research concerning smoking and relationship factors, we can begin to outline the ways in which a partner might affect an individual's smoking over the course of cessation. In the initial stage of cessation (i.e., a decision to quit and initial behavior change), it is important that partners provide support for quitting as well as more general support, which can serve as a stress buffer. In relation to smoking-specific support, partners should place emphasis on avoiding negative behaviors, which can impede attempts at cessation. Placing emphasis on avoiding negatives is particularly important for nonsmoking partners, who may not understand the difficulties associated with quitting. In addition to avoiding negatives, increases in positive support will increase the positive-to-negative ratio, which predicts successful cessation.

Once a person has begun the cessation process, it appears that partner smoking is a significant threat to continued abstinence. Perhaps by affecting several factors related to smoking cessation, partner smoking can have a consistent negative impact on long-term cessation. Given that the majority of smokers live with other smokers, attention to partner smoking is an important contribution from a couple perspective. Although there is little research concerning the conditions under which these variables operate and the mechanisms through which they have influence, partner smoking and partner support have emerged as clear targets for couple interventions around smoking cessation.

To our knowledge, no research exists concerning the links between smoking and more general relationship functioning. For example, to what degree does relationship conflict influence smoking behavior? Likewise, to what degree does smoking behavior or disputes about smoking habits affect relationship quality? Related to Doherty and Whitehead's (1986) family systems view, a couple intervention would benefit from knowing how and to what degree smoking becomes ingrained into partner interactions. Such investigations would enrich our understanding of smoking and smoking cessation for a couple.

COUPLE- AND PARTNER-BASED INTERVENTIONS

Previous Treatments

Several outcome studies have compared treatments involving a partner with treatments focusing on the individual. These studies have been variously reviewed by Campbell and Patterson (1995) and Lichtenstein et al. (1986). In general, previous interventions have focused on increasing support for the individual's quitting smoking, and they have used a variety of persons to provide support. As a result, partners in these interventions have included a variety of individuals in the process of cessation (e.g., coworkers or friends as well as partners). We review previous treatments involving any type of partner for two reasons. First, previous interventions involving friends or coworkers have typically used formats similar to those used in interventions involving partners. Thus, there is some basis for comparing treatment components across these studies. Second, because of a lack of direct comparisons, there is currently no evidence to suggest that involving a partner in cessation efforts is superior to involving some other kind of acquaintance. Given the evidence concerning a partner's impact on cessation reviewed earlier in the chapter, a couple approach to smoking cessation seems reasonable. We must acknowledge, however, the potential benefits of support from individuals outside of a marriage or intimate relationship.

Two treatment-outcome studies have demonstrated benefits for involving partners in an individual's smoking-cessation efforts. In Janis and Hoffman's (1970) investigation, 30 participants in a smoking-cessation program were paired and assigned to one of three partner conditions. All participants attended five weekly meetings, during which they were instructed about the cessation process and then given an opportunity for open discussion about their experiences. In the high-contact partner condition, participants were assigned a steady partner from the group and instructed to talk daily on the phone in addition to attending the weekly sessions. Partners were not given any instructions concerning the content of these calls. In the low-contact partner condition, participants were assigned a steady partner whom they spoke with only during the weekly meetings. In the control condition, participants were assigned to a different partner each week, and there was no contact outside of sessions. By the final session, partners in the high-contact condition had more unfavorable attitudes toward smoking, more favorable attitudes toward their partner and the clinic, and fewer symptoms of anxiety than did participants in the other two groups. In addition, participants in the high-contact condition demonstrated less smoking at 6-month and 1-year follow-up than did participants in the other two conditions, despite the fact that they were no longer in contact with their partners. The results of this study indicate the potential benefits of supportive contact between two individuals who have decided to change their smoking behavior. The nature of the study makes it difficult, however, to isolate the kind of support that was beneficial during the cessation process.

Gruder et al. (1993) examined a more structured approach to involving a partner in smoking cessation. In this investigation, smokers who were interested in a televised cessation program and who had a nonsmoking "buddy" willing to participate in treatment were randomly assigned to one of three conditions. All participants received a self-help cessation manual and were encouraged to watch 20 televised segments concerning smoking cessation. These components constituted the control condition. Participants in the discussion and social support conditions also attended three weekly group meetings, during which they discussed how to obtain effective support around quitting, and they received supportive phone calls from a counselor 1 and 2 months after the program ended. Partners in the social support condition also received a support guide and attended the second weekly meeting, where they met as a separate group and discussed specific ways to assist their partner. At the end of treatment, Gruder et al. observed significantly higher ratios of positive to negative behaviors (as measured by the PIQ) in the social support condition than in the other conditions. More specifically, levels of positive behaviors did not differ among the conditions, suggesting that the social support condition was most effective in decreasing negative behaviors from the support partner. Gruder et al. also found that participants in the social support condition used the cessation materials and watched the television programs more frequently than did participants in the other conditions. In line with this increased support and increased use of materials, participants in the social support condition demonstrated the highest levels of cessation at 6- and 12- month follow-up. Thus, it appears that participants with a trained and supportive partner were more involved in the program and more likely to quit smoking than participants without such a partner. Unfortunately, although the social support condition significantly enhanced initial cessation rates, it did not improve maintenance of cessation. By 24 months, participants in the social support condition evidenced cessation rates similar to those observed in the discussion condition. Although Gruder et al. did not present data to explain the findings concerning maintenance, the literature on prediction of cessation suggests that the presence of smokers in the participants' environments and decreases in support over time could have contributed to the findings.

In contrast to the findings of Janis and Hoffman (1970) and Gruder et al. (1993), several programmatic attempts to involve partners in cessation have not supported the benefits of this approach. In one such investigation, Abrams et al. (1985) assigned participants in a work-site cessation program to one of three conditions. As part of a cognitive–behavioral management condition, individuals were taught cognitive–behavioral coping strategies such as stimulus control, relaxation training, and cognitive restructuring. In a social skills–support treatment, individuals were taught to cope with interpersonal aspects of smoking (i.e., develop a nonsmoking support network) and were encouraged to identify a nonsmoking individual who could provide consistent support. In the health education–nonspecific-support condition, participants attended nondirective support groups and received information about the health consequences of smoking. At 6-month follow-up, general support and negative smoking-specific support were related to cessation across treatments. However, Abrams et al. did not observe differences in cessation rates or support among treatments. Thus, they concluded that social support treatment was not superior to individual treatment in helping individuals quit smoking. Note that the social support treatment was the least structured of any of the partner models that have been investigated in that it did not require the participation of a steady partner. In addition, all individual cessation training was eliminated from the social support condition. Our view, and the view expressed more consistently in the literature, is that partner involvement is a supplement to individual cessation programs rather than a replacement.

In another work-site study, Malott, Glasgow, O'Neill, and Klesges (1984) evaluated the effects of adding a coworker support program to an individual cessation intervention. Participants in the individual condition attended six weekly group meetings, during which they were presented with strategies for reducing their nicotine intake and controlling their access and exposure to smoking. Participants in the support condition participated in these same meetings but were placed in pairs and instructed to discuss their progress with their partner daily. In addition, individuals in the support condition received weekly installments of a support guide. To ensure that partners were performing helpful behaviors, individuals in each pairing exchanged a partner-support checklist, on which they indicated the behaviors that would be most helpful to them. Partners monitored their performance of these behaviors over the course of treatment. Individuals in the support condition did not demonstrate higher cessation rates than those in the control condition at 6-month follow-up. At the end of treatment, Malott et al. also observed no group differences in positive support. Two characteristics of the support condition may have contributed to these findings. First, participants rated the support condition as a less credible treatment than the individual condition. This finding suggests that individuals in the support condition may not have understood or agreed with the rationale for involving a fellow worker in their cessation efforts. Second, the materials that partners received focused only on increasing positive support behaviors. Lack of negative support was related to cessation, but positive support was not. Thus, Malott et al. concluded that an intervention that focused on decreasing negatives in support interactions rather than increasing positives might be more effective.

Glasgow et al. (1986) examined this possibility in a follow-up study of a work-site cessation program. Again, participants in the program were assigned to the individual cessation condition or to a support condition. However, two changes were made to the program. First, the support manual that partners received discussed increasing positive behaviors and decreasing negative behaviors. Second, participants in the support condition chose a significant other as a partner rather than including another participant as the support partner. This partner attended two of the six weekly meetings and received two phone calls during the program, which assisted him or her in providing support for the participant. As in the previous study, Glasgow et al. did not observe higher cessation rates in the support condition as compared with the control condition. Also similar to the previous study, they observed that negative behaviors were related to cessation but positive behaviors were not. In addition, no between-groups differences in supportive behaviors were observed.

A similar effort to involve an individual's partner or significant other in cessation was evaluated by McIntyre-Kinsolver, Lichtenstein, and Mermelstein (1986). Participants in this study were assigned to a cognitive–behavioral treatment condition or a combination of this treatment with a partner-support component. All participants attended six weekly group sessions covering issues including nicotine fading, self-management, and relapse prevention. Partners in the support condition attended the weekly meetings with the participants; they participated in the basic treatment plus group discussions about helpful and unhelpful support behaviors. Although trends in cessation rates at the end of treatment and over 1-year follow-up favored the support condition, the differences were not significant. In addition, although partner support was related to cessation over the first 3 months, there were no significant group differences on this variable. Thus, McIntyre et al. concluded that partner support was related to cessation but that the intervention was not successful in modifying partner support.

Perhaps most relevant to our discussion of a couple approach to smoking cessation is Nyborg and Nevid's (1986) comparison of couple and individual treatment. In this study, 40 couples in which both partners smoked were assigned to one of five conditions: a no-contact control condition or four treatment conditions that varied by therapist involvement (therapist administered vs. self-administered) and partner involvement (couples training vs. individual training). Participants in the therapist-administered treatments received eight weekly treatment sessions, whereas those in the self-administered conditions received self-help materials and weekly phone contacts. Participants in the individual treatments received a behavioral smoking-cessation manual and weekly contacts, in which the importance of individual coping was emphasized. Participants in the couple treatments received the cessation materials and, in addition, a support manual that included strategies such as mutual modeling of nonsmoking behavior, mutual monitoring, and partner or couple reinforcements for decreases in smoking. At the end of treatment and across 6 months of follow-up, participants in the couple treatments demonstrated the highest rates of cessation; however, the group differences were not significant. Several possibilities can be offered for the lack of significance in these findings. First, small sample sizes may have impaired the detection of group differences. Second, some components of the couple treatment (e.g., mutual monitoring of smoking) may have been experienced as negative or coercive, which may have lessened the impact of the intervention. Such an explanation is supported by significant decreases in couples' relationship adjustment across treatment. The observed decrease in relationship adjustment also could suggest that changes in couples' smoking patterns introduced conflict or strain that needed to be addressed in treatment. Finally, Nyborg and Nevid did not examine levels of support over time, leading them to suggest that mutual support may have attenuated or become more negative over time.

Summary

Previous attempts to involve a partner in cessation programs typically have not supported the benefits of such an approach in comparison with individual treatments. However, the consistent finding that partner support is related to cessation suggests that these interventions have lacked the intensity needed to modify smoking behavior and support within an interpersonal context. Review of the treatment literature and the literature on interpersonal predictors of smoking cessation suggest several ways that previous interventions may be improved.

First, previous studies have assessed neither the smoker's nor the partner's motivation with regard to treatment. As previously described, individuals often possess barriers to cessation. In addition, partners may be skeptical about their need to become involved in treatment and, as a result, may not be adequately motivated to provide support. One solution to this problem is to involve couples in smoking cessation at particularly relevant or "teachable" periods in their lives. Such periods may occur, for example, after significant health threats to one partner, such as a heart attack or development of cancer. In this context, both partners are likely to be motivated to change their smoking for the good of one or both partners. Another example is pregnancy, when smokers are likely to think about the harmful effects that smoking may have on the child and on their ability to be healthy parents (e.g., Haug, Aaro, & Fugelli, 1992). Pregnancy also typically occurs early in couples' lives together, so the cumulative effects of their smoking can be minimized. Our current efforts at involving the couple in smoking cessation are targeted at this teachable period of pregnancy. In general, it appears that couple interventions should take steps to maximize couples' motivations for involvement.

Second, the majority of previous interventions have not accounted for or addressed the smoking status of the supporting partner. Review of the literature on predictors of cessation indicates that partner smoking is an important, if not the most important, variable to consider. In particular, interventions targeting couples in which both individuals smoke need to incorporate a quitting process for both partners. Otherwise, attempts to increase support may be overridden by continued exposure to a partner's smoking. Along these lines, it is interesting that the two treatment studies showing significant effects specified the choosing of a nonsmoking partner or a partner who was quitting (Gruder et al., 1993; Janis & Hoffman, 1970).

Third, previous interventions have consistently used group formats for both individuals and couples. Although such interventions are highly efficient, these programs are least preferred by smokers, resulting in low participation and high attrition rates. Moreover, these interventions have placed little emphasis on tailoring program components to fit the needs of individual couples. In some interventions (e.g., Gruder et al., 1993), partners did not even meet in the same group as the individuals they were supporting. Perhaps a more appropriate technique from a couple perspective is to help individual couples reach a personalized agreement about support behaviors. In the context of an ongoing therapeutic relationship, couples can then be contacted at several points, both individually and together, to help solve any problems that have arisen in their support efforts. Such an approach maximizes the likelihood that general support principles will be applied appropriately to a given couple. These approaches can be adapted for use in state-of-the-art self-help cessation interventions that include follow-up telephone counseling.

Fourth, previous interventions have varied in their emphasis on decreasing negative behaviors versus increasing positive behaviors. Findings from both basic research and from treatment-outcome studies demonstrate that emphasis must be placed on decreasing negative behaviors in relation to smoking. Behaviors such as nagging, criticizing, and policing are impediments to cessation. Positive behaviors, such as rewarding and praising, are not unimportant, but they have a less consistent relation to cessation. Therefore, increasing positives should be emphasized only to the degree that such emphasis does not weaken attention to the negatives. The same is true for enhancement of more general social support. Although such support is important for general life and relationship functioning and may benefit cessation, it should not dilute a focus on reducing negative behaviors around smoking.

In conclusion, although the results of previous treatment studies provide inconsistent support for the benefits of involving a partner, the results of these studies in conjunction with findings from basic research lay the groundwork for the next series of investigations. What we have learned about couple functioning and smoking, along with the use of more recent conceptual models for couple interventions, may increase the efficacy of couple approaches to smoking cessation.

PROPOSED MODEL

Taking into account the findings regarding predictors of cessation along with the results of previous treatment studies, we propose a framework for working with couples around smoking cessation. This framework uses the different ways of including a partner in treatment of an individual outlined by Baucom, Shoham, Mueser, Daiuto, and Stickle (1998). Therefore, we discuss three conceptual models for involving partners in smoking-cessation interventions: partner assisted, disorder specific, and general couples therapy. We then discuss how these three approaches can be included in a comprehensive intervention framework. The appropriateness of these different intervention approaches is likely to vary as a function of the couple's needs and the setting within which the intervention is offered. For example, the three approaches differ in the degree to which the couple is asked to change aspects of their relationship to promote smoking cessation. In some instances, couples might need to restructure certain aspects of their interaction (e.g., not going to smoke-filled nightspots) to assist the smoker, whereas other couples might not need to alter many aspects of their couple functioning. In addition, persons who seek intervention for smoking cessation per se might not wish to explore their relationship with their partners; similarly, the partners of these individuals might not be willing to be involved in such an intervention. However, couples who are seeking intervention for relationship distress and who also wish to quit smoking might be open to exploring their relationship more fully. Similarly, some intervention settings are focused on helping persons to quit smoking and might not have personnel appropriately trained to intervene more fully on couples' relationships. Furthermore, at present there is no evidence concerning the efficacy of the full model in comparison with more limited interventions. Therefore, we recommend that the proposed approaches be incorporated into cessation interventions and sequenced according to clinical indications (e.g., need for disorder-specific or general relationship work) and feasibility (e.g., clinical resources, opportunity for contact with couples over time). In addition, the general therapeutic guidelines presented here should be individually tailored to meet the needs of a given couple.

Given that self-help approaches are currently state-of-the-science with respect to smoking cessation, clinicians may face issues around justifying the involvement of a partner to an individual quitting smoking. If one or both partners express a desire to quit smoking within the context of ongoing couples work, this issue may be minimal. If an individual presents seeking help with smoking cessation, however, justifying a couple perspective may be necessary. Two lines of evidence contribute to this justification. First, strong evidence suggests that a partner's behavior affects an individual's cessation efforts. Second, interventions involving partners have been effective with regard to individual behavior changes such as weight loss (Black, Gleser, & Kooyers, 1990) and reduction of problem drinking (McCrady, Stout, Noel, Abrams, & Nelson, 1991). Thus, similar to other difficult behavior changes, it is anticipated that changes in smoking behavior can be influenced by a partner. Such reasoning can be conveyed to individuals or couples in a clinically meaningful way.

Partner-Assisted Interventions

In a partner-assisted approach to smoking cessation, the partner serves primarily as an assistant therapist or coach in the individual's cessation efforts. In this context, partner support is primarily smoking specific in that the partner helps the individual to construct and implement his or her strategies for quitting smoking. In such an approach, it is important that the smoker dictates the choice of individual coping strategies that will be most helpful, along with identifying behaviors from the partner that will be most supportive. In this way, the smoker can maintain a sense of efficacy in relation to quitting, which is an important predictor of cessation (e.g., DiClemente, 1981; Muddle, Kok, & Strecher, 1995). Following this general principle, a partner can assist an individual's efforts to quit smoking by avoiding negative–coercive behaviors, performing supportive behaviors with respect to cessation, helping the individual plan for high-risk situations, and by quitting smoking if she or he smokes.

Avoiding Negative–Coercive Behaviors

As outlined previously, the basic literature on predictors of cessation indicates that negative behaviors from a partner with respect to smoking are impediments to cessation. Therefore, it is important to help partners of smokers identify and avoid such behaviors. This aspect of treatment may be particularly relevant for nonsmoking partners, who tend to be more negative with respect to their partner's smoking. Examples of negative behaviors that should be avoided are nagging the partner to quit smoking, criticizing the partner's efforts to quit, checking the partner and the house for signs of smoking (e.g., smelling hair or breath, looking for cigarettes), and counting the number of cigarettes the partner has smoked (e.g., "Haven't you already had two today?"). On the surface, such behaviors appear easy for a couple to identify and label as unhelpful. However, partners often perform such behaviors in a good-faith attempt to help the partner stay motivated or committed during the cessation process. Therefore, it is important to engage the couple in discussion about the intentions behind such behaviors and the impact that they have on the smoker. Then, the partners should be assisted in finding ways to avoid negative behaviors or to find more positive ways of expressing their concerns.

Supportive Behaviors

In addition to avoiding negative behaviors with respect to smoking, partners can be helpful by giving positive support to the individual's cessation efforts. One form of such support is for the partner to find ways of effectively prompting or reminding the smoker to use his or her individual coping strategies. For example, if the individual is experiencing cravings for a cigarette, the partner may ask or remind the individual about relaxation strategies or cigarette substitutes that the individual had decided to use. Again, it is important that such prompting be done without criticism or negativity and with respect for the smoker's autonomy. Along the same lines, a partner may help the individual avoid smoking by taking a walk or playing a game. In general, the partner is making positive contributions to the individual's use of coping strategies.

Another form of support with respect to smoking involves reward, reinforcement, or praise for the individual's cessation efforts. Along these lines, a partner may offer verbal reinforcement (e.g., "I'm really impressed by the way you have been handling smoking lately") or some tangible reward (e.g., a surprise gift). It is important that such support be directed toward efforts rather than outcome, so that slips in the cessation process do not lead to a decrease in support. It is also important for the couple to decide on the kinds of reinforcement that will seem comfortable, as well as the timing of such reinforcement. Our experience suggests that smokers do not necessarily want to be praised every day for their cessation efforts. In addition, partners may not perform the supportive behaviors if they do not feel comfortable or natural. Thus, it is important to help the couple agree on effective support strategies.

High-Risk Situations

Another way that partners can assist in the cessation process is by helping individuals to plan for and cope with high-risk situations. These situations are ones in which the individual will feel particularly tempted to smoke. Within a partner-assisted approach, high-risk situations are confined to situations that do not involve aspects of the couple's relationship. For example, a partner may help the smoker plan for a long car trips if that is a situation where the individual typically smokes. (Within the disorder-specific approach, we address high-risk situations related to relationship habits or patterns.)

There may be two types of high-risk situations for the smoker as an individual; those where the partner is present (e.g., a cookout with friends) and those where the partner is absent (e.g., smoker goes to another smoker's house alone). In both situations, partners may contribute to a process of dealing with high-risk situations that involves several steps. First, the couple can work together to identify the situations that put the smoker at risk. Second, the partner can help the individual plan for coping with urges to smoke in those situations. Third, the partner can help the smoker evaluate her or his coping in the situation, provide praise and reinforcement, and help plan any changes for the future. When the high-risk situation involves both partners, a partner also can support the individual's coping during the situation. Such support can be handled as previously described. In presenting this model to the couple, it is important to emphasize that dealing with high-risk situations is a dynamic and changing process that requires consistent communication and planning.

Partner Smoking

Finally, but perhaps most important, smoking by the partner should be addressed with respect to helping a person quit smoking. Emphasis on the partner's smoking is a somewhat difficult topic when the partner has not requested help with cessation. Nevertheless, partner smoking is a powerful predictor of relapse, and this fact should be presented to the couple from an educational and motivational standpoint. Thus, the first step in addressing partner smoking is educating the partner about the effects of his or her smoking on the individual who is trying to quit. Then the partner's readiness to quit smoking should be assessed, and intervention should be planned appropriately.

If a partner is not ready to quit smoking, it may be most appropriate to help the couple find ways of keeping the partner's smoking away from the individual and the household. In essence, the sights and smells of smoking should be removed from the individual's environment (e.g., cars, clothes, breath, house). Although such a strategy may be the only reasonable approach, our experience suggests that it is difficult to implement completely and, over time, carelessness may lead to exposure of the individual to smoking. As a result, partner quitting is the most desirable outcome. Furthermore, partner quitting may provide several valuable contributions to an individual's cessation process. First, it reduces the health risks associated with direct and passive smoking for both partners. Second, it may increase empathy and support for quitting from the partner while serving as an example of support. Third, as we have alluded to, it provides effective removal of an important and ongoing high-risk situation. Thus, partner quitting may be a powerful contributor to an individual's cessation process. One possible caveat to this approach is that it may increase the likelihood that partners will relapse together. However, no data exist regarding this issue. Therefore, given the impact of partner smoking on cessation, partner quitting currently appears to be an important goal of a couple approach to cessation.

Disorder-Specific Interventions

A disorder-specific approach to smoking cessation involves helping the couple identify and address interactions or aspects of the relationship that may contribute to smoking. This is in contrast to a partner-assisted approach, in which the partner serves as a coach or substitute therapist without attempting to alter his or her own relationship with the smoker. Thus, a disorder-specific approach targets more general aspects of the relationship that are related to smoking cessation. Common areas involved in a disorder-specific approach to smoking cessation are high-risk couple routines and more general aspects of support.

High-Risk Couple Routines

In the context of a partner-assisted approach, we outlined a process by which partners can help individuals cope with high-risk situations. In the disorder-specific context, we focus on couple interactions or relationship patterns that constitute or contribute to high-risk situations. For example, a person may be tempted to smoke whenever she or he is driving. A partner-assisted approach to this issue concerns ways that the partner may help the individual prepare for and cope with these cravings. A disorder-specific approach to the same issue might involve rearranging the couple's division of labor so that the smoking individual is not heavily relied on to drive. Other examples of couple routines related to smoking are coffee and cigarettes after meals, couple time around smoking before bed, or regular outings to smoke-filled clubs.

In essence, addressing high-risk couple routines involves helping the couple to modify patterns that contribute to smoking through problem solving (i.e., Baucom & Epstein, 1990). In some cases, it may make sense for the couple to avoid situations or devise new activities to replace the old ones (e.g., walking instead of smoking before bed, going to movies rather than clubs). In other instances, it may be most appropriate to modify the existing situations to decrease the likelihood of smoking (e.g., sitting in the non-smoking section of restaurants and walking after a meal instead of having dessert or coffee). Thus, partners should identify high-risk situations and develop appropriate and mutually acceptable solutions.

General Support

Partners may contribute to cessation directly by providing smoking-specific support in a partner-assisted manner. However, couples also can increase patterns of general support in the relationship in ways that decrease stress on the individuals. Thus, general support from a partner may benefit cessation indirectly through stress reduction. In helping couples increase general support in the relationship, we focus on two primary categories of support. First, partners can provide emotional support by listening to a variety of problems, expressing empathy and understanding, and providing general praise and encouragement. Second, partners can provide instrumental support, such as helping with household chores or tasks. As with partner-assisted support, it is important to engage the couple in discussion about the ways in which general support can be provided most effectively. This discussion may involve sharing feelings about desired support and problem solving around how support will be provided (i.e., Baucom & Epstein, 1990).

To create stable mechanisms for general support, it seems important to make the support as reciprocal as possible. Obviously, the goal of general support is to assist the smoker in the process of cessation. However, unless the partner is adequately reinforced for support or unless support is somewhat reciprocal, it may decline over time. Therefore, it seems important to help the couple think about ways to support or reinforce the supporter. This issue is somewhat more straightforward when both partners are quitting. In that case, general support should be mutual and reciprocal.

General Couples Therapy

A final model for involving the partner in smoking cessation is through general couple therapy. The logic behind such an approach is that relationship distress or conflict provides a general stressor that affects individual functioning (Baucom et al., 1998). Thus, relationship conflict or dissatisfaction might increase a person's stress level and subsequent smoking behavior. In addition, it is likely to be difficult for individuals in a distressed relationship to give and receive support effectively. As a result, relationship distress may decrease the efficacy of the interventions we have described thus far. Therefore, when clinically indicated, it may be beneficial to work with the couple around general relationship issues before or along with smoking-specific interventions. For example, couples might be taught communication skills that they apply to issues in the relationship before applying them to smoking-related concerns.

Couple therapy also might serve as an important adjunct to more specific interventions. As Nyborg and Nevid's (1986) findings suggest, alteration of smoking patterns in a relationship may produce relationship distress or conflict. In particular, smoking behaviors may serve important needs within the relationship that must be renegotiated when smoking patterns change (e.g., Doherty & Whitehead, 1986). For example, smoking may be a way for a partner to communicate their need for time alone (e.g., "I am going out back to have a cigarette"). When this behavior is removed, the partner may benefit from finding new ways to express that need effectively.

Despite its possible contribution within a couples approach to smoking cessation, general couples therapy will be an infrequent intervention. If a couple presents for general couples therapy and smoking cessation is raised during that process, then it may be relatively easy to address both issues. It is less likely, however, that an individual presenting for assistance with cessation will be interested in general couples therapy. The first step in this latter case is to determine the partner's involvement in smoking-specific interventions. If a partner becomes involved in cessation and general couples therapy seems indicated, then the couple may be presented with the rationale that relationship stress can increase an individual's smoking. Such a rationale may help the couple justify attention to more general relationship issues in relation to smoking cessation.

CONCLUSIONS AND FUTURE DIRECTIONS

Couple approaches to smoking cessation remain in their infancy. Despite strong evidence that a partner's behavior can affect an individual's success with cessation, investigators have yet to develop highly effective strategies that consistently increase partner support for an individual's cessation attempts. Smoking cessation is a difficult behavior change to induce and perhaps even more difficult to maintain over a long time period. Successful couple-based interventions likely will require that both individuals be motivated at the same time period, along with receiving helpful strategies for support and stopping smoking. We believe that certain time periods or phases in a couple's life cycle are likely to contribute to this joint, high level of motivation. In essence, there might be teachable moments that increase the couple's likelihood of working together productively. As noted earlier, such times might occur after one individual has experienced a serious illness or disease, such as cancer or heart disease. On a more normative basis, couples also might be motivated to quit smoking when the woman is pregnant. At present, we are conducting a brief, partner-assisted and disorder-specific intervention following the principles outlined in this chapter to assist pregnant women and their partners in smoking cessation. We hope that with the benefit of findings from previous investigations and this time of high motivation for both men and women, we can assist couples with this important, yet complex and difficult behavior change.

REFERENCES

Aaronson, L. S. (1989). Perceived and received support: Effects on health behavior during pregnancy. *Nursing Research, 39,* 4–9.

Abrams, D. B., Pinto, R. P., Monti, P. M., Jacobus, S., Brown, R., & Elder, J. P. (1985, March). *Health education vs. cognitive stress management vs. social support training for relapse prevention in worksite smoking cessation.* Paper presented at the annual convention of the Society for Behavioral Medicine, New Orleans, LA.

Baucom, D. H., & Epstein, N. (1990). *Cognitive behavioral marital therapy.* New York: Brunner/Mazel.

Baucom, D. H., Shoham, V., Mueser, K. T., Daiuto, A., & Stickle, T. R. (1998). Empirically supported couple and family interventions for marital distress and adult mental health problems. *Journal of Consulting and Clinical Psychology, 66,* 53–88.

Black, D. R., Gleser, L. J., & Kooyers, K. J. (1990). A meta-analytic evaluation of couples weight-loss programs. *Health Psychology, 9,* 330–347.

Burchfiel, C. M., Higgins, M. W., Keller, J. B., Howatt, W.F., Butler, W. J., & Higgins, I. T. (1986). Passive smoking in childhood. *American Review of Respiratory Disease, 133,* 966–973.

Campbell, T. L., & Patterson, J. M. (1995). The effectiveness of family interventions in the treatment of physical illness. *Journal of Marital and Family Therapy, 21,* 545–583.

Centers for Disease Control. (1992). Cigarette smoking among adults—United States, 1990. *Morbidity and Mortality Weekly Reports, 41,* 354–355.

Cohen, S., & Lichtenstein, E. (1990). Partner behaviors that support quitting smoking. *Journal of Consulting and Clinical Psychology, 58,* 304–309.

Collins, N. L., Dunkel-Schetter, C., Lobel, M., & Scrimshaw, S. C. M. (1993). Social support in pregnancy: Psychosocial correlates of birth outcomes and postpartum depression. *Journal of Personality and Social Psychology, 65,* 1243–1258.

Coppotelli, H., & Orleans, C. T. (1985). Partner support and other determinants of smoking cessation maintenance among women. *Journal of Consulting and Clinical Psychology, 49,* 648–658.

Curry, S. J. (1993). Self-help interventions for smoking cessation. *Journal of Consulting and Clinical Psychology, 59,* 318–324.

DiClemente, C. C. (1981). Self-efficacy and smoking cessation maintenance: A preliminary report. *Cognitive Therapy and Research, 5,* 175–187.

Doherty, W. J., & Whitehead, D. (1986). The social dynamics of cigarette smoking: A family systems perspective. *Family Process, 25,* 453–459.

Environmental Protection Agency, Office of Health and Environmental Assessment. (1992). *Respiratory health effects of passive smoking: Lung cancer and other disorders* (Report No. EPA/600/60-90/100 F). Washington, DC: Author.

Fingerhut, L. A., Kleinman, J. C., & Kendrick, J. S. (1990). Smoking before, during, and after pregnancy. *American Journal of Public Health, 80,* 541–544.

Floyd, R. L., Rimer, B. K., Giovino, G. A., Mullen, P. D., & Sullivan, S. E. (1993). A review of smoking in pregnancy: Effects on pregnancy outcomes and cessation efforts. *Annual Review of Public Health, 14,* 379–411.

Garvey, A. J., Bliss, R. E., Hitchcock, J. L., Heinhold, J. W., & Rosner, B. (1992). Predictors of smoking relapse among self-quitters: A report from the normative aging study. *Addictive Behaviors, 17,* 367–377.

Ginsberg, D., Hall, S. H., & Rosinsky, M. (1991). Partner interaction and smoking cessation: A pilot study. *Addictive Behaviors, 16,* 195–202.

Glasgow, R. E., Klesges, R. C., & O'Neill, H. K. (1986). Programming social support for smoking modification: An extension and replication. *Addictive Behaviors, 11,* 329–345.

Graham, S., & Gibson, R. W. (1971). Cessation of patterned behavior: Withdrawal from smoking. *Social Science and Medicine, 5,* 319–337.

Gruder, C. L., Mermelstein, R. J., Kirkendol, R. H., Hedeker, D., Wong, S. C., Schreckengost, J., Warnecke, R. B., Burzette, R., & Miller, T. Q. (1993). Effects of social support and relapse prevention training as adjuncts to a televised smoking cessation intervention. *Journal of Consulting and Clinical Psychology, 61,* 113–120.

Gunn, R. C. (1983). Does living with smokers make quitting cigarettes more difficult? *Addictive Behaviors, 8,* 429–432.

Haug, K., Aaro, L. E., & Fugelli, P. (1992). Smoking habits in early pregnancy and attitudes toward smoking cessation among pregnant women and their partners. *Family Practice, 9,* 494–499.

Janis, I. L., & Hoffman, D. (1970). Facilitating effects of daily contact between partners who make a decision to cut down on smoking. *Journal of Personality and Social Psychology, 17,* 23–35.

Jarvik, M. E., & Henningfield, J. E. (1993). Pharmacological adjuncts for the treatment of tobacco dependence. In C. T. Orleans & J. Slade (Eds.), *Nicotine addiction: Principles and management* (pp. 245–261). New York: Oxford University Press.

Kottke, T. E., Battista, R. N., DeFriese, G. H., & Brekke, M. L. (1988). Attributes of successful smoking interventions in medical practice: A meta-analysis of 39 controlled trials. *Journal of the American Medical Association, 259,* 2883–2889.

Lando, H. A. (1993). Formal quit smoking treatments. In C. T. Orleans & J. Slade (Eds.), *Nicotine addiction: Principles and management* (pp. 221–244). New York: Oxford University Press.

Lichtenstein, E. (1982). The smoking problem: A behavioral perspective. *Journal of Consulting and Clinical Psychology, 50,* 804–819.

Lichtenstein, E., Glasgow, R. E., & Abrams, D. B. (1986). Social support in smoking cessation: In search of effective interventions. *Behavior Therapy, 17,* 607–619.

Malott, J. M. Glasgow, R. E., O'Neill, H. K., & Klesges, R. C. (1984). Co-worker social support in a worksite smoking control program. *Journal of Applied Behavior Analysis, 17,* 485–495.

Martinez, F. D., Cline, M., & Burrows, B. (1992). Increased incidence of asthma in children of smoking mothers. *Pediatrics, 89,* 21–26.

McBride, C. M., Curry, S. J., Grothaus, L. C., Nelson, J. C., Lando, H., & Pirie, P. L. (1998). Partner smoking status and pregnant smoker's perceptions of support for and likelihood of smoking cessation. *Health Psychology, 17,* 63–69.

McBride, C. M., Pirie, P. L., & Curry, S. (1992). Postpartum relapse to smoking: A prospective study. *Health Education Research: Theory and Practice, 7,* 381–390.

McCrady, B. S., & Epstein, E. (1995). Couples therapy in the treatment of alcohol problems. In N. S. Jacobson & A. S. Gurman (Eds.), *Clinical handbook of couple therapy* (pp. 369–393). New York: Guilford Press.

McCrady, B. S., Stout, R., Noel, N., Abrams, D., & Nelson, H. F. (1991). Effectiveness of three types of spouse-involved behavioral alcoholism treatment. *British Journal of Addiction, 86,* 1415–1424.

McIntyre-Kingsolver, K., Lichtenstein, E., & Mermelstein, R. J. (1986). Spouse training in a multi-component smoking-cessation program. *Behavior Therapy, 17,* 67–74.

Mermelstein, R., Cohen, S., Lichtenstein, E., Baer, J. S., & Kamarck, T. (1986). Social support and smoking cessation and maintenance. *Journal of Consulting and Clinical Psychology, 54,* 447–453.

Mermelstein, R., Lichtenstein, E., & McIntyre, K. (1983). Partner support and relapse in smoking-cessation programs. *Journal of Consulting and Clinical Psychology, 50,* 465–466.

Muddle, A. N., Kok, G., & Strecher, W. J. (1995). Self-efficacy as a predictor for the cessation of smoking: Methodological issues and implications for smoking cessation programs. *Psychology and Health, 10,* 353–367.

Murray, R. P., Johnston, J. J., Dolce, J. J., Lee, W. W., & O'Hara, P. (1995). Social support for smoking cessation and abstinence: The lung health study. *Addictive Behaviors, 20,* 159–170.

Nyborg, K. F., & Nevid, J. S. (1986). Couples who smoke: A comparison of couples training versus individual training for smoking cessation. *Behavior Therapy, 17,* 620–625.

Ockene, J. K., Benfari, R. S., Nuttal, R. L., Hurwitz, I., & Ockene, I. S. (1982). Relationship of prosocial factors to smoking behavior changes in an intervention program. *Preventive Medicine, 11,* 13–28.

Ockene, J. K., Nuttal, R. L., Benfari, R. S., Hurwitz, I., & Ockene, I. S. (1981). A psychosocial model of smoking cessation and maintenance of cessation. *Preventive Medicine, 10,* 623–638.

Orleans, C. T., Schoenbach, V. J., Wagner, E. H., Quade, D., Salmon, M. A., Pearson, D. C., Fiedler, J., Porter, C. Q., & Kaplan, B. H. (1991). Self-help quit smoking interventions: Effects of self-help materials, social support instructions, and telephone counseling. *Journal of Consulting and Clinical Psychology, 59,* 439–448.

Pollak, K. I., & Mullen, P. D. (1997). An exploration of the effects of partner smoking, type of social support, and stress on postpartum smoking in married women who stopped smoking during pregnancy. *Psychology of Addictive Behaviors, 11,* 182–189.

Price, R. A., Chen, K., Cavalli-Sforza, L. L., & Feldman, M. W. (1981). Models of spouse influence and their applications to smoking behavior. *Social Biology, 28,* 14–29.

Roski, J., Schmid, L. A., & Lando, H. A. (1996). Long-term associations of helpful and harmful spousal behaviors with smoking cessation. *Addictive Behaviors, 2,* 173–185.

Shopland, D. R., & Burns, D. M. (1993). Medical and public health implications of tobacco addiction. In C. T. Orleans & J. Slade (Eds.), *Nicotine addiction: Principles and management* (pp. 105–128). New York: Oxford University Press.

Stevens, P. A., Greene, J. G., & Primavera, L. H. (1982). Predicting successful smoking cessation. *Journal of Social Psychology, 118,* 235–241.

Sutton, G. (1980). Assortative marriage for smoking habits. *Annals of Human Biology, 7,* 449–456.

Surgeon General. (1986). *The health consequences of involuntary smoking: A report of the Surgeon General* (DHHS Publication No. CDC 87–8398). Washington, DC: U.S. Government Printing Office.

Venters, M. H., Jacobs, D. R., Luepker, R. V., Maiman, L. A., & Gillium, R. F. (1984). Spouse concordance of smoking patterns: The Minnesota heart survey. *American Journal of Epidemiology, 120,* 608–616.

Warner, K. E. (1993). The economics of tobacco. In C. T. Orleans & J. Slade (Eds.), *Nicotine addiction: Principles and management* (pp. 46–58). New York: Oxford University Press.

West, D. W., Graham, S., Swanson, M., & Wilkinson, G. (1977). Five year follow-up of a smoking withdrawal clinic population. *American Journal of Public Health, 67,* 536–543.

Whitehead, D., & Doherty, W. J. (1989). Systems dynamics in cigarette smoking: An exploratory study. *Family Systems Medicine, 7,* 264–273.

Wright, A. L., Holberg, C. J., Martinez, F. D., Halonen, M., Morgan, M., & Taussig, L. M. (1994). Epidemiology of physician-diagnosed allergic rhinitis in childhood. *Pediatrics, 94,* 895–901.

12

WHEN THE BOUGH BREAKS: THE RELATIONSHIP BETWEEN CHRONIC ILLNESS IN CHILDREN AND COUPLE FUNCTIONING

REBECCA GAITHER, KRISTIN BINGEN, AND JOYCE HOPKINS

BACKGROUND

This chapter focuses on the relationship between couple functioning and chronic illness in children. Unlike the other chapters in this volume, therefore, this chapter examines the reciprocal relationship between illness and couple functioning in a triadic rather than a dyadic relationship. Another unique aspect of this chapter is the developmental issues that affect these relationships because children vary in their ability to understand their illness and to participate in their own care at different developmental stages. The developmental stage of the child, therefore, may play an important role in the impact of the illness on the couple. Families also have developmental stages that serve as important factors in the response to the child's illness. For example, if the child with chronic illness is a firstborn infant, the couple has to learn to cope with caring for a chronically ill child while they are adjusting to the transition to parenthood. If the illness occurs in a family with more than one child, then parents have to cope with caring for the sick child as well as balancing the needs of other children at different developmental stages.

Chronic illness occurs in approximately 10% to 25% of children (Midence, 1994; Perrin, 1986) and consists of a large number of illnesses that vary in prevalence from being extremely rare to quite common. For example, asthma, which is considered to be the most common childhood illness, has a prevalence rate of 7% (Northey, Griffin, & Krainz, 1998), whereas cystic fibrosis (CF) has a prevalence rate of 0.05% (Thompson & Gustafson, 1996). Although it has been estimated that medical expenses are up to six times higher for a family with a chronically ill child compared with a healthy child (Northey et al., 1998), the total economic impact of chronic childhood illness is difficult to estimate. Medical costs may include expenses for extended hospital stays for acute phases of illness, home nursing care, daily medication regimens, and physical therapies. With managed care limiting cost coverages, families may have to cover a large portion of these expensive procedures themselves, resulting in severe financial strain. In addition to the medical expenses directly incurred as a result of the illness, there also may be hidden costs. For example, there are no data on the loss of family income as a result of one parent voluntarily leaving employment to care for the chronically ill child. Socially, families may become constricted in their activities because they mobilize around caring for the ill child and severely limit their social and recreational activities.

In addition to the social and financial pressures, the emotional cost of caring for an ill child affects each member of the parental dyad differently, and this often leads to conflict or strain between the couple. The conflict or strain, in turn, may have a negative impact on the child's adjustment to the illness. Conversely, caring for a chronically ill child brings some couples closer together, and the strong positive relationship in the parental dyad may serve as a protective factor in the child's adjustment to the illness. The following case examples illustrate these two sides of the coin. In one family, the child's chronic illness led to couple distress and severe family problems, which, in turn, led to behavioral problems in the child. In the other family, caring for their child with a chronic illness had a positive impact on the couple's functioning, and the child's outcome was positive as well.

Case Example 1: A Family in Trouble

Raphael, a 6-year-old Hispanic boy, was diagnosed with hepatoblastoma, or cancer of the liver. Immediately after the diagnosis, Raphael underwent surgery to remove the cancerous cells and began weekly chemotherapy. When Raphael and his mother, Maria, initially came to the oncology clinic at a metropolitan hospital for treatment, Raphael's oncologist referred the family to the pediatric psychology service due to concerns regarding the family's adjustment to Raphael's unexpected and life-threatening illness. During the intake interview with Raphael and his mother, Raphael clung to his mother's side, often hiding behind her, to avoid interaction with the therapist. He appeared sad and withdrawn and would not verbally respond to the therapist. Maria was guarded, initially. However, as the session progressed, she began to tearfully disclose the struggles her family had endured since receiving Raphael's diagnosis.

She described the family composition as including herself, Raphael's father, Carlos, and Raphael's three younger sisters, a 4-year-old and 3-year-old twins. Since Raphael's diagnosis, Maria had been the sole caregiver of her four children while Carlos began to work overtime hours to support the family and pay for Raphael's mounting medical bills. Maria described that she was becoming overwhelmed with caring for her sick child and felt guilty for neglecting Raphael's siblings. Unfortunately, Maria had no social support available to assist her in caregiving because relatives mainly lived in Mexico. Additionally, Maria described feeling lonely and depressed due to being apart from her partner, and she felt that she had no one to talk to about her fears and worries related to Raphael's illness. At the same time, Raphael also was struggling to cope with his diagnosis and frightening visits to the hospital. He began to withdraw from his friends in the neighborhood and clung to his mother's side at home. Raphael began to quarrel with his siblings when his mother would divide her attention and had temper tantrums when he did not get his way.

Raphael's outpatient treatment consisted of weekly blood drawings and chemotherapy as well as a 4-day inpatient stay at the hospital for intravenous chemotherapy. During initial outpatient visits, Raphael would hide behind his mother and would become limp in her arms during the blood drawing and chemotherapy. He also avoided interacting with other children who visited the oncology clinic on a weekly basis. However, he participated in group art therapy at the clinic alongside his mother and with encouragement from his therapist, whom he had warmed up to. Maria often would cry while Raphael was receiving treatment and often struggled with managing Raphael's emotional and behavioral difficulties.

As treatment progressed, Maria began to report increasing relationship strain, stating that Carlos avoided the family's difficulties by working overtime. The couple did not spend any time alone together at home because their leisure time was spent caring for Raphael, and their relationship lacked the intimacy it once had. In addition, Maria spent many hours with Raphael during his inpatient visits, caring for him when he was getting sick from the chemotherapy, and she often felt too tired and depressed to interact with her partner. They frequently argued about how to manage Raphael's behavior problems as well. While Maria and Carlos would argue, Raphael often would withdraw to his room.

As family tension increased, Raphael's emotional and behavioral problems escalated. His temper tantrums and fights with siblings at home became more frequent, and he often would refuse to go to school. During clinic visits, he began to cry uncontrollably, while huddled in a corner of the room, and would physically attempt to refuse treatment. Attempts to soothe Raphael by his mother, therapist, and other physicians were often futile. Concerns were mounting regarding Raphael and his family's difficulties in adapting to his chronic illness.

Case Example 2: Resilience and Support

Jason, the firstborn in his Black family, was born with a congenital heart disease. After his birth, Jason spent his first 2 months of life in a neonatal intensive care unit in an incubator attached to heart monitors. Jason's mother, Cherisse, and father, Raymond, spent many hours visiting their newborn son together in the hospital. In addition to adjusting to parenthood, they were also coping with a life-threatening diagnosis in their firstborn. During this stressful time, the couple was referred by a neonatal nurse to a therapist within the hospital to help them cope with their son's illness and prognosis.

During his early years, Jason required a heart monitor while he slept, which, on many occasions, alerted his parents that his heart had arrested. Cherisse and Raymond made many frightening trips to the hospital emergency room, not knowing if their son would survive this particular crisis. Additionally, Jason had to visit his pediatrician frequently because every time he had even the slightest cold, he required medical treatment to prevent any more serious problems that might have further weakened his heart. While Cherisse and Raymond were increasingly becoming distressed with caring for their sick child, their relatives and friends rallied to provide much needed support by preparing meals for the couple, as well as listening to their troubles and concerns. In addition, Jason's grandparents cared for Jason for a few precious hours each week, during which time Cherisse and Raymond were encouraged by the therapist to see a movie or "get a bite to eat together." Although the couple felt guilty initially for leaving their sick child, they cherished the time they spent alone together and reported that it rejuvenated their strength and resilience in coping with their child's illness.

As Jason matured, his emotional strength grew as well. He often cried during his frequent doctor visits. However, he coped well with the intrusive medical treatments, including three corrective heart surgeries. During these times, Jason's parents attempted to lift his spirits by taking him on family outings (a younger sister was born when he was 4), such as a trip to the zoo or a sports event, whenever his strength permitted. Jason's parents alternated taking time off from work to transport him to the doctor. Whenever his health permitted, Jason enjoyed attending school and interacting with his peers, although he could not participate in sports because of his weakened condition.

Although doctors told Cherisse and Raymond that their infant probably would not live, Jason is now a well-adjusted 8-year-old. Cherisse and Raymond report that caring for a chronically ill child was extremely stressful, and they continually worry about Jason and his health, along with caring for his younger sister. However, the couple describes their struggles as bringing them closer, and they now cherish every moment they have together.

There are some obvious factors, specifically social support and financial resources, that may account for the dramatically different outcomes in each of these children and their parents. However, as the following review of the extant literature on the effects of chronic childhood illness on couple functioning will show, the empirical literature does not provide a clear answer as to what factors predict a positive versus a negative outcome.

ASSOCIATION OF ILLNESS AND COUPLE FACTORS

Effects of Childhood Illness on the Couple's Relationship

Given that caring for a child with a chronic illness is considered to be a major stressor (Gordon Walker, Johnson, Manion, & Cloutier, 1996; Sabbeth & Leventhal, 1984), it is generally assumed that the child's illness will have a negative impact on the couple's relationship. It is somewhat surprising, then, to find that the empirical literature does not necessarily support this view. Indeed, while some data indicate that having a child with a chronic illness has a negative impact on the couple's relationship (e.g., Allen, 1993; Tew, Payne, & Laurence, 1974; Whyte, 1992), results from other studies indicate that there are either no effects (Cappelli, McGrath, Daniels, Manion, & Schillinger, 1994; Kazak, Reber, & Snitzer, 1988; Nishiura & Whitten, 1980; Spaulding & Morgan, 1986; Taanila, Kokkonen, & Jarvelin, 1996) or positive effects (e.g., Barbarin, Hughes, & Chesler, 1985; Chang, 1991; Koocher & O'Malley, 1981; Mahlmann, 1994; Martin, 1975; Nulsen, 1990; Perrin & MacLean, 1988; Sabbeth & Leventhal, 1984; Vance, Fazan, Satterwhite, & Pless, 1980; Zimand & Wood, 1986). Specific negative effects that have been reported include lack of time with partner (Turk, 1964); communication problems (Turk, 1964; Whyte, 1992); higher divorce rates (Denning, Gluckson, & Mohr, 1976); increased relationship conflict (Crain, Sussman, & Weil, 1966); increased role strain (Crain et al., 1966; Quittner et al., 1998); and decreased relationship satisfaction (e.g., Cappelli et al., 1994; Hauenstein, 1990; Kazak, 1989; Kazak et al., 1988; Michael & Copeland, 1987; Quittner, DiGirolamo, Michel, & Eigen, 1992; Reynolds, Garralda, Jameson, & Postlethwaite, 1988; Sheeran, Marvin, & Pianta, 1997; Tew et al., 1974; Whyte, 1992).

Sabbeth and Leventhal (1984) were among the first to debunk the myth that having a child with chronic illness places a significant risk on the couple's relationship. In their review of 34 studies, they found low rates of divorce among parents of children with a chronic illness. However, they also found indications that parents of chronically ill children experienced more couple distress than parents of healthy children. More unexpectedly, other investigators have found an association between having a child with a chronic illness and positive effects on the couple such as increased closeness (Barbarin et al., 1985; Chang, 1991; Martin, 1975; Taanila et al., 1996), greater cohesion (Quittner, DiGirolamo, et al., 1992), and increased support (Barbarin et al., 1985).

One factor that may account for these apparently contradictory findings is that researchers have studied the impact of a wide range of different disease processes on the couple's relationship under the rubric of "the effects of chronic childhood illness." These diseases include illnesses as varied as CF, cancer, spina bifida, diabetes, and sickle-cell anemia. Although each of these illnesses shares common factors that might affect the couple relationship, such as burden of care and family stress, they also vary in terms of severity, course, and prognosis, which would obviously have a different affect on the couple relationship across different illnesses. Therefore, to integrate the findings and draw meaningful conclusions, this chapter presents the data that are specific to each particular illness.

Cystic Fibrosis

CF is an autosomal recessive genetic illness involving the mucus-secreting glands of the lungs, pancreas, liver, intestines, and genitals. This disease occurs in 1 in 2,000 live births in the White population, only about 1 in 17,000 births in the Black population, and extremely rarely in the Asian population (Thompson & Gustafson, 1996). CF leads to multiple physical problems, including chronic bronchial airway obstruction, gastrointestinal complaints, and maldigestion. Although CF is a lethal illness, recent advances in medical treatment have dramatically increased life expectancy to approximately 29 years (Ievers & Drotar, 1996). The medical management of children with CF requires an intense daily regimen of percussive therapy, dietary management, multiple and complex medication administrations, and physical therapy (Mrazek, 1991). As a result, the burden of care for a child with CF is stressful and demanding for the parents.

Descriptive studies that do not use a control group have found negative effects from the impact of CF on couple functioning. Whyte (1992) described several case studies of parents caring for a child with CF. These parents reported guilt feelings due to genetic transmission of the illness, fear of pregnancy, stress due to the chronic burden of care, and poor couple communication. Turk (1964) administered a questionnaire to 25 families of children with

CF and found that parents reported a decrease in time available for partner, less time and energy for sexual relationship, financial stressors that affected the relationship, and communication problems. Another study of 103 families (Denning et al., 1976) found that the burden of caring for a child with CF causes continual couple stress resulting from the home treatment program, burden of care falling on one parent, financial strains, fear of the child dying, pressure from relatives, the hereditary nature of the disease, and fear of pregnancy. They also found a 9.5 times greater divorce rate among the families of children with CF compared with the general population. Although these studies suggest areas of negative impact on couples with a child with CF, the lack of a control group, use of unstandardized assessment measures such as survey-type questionnaires and unstructured interviews, and use of descriptive rather than quantitative data bring into question the validity of the results.

Other studies have incorporated widely used, well-validated assessment instruments and healthy comparison groups. In one study (Quittner, DiGirolamo, et al., 1992), data indicated that parents of children with CF report lower couple satisfaction than parents of healthy children. Recently, Quittner et al. (1998) examined role strain, parenting stress, social and recreational time, couple satisfaction, intimacy, and depression in a well-controlled study of 33 couples caring for a young child with CF. These parents reported greater couple role strain on measures of conflict over child rearing issues, child care duties, and exchanges of affection compared with a matched group of parents caring for healthy children. In addition, the parents in the CF group spent less time in social and recreational activities than the parents in the comparison group. No differences were found in couple satisfaction or parental depression between the two groups.

To summarize, studies on CF in children have generally found a negative impact on the parents' relationship. Specific aspects of the relationship such as role strain, decreased time in social and recreational activities, greater time spent in medical caregiving activities, and decreased intimacy may lead to problems in couple functioning. Inconsistent results on the effects of CF on couple satisfaction may be due to differences in the age of the child population studied. It may be that parents of older children with CF have experienced a longer period of chronic stressors related to the child's illness, leading to less couple satisfaction over time.

Cancer

Childhood cancer consists of a variety of diseases, including leukemias, lymphomas, and cancers of the brain and central nervous system. Approximately 6,000 children are diagnosed with cancer in the United States each year (Chang, 1991). Children with cancer often require frequent hospitalizations for surgery and medical treatments, such as chemotherapy and radiation, and secondary complications. The course of the illness tends to change significantly across time, with recurrent remissions, relapses, and intermittent crises. Although cancer may be terminal, advances in treatment have led to increased long-term survival rates and cures, thus bringing cancer into the realm of chronic rather than acute illness (Mrazek, 1991).

Clinical anecdotal data reported by parents of children with leukemia who participated in weekly group sessions over the course of a year indicated that they experienced relationship difficulties consistent with role strain (Heffron, Bommelaere, & Masters, 1973). Specifically, mothers reported resentment toward the fathers, who could escape to jobs where they often worked long overtime hours, while mothers were left to handle the details of management of the ill child.

However, results from empirical studies are not nearly as clear-cut. For example, Lansky, Cairns, Hassanein, Wehr, and Lowman (1978) studied 188 families in which one or more children had a malignant neoplasm. There was a lower divorce rate among these families than in the normal population for the same time period. In a subset of these families, they found that 38 couples with a child with cancer experienced significant couple stress compared with 23 couples with a child with hemophilia. However, there was less relationship stress in the parents of children with cancer than in a standardization group of couples in couple counseling. Additionally, when the length of survival time since diagnosis was taken into consideration, there was not a corresponding increase in couple stress. These data suggest that although there may be some degree of couple distress associated with having a child with cancer, the distress may be relatively mild.

Furthermore, Barbarin et al. (1985) found that caring for a child with a variety of different cancer diagnoses had either a positive impact or no impact on the relationship of 32 couples. The parents of the children in this study reported feeling increased closeness and support from their partner since the child's diagnosis. Factors that influenced perception of relationship quality differed between men and women. Women who perceived their partner as actively involved in the medical care of their child tended to rate their relationship quality higher than women whose partner was not as involved. On the other hand, men rated their partner as less supportive, the more time she spent in the hospital with the sick child. Barbarin et al. also found a significant negative correlation between the length of the child's illness and the quality of the parents' relationship. On the basis of these results, they concluded that the burden of caring for a child with cancer serves as a chronic stressor, which may have a mounting impact over time.

Although it is clear from these studies that caring for a child with cancer is a stressful event for parents, it does not necessarily have a detrimental effect on the couple relationship. When distress occurs within the relationship, it does not appear to significantly affect functioning, because these couples report less distress than couples seeking counseling and divorce rates appear to be lower in the parents of children with cancer than in the general population. In fact, many couples report that having a child with cancer has brought them closer together (Chang, 1991). It appears that the positive impact on the couple relationship is mediated by the male partner's involvement in the various aspects of caring for the ill child and the woman spending more time with her partner. Although the data generally indicate that having a child with cancer has a minimal negative impact, or, in some cases, a positive impact, on the couple relationship, note that stage of the illness and length of time since diagnosis may be important factors in how cancer affects the quality of the relationship. However, these data all are based on retrospective or cross-sectional studies. Therefore, prospective studies that establish baseline functioning at the time of diagnosis and then follow families longitudinally are needed to determine the long-term impact of caring for a child with cancer on couple functioning.

Spina Bifida

Spina bifida is a congenital birth defect resulting from the malformation of the neural tube, which results in physical impairments ranging from paralysis to poor muscle control and scoliosis. Spina bifida occurs in approximately 1 in 1,000 live births in the United States (Thompson & Gustafson, 1996). The course of the defect itself is generally static, but common sequelae include incontinence, chronic renal infections, hydrocephaly, and physical deformities in the lower extremities (Spaulding & Morgan, 1986; Thompson & Gustafson, 1996). Treatment regimens can include surgical closure of the spine, shunting for prevention of hydrocephalus, and bladder and bowel treatment including periodic catheterization.

In general, the literature on the relationship between having a child with spina bifida and couple satisfaction suggests that this disorder has minimal impact on a couple's functioning. There is only one study in which the data have suggested that there is a negative association between couple functioning and having a child with spina bifida. Specifically, Tew et al. (1974) conducted a prospective, longitudinal study of 59 families with a child with spina bifida and 58 families of healthy children. The results indicated that about 70% of mothers of children with spina bifida and mothers of healthy children reported that they had a satisfactory relationship with their partner at the time of their child's birth. However, at the 9-year follow-up, only 46% of mothers of children with spina bifida reported having a satisfactory relationship, compared with 79% of the control group. Additionally, the divorce rate for the parents of children with spina bifida was higher than both the national average and the divorce rate in the control group. However, it is difficult to generalize from the results of this study because of the reliance on maternal report alone and the failure to use standardized assessment measures. Furthermore, results from several other studies failed to find a negative impact on couple functioning related to having a child with spina bifida. Specifically, Martin (1975) did not find greater divorce or separation rates in parents of children with spina bifida compared with either parents of healthy controls or parents of children with diabetes. In addition, 75% of those parents who divorced reported that their relationship was unsatisfactory before the birth of their child, whereas the mothers who remained married reported that their relationship with their partner had improved after the birth of their child.

Two other studies that used standardized, validated assessment measures and matched control groups also found no effects of caring for a child with spina bifida on the couple's relationship (Cappelli et al., 1994; Spaulding & Morgan, 1986). Spaulding and Morgan found no differences between 38 parents of children with spina bifida compared with a matched control group of 38 parents of healthy children on measures of parenting attitudes, relationship adjustment, stress, and family functioning. Also, parents of children with spina bifida reported having a relationship quality similar to parents of healthy children. Cappelli et al. reported that 46 couples with a child with spina bifida had lower divorce–separation rates than are found in the general population. However, although these studies were methodologically sound, they did not use a longitudinal design, and the possibility remains that over time having a child with spina bifida does have a negative impact on couple functioning, as indicated by the data in the Tew et al. (1974) study. To address this issue, a replication of this study, using both maternal and paternal report, as well as standardized, well-validated assessment measures, is needed. At the present time, the only conclusion that can be drawn from the literature is that having a child with spina bifida does not seem to have a negative impact on couple functioning in the short term.

Diabetes

Juvenile-onset diabetes is a disease caused by deficient production of insulin resulting in dysregulation of blood sugar levels. Approximately 1.6 per 1,000 school-age children are affected by this disorder (Thompson & Gustafson, 1996). Treatment of diabetes involves a daily regimen of insulin injections, blood sugar monitoring, and dietary and activity restrictions. Although diabetes can be life-threatening, children generally survive well into adulthood with careful adherence to daily treatment routines. However, hypoglycemic or hyperglycemic coma, ketoacedotic episodes, and vascular complications can occur (Mrazek, 1991).

Crain et al. (1966) found that parents of 54 children with diabetes had a significantly lower consensus on goals of family life and significantly greater role tension compared with parents of 76 healthy children. Additionally, there was a statistical trend for mothers of children with diabetes to report more couple conflict than mothers in the control group.

Descriptive data from a study on the effects of early-onset disability in their offspring on the couple relationship in parents of children with juvenile-onset diabetes, parents of children with mental retardation, and parents of children with motor impairment (Taanila et al., 1996) indicated mainly positive effects. Seventy percent of all the parents reported that having a child with an illness or disability did not affect their couple relationship at all, 23% reported feeling closer to their partner, and only 7% reported being drawn apart from each other. The authors reported that factors that were associated with a good outcome were the parents receiving adequate information about their child's illness or disability and parents having enough time for themselves.

Similarly, Nulsen (1990) found that parents of children with diabetes and parents of children with CF reported both good communication and couple satisfaction. However, both of these studies suffer from the lack of a comparison group of parents of healthy children, which makes it difficult to derive any conclusions from the findings. The only study that did include an appropriate control group (Crain et al., 1966) indicated that there were some negative effects on couple satisfaction associated with having a child with diabetes. Therefore, further research using standardized assessment measures, healthy comparison groups, and a prospective longitudinal design is needed to determine how caring for a child with diabetes affects the parental relationship over time.

Sickle-Cell Anemia

Sickle-cell anemia is a genetic disorder characterized by chronic hemolytic anemia and vasculopathy. Specifically, red blood cells in individuals with sickle-cell anemia contain an abnormal form of hemoglobin that forms long polymers as it gives up oxygen. These polymers cause the cell to bend out of a normal disc or donut shape into a crescent shape, like a sickle. When these abnormally shaped red cells go through the small blood vessels, they clog the flow and break apart. This can cause pain, damage, and a low blood count, or anemia. Sickle-cell anemia occurs in about 50,000 people in the United States, predominantly among the Black population. The symptoms include recurrent pain crises resulting from obstruction of blood flow due to the sickling of cells. The pain crises generally last 4–6 days but may last for weeks. Complications include occlusive strokes, intracranial hemorrhage, organ failure, cardiac complications, and immunologic complications. Treatment typically includes management of pain through hydration and analgesia. In addition, blood transfusions are used to treat acute complications (Thompson & Gustafson, 1996).

In a study of families with children with sickle-cell anemia between infancy and 17 years of age, few parents reported that their child's illness had negative effects on their relationship with their partner (Nishiura & Whitten, 1980). However, this study reported only descriptive statistics based on structured interviews and lacked a control group. In addition, slightly over one half of the families had only one parent in the home, and these parents were not asked about their couple relationships. The failure to assess the impact of having a child with sickle-cell anemia on the couple relationships among the single parents, whose relationships either had dissolved or never had occurred, may have prevented finding any negative effects.

Results from a study that did include a comparison group of 72 parents of healthy children (Evans, Burlew, & Oler, 1988) indicated that 78 Black parents of young children with sickle-cell anemia reported significantly less positive affect in their couple relationship than did the comparison group. However, although this study used an appropriate control group, the lack of standardized assessment measures also makes it difficult to draw meaningful conclusions from these data. Again, it is clear that further research is needed in this area to determine how having a child with sickle-cell anemia affects the couple's functioning.

Other Chronic Illnesses

Researchers have studied families of children with a variety of other chronic illnesses, including asthma, renal and gastrointestinal disorders, and phenylketonuria. Generally, results from these studies suggest that the divorce rate among parents of children with a chronic illness is similar to, or lower than, parents with a healthy child or the general population (Reynolds et al., 1988; Zimand & Wood, 1986). Similar to the finding presented in relation to specific childhood disorders, results of some of these studies indicate that having a child with a chronic illness negatively affects the parent's dyadic relationship (Allen, 1993; Reynolds et al., 1988), whereas others indicate positive or no effects (Kazak et al., 1988; Vance et al., 1980; Zimand & Wood, 1986).

Summary

Although there are a plethora of studies examining the relationship between couple functioning and having a child with a variety of chronic illnesses, results of these studies are often contradictory, even when assessing the effects of the same illness on couple functioning. These conflicting results may be due, in part, to the fact that many of these studies suffer from substantive methodological problems. Sampling problems include the lack of fathers in many studies, resulting in an overreliance on maternal report. Also, many studies include children who vary widely in age, so that children with diverse developmental capacities are collapsed into one group. Although some researchers have included unmarried parents, they consistently fail to assess relationship issues in these individuals, as though their lack of a marital partner is irrelevant. Many studies fail to use appropriate control groups or any comparison groups at all, making it impossible to determine if the couple distress is related to the child's illness or is typical of families at this particular developmental stage. Another problem is the use of unstandardized assessment measures to assess couple functioning and the lack of consensus between studies as to what domains should be measured to assess couple functioning, so that it is difficult to determine whether different researchers are even assessing the same construct. Finally, much of the research has relied on retrospective data. There is a serious lack of prospective longitudinal studies that assess couple functioning across the course of the child's illness, although length of time spent caring for an ill child has been shown to be a significant factor in determining how the child's illness affects the parents' functioning.

Despite these methodological problems, it is clear that having a child with a chronic illness does not necessarily have a negative impact on couple functioning. Although results from some studies indicate that there are negative effects, other data suggest that there are minimal, or even positive, effects. Also, there are no data that suggest that divorce rates are higher in families with a chronically ill child, and in fact, divorce rates tend to be lower than in the general population. To draw conclusions from these diverse findings, it seems necessary not just to assess the impact of a particular type of illness in their offspring on couple functioning, but to simultaneously examine how other factors related to that specific illness may interact with or serve as a mediator or a buffer in the relationship between chronic childhood illness and couple functioning. One such factor that should be considered in future research designs is the severity of the illness or health status of the child at a given point in time. Children with CF have a poorer prognosis, with a variety of severe medical complications, than do children with the other chronic childhood illnesses studied. However, to date, there are no studies that include severity of the illness as a possible mediator in the relationship between childhood illness and couple functioning.

Another factor that would be likely to affect the impact of the child's illness on the couple's functioning is the length of time the parents care for a child with a chronic illness. Several studies (Barbarin et al., 1985; Dahlquist, Czyzewski, & Jones, 1995; Tew et al., 1974) have indicated that the longer parents have been caring for a child with chronic illness, the greater the distress reported in the couple's relationship. Thus, the burden of caring for a child with a chronic illness may serve as a long-term stressor that has a mounting impact over time.

Several aspects of family functioning appear to mediate the relationship between caring for a child with a chronic illness and couple functioning. The parents' resolution of their child's diagnosis has been shown to affect the couple's relationship (Sheeran et al., 1997), so that when mothers are unresolved with regard to the diagnosis, their partners report lower relationship

satisfaction. Also, converging data suggest that the emotional and time demands of caring for a child with a chronic illness affect performance of social
roles within the family. Specifically, results from several studies indicate that
mothers often feel overwhelmed with the burden of being the primary care-
taker of the ill child and also feel resentment toward the father who is away
at work. Fathers report not having enough time to spend with the mother,
who is preoccupied with caring for the child. Thus, the reorganization of familial roles and the lack of time for social and recreational activities for the
couple may lead to significant stress in the couple relationship. Therefore,
further research using a prospective, longitudinal design is needed to determine what factors predict a positive versus a negative outcome.

Effect of the Couple's Relationship on the Child's Illness

There is a dearth of data on the how couple functioning affects the
course and outcome of the child's illness because most of the studies that
have addressed this issue have examined the effects of family rather than couple functioning. There are frequent reports in the pediatric chronic-illness
literature that family environment has a significant impact on the child's psychological functioning and, in some cases, health status (Patterson, Budd,
Goetz, & Warwick, 1993; Varni et al., 1996). Researchers have examined
such diverse variables as parent–child relationships, couple functioning, sibling relationships, and parental psychological functioning under the rubric of
"family environmental variables." High family stress has been shown to have
a negative impact on child psychological functioning and adaptation to
chronic illness (Burlew, Evans, & Oler, 1989; Drotar, 1997; Wallander &
Thompson, 1995; Wallander & Varni, 1992). Wallander and Thompson
reviewed several studies on the effects of family functioning on the child's
psychological adjustment and concluded that the data indicate that less cohesion and support in families are associated with poor psychological adjustment in children with chronic illnesses. A review of the sickle-cell anemia
literature revealed that the greater the family stressors, the poorer the child's
psychosocial adjustment to the illness (Burlew et al., 1989).

In a longitudinal study that monitored health status in 91 children
with CF over a 10-year period, Patterson et al. (1993) found that compliance with home treatment, balanced family coping, and a low emphasis on
personal growth within the family accounted for one third of the variance
in pulmonary functioning in these children. There also are data that suggest
that recurrent pain problems in children may be a response to family stressors (Goodman, Gidron, & McGrath, 1994).

Asthma researchers also have examined the effects of various aspects
of family functioning on asthma onset and course with mixed results.
Mrazek, Klinnert, Mrazek, and Macey (1991) followed a group of families
with children genetically at risk for asthma from birth to age 2. Mothers who

were rated as having early parenting or coping difficulties were more likely to have an infant who later developed asthma. On the other hand, low couple satisfaction in these families was not associated with a later onset of asthma. Similarly, there were no differences in self-reported relationship adjustment between parents of children without asthma and parents of children who developed asthma based on a prospective longitudinal study (Askildsen, Watten, & Faleide, 1993).

There are data that indicate that good family functioning is associated with a higher quality of psychological adjustment and physical outcome in the chronically ill child (Tansella, 1995; Varni, Wilcox, & Hanson, 1988). Chronic illness in children may serve to mobilize increased social support through the family's rallying around the ill child (Garralda, 1994). This increased family support, in turn, serves as a psychosocial buffer for the child. In particular, good family relationship functioning has been associated with positive psychological adjustment in chronically ill children. For example, Varni et al. (1988) found that families with high levels of cohesion and expressiveness and low levels of conflict were more likely to have children with good psychological adjustment to juvenile rheumatoid arthritis.

Due to the correlational nature of most studies that assess the impact of family functioning on child health status, it is difficult to determine the direction of effects, that is, whether greater family stress leads to poorer health status in the child, or poorer health status in the child leads to greater family stress. More likely, there is a reciprocal relationship in which greater stress leads to poorer health status, which in turn further increases family stress. However, the precipitating event (poor health status or family stress) may vary from one family to another. For example, one case study of a family with a child with sickle-cell anemia revealed that when the parent's relationship conflicts increased, the child's illness episodes subsequently increased (Graham, Reeb, Levitt, Fine, & Medalie, 1982). There also was a brief couple separation after one of the child's hospitalizations, suggesting that the increased stress of the child's illness may have affected the couple's functioning.

To summarize, it is apparent that the family is the primary environment in which the child functions and can serve either as a source of stress or a source of support for the child with a chronic illness. Family environmental factors that have been identified as stressors for children include lack of cohesion and support within the family, parental psychopathology, and couple conflict. Data indicate that these variables affect the child's psychosocial adjustment to the illness and also have a direct impact on the child's health status. However, to date, there are only a few studies that have directly examined the effects of the parental relationship, rather than various aspects of family functioning, on the child's health status. This is surprising given that it is well known that there is a significant association between stress and children's health status (Boyce et al., 1995; Jemerin & Boyce, 1990) and couple distress has been shown to be a major stressor for children (Cummings & Davies, 1994). Furthermore, there are extensive data that suggest that couple functioning has a significant effect on the partner's health status in a variety of adult disorders, including chronic pain, cancer, asthma, and arthritis (see other chapters, this volume). Therefore, further research is needed to address this gap in the literature. Because of the reciprocal nature of the relationship between couple functioning and children's health status, it is important to design prospective, longitudinal studies that assess couple functioning and child health status and psychosocial adjustment over time.

ASSESSMENT

Although there are some cases in which caring for a child with a chronic illness results in increased couple intimacy, data indicate that caring for a child with a chronic illness frequently is associated with increased couple stress. In addition, family stress has been associated with poorer adjustment to chronic illness in children. Thus, it is critical for health care providers who are responsible for the care of children with chronic illnesses to carefully monitor the functioning of the child's parents, in addition to the child's health status and psychosocial adjustment. Assessment of the parental relationship and the child's medical and psychological functioning over time will enable the health care provider to intervene early if problems begin to develop in any of these areas. In the next section of this chapter, therefore, we provide a brief overview of the standardized assessment instruments that can be used to assess parent, as well as child, functioning.

Couple Functioning

The Dyadic Adjustment Scale (DAS; Spanier, 1976) is the measure most commonly used to assess satisfaction in couple relationships. The measure consists of four factor analytically derived subscales: Dyadic Consensus, Cohesion, Satisfaction, and Affection. The DAS also yields a total score of couple satisfaction. It has been shown to differentiate between married and divorced couples and is considered to be a reliable and valid instrument for the assessment of couple satisfaction in the normal population. However, Gordon Walker, Manion, Cloutier, and Johnson (1992) have criticized the use of the DAS as a measure of couple satisfaction in couples with a chronically ill child because they found that these couples had significantly higher mean DAS scores than Spanier's normative sample. In addition, parents of children with chronic illness who reported that they were experiencing couple distress scored higher than Spanier's recommended cutoff score for identifying distressed couples, although their scores were significantly lower than those of nondistressed couples with healthy children. This indicates that using the cutoff score recommended by Spanier for identifying distressed couples may lead to an underestimate of distress in couples with a chronically ill child. Nevertheless, the DAS was useful in predicting which couples would request therapy for couple distress. Therefore, it seems that the DAS can still be considered a useful instrument for assessing couple satisfaction in couples with chronically ill children if a few caveats are kept in mind. Specifically, Gordon Walker et al.'s (1992) recommendation that a higher cutoff score for couple distress (109.7 vs. 97) should be used to identify distress in couples with a child with a chronic illness. Also, a multimethod assessment strategy, including interview, rather than the DAS as the sole measure of couple satisfaction, is recommended.

Other variables that may affect the couple's relationship and, therefore, are important to assess include role strain and parental psychological functioning. Researchers who have examined the effects of role strain on couples with chronically ill children have used daily diaries to assess the amount of time each parent spends in household and child-care tasks versus time for recreational and leisure activities (Quittner, DiGirolamo, et al., 1992; Quittner et al., 1998; Quittner, Opipari, Regoli, Jacobsen, & Eigen, 1992). These studies have indicated that when there is an imbalance between the partners regarding who is responsible for child-care and household tasks, couples tend to experience more relationship distress. An imbalance in the amount of time spent in child-care tasks versus recreational or leisure activities also is predictive of greater couple distress. Therefore, monitoring of role strain is an important aspect of assessment for parents of chronically ill children. In addition to the use of diaries, Quittner, DiGirolamo, et al. found that an interview format was useful in assessing role strain in parents of children with chronic illness.

Depression and other forms of parental psychopathology have been associated with both parental dyadic functioning and child psychological functioning. Therefore, it is important to assess the psychological functioning of each parent. Several assessment tools are commonly used to assess parental psychological functioning, including the Beck Depression Inventory (Beck, Ward, Mendelson, Mock, & Erbaugh, 1961), the Center for Epidemiological Studies Depression Scale (Radloff, 1977), and the Symptom Distress Checklist—Revised (Derogatis, 1983).

Child Functioning

Psychosocial adjustment to the illness has a significant impact on the child's health status and is obviously an important variable in its own right. It is particularly important to assess those aspects of child functioning that may affect the disease process. For example, externalizing behavior problems may interfere with a child's compliance with medical treatment regimens, which may have a negative impact on the course of the illness. The Child

Behavior Checklist (CBCL; Achenbach, 1991; Wallander & Thompson, 1995) is considered to be the gold standard for the assessment of behavior problems in children between the ages of 4 and 18 years. The CBCL consists of 118 items rated on 3-point scales, with forms available for multiple informants, including parent, youth, and teacher. Two broad scales, Internalizing and Externalizing, were formed by second-order factor analysis. The CBCL also yields a Total Behavior Problems score. Several subscales yield scores regarding specific areas of child functioning. The CBCL has been criticized for its use as a measure of behavior problems with chronically ill children because endorsement of the physical symptom items may falsely elevate the Total Behavior Problems scale. Furthermore, the CBCL may underestimate the existence of less serious problems of adjustment (Harris, Canning, & Kelleher, 1996; Wallander & Thompson, 1995). In spite of these limitations, the CBCL is a valid, reliable measure that would serve as a useful screening instrument for assessing behavior problems in chronically ill children. A particular advantage of the CBCL is its multiple-informant design, which allows for the assessment of the child's behavior from several perspectives.

For younger children, there is another version of the CBCL, the Child Behavior Checklist for Ages Two-to-Three (CBCL 2–3; Achenbach, 1992). It consists of 100 parent-report items, rated on a 3-point scale, which yield six factor analytically derived subscales: Social Withdrawal, Depressed, Sleep Problems, Somatic Complaints, Aggressive, and Destructive. Two broad scales, Internalizing and Externalizing, were formed by second-order factor analysis. Adequate reliability and excellent construct validity have been demonstrated for the CBCL 2–3 (Achenbach, Edelbrock, & Howell, 1987).

Assessment of the couple relationship in the parental dyad and the child's psychosocial adjustment requires the health care provider to monitor the functioning of all parties during the various phases of the child's illness to detect changes that may occur over the course of the illness. The extant literature suggests that the stress of coping with a child's chronic illness increases over time and that couples who appear to be functioning well early in the disease process sometimes develop maladaptive patterns of functioning over the long course of the illness (Barbarin et al., 1985). As the child develops, the illness takes on new meanings and requires different challenges for both the child and the parents (Kazak, 1989). Therefore, ongoing assessment of parental and child functioning should be considered an essential part of the child's treatment program.

INTERVENTION

Treatment of couples with a chronically ill child means that in addition to the couple, there are three individual patients—the mother, the father, and the child—each of whom may be viewed as therapeutic targets. Thus, a family with a chronically ill child may require several different types of interventions, targeted at different individuals, to address the range of problems encountered. For example, in the first case presented at the beginning of this chapter, it seems likely that the family would benefit from a comprehensive treatment approach that would include individual therapy for Maria to help her deal with her depression, couple's therapy for the parents to reduce couple distress, and either parent training or individual therapy for Raphael to deal with his behavior problems and school difficulties. In the second case, brief couples therapy was the only intervention required. The range of treatment options available highlights the importance of ongoing assessment to determine which treatment modalities are indicated for a particular family at a specific point in time. The next section consists of an overview of the treatment strategies that have been recommended in the literature.

Interventions Targeted at the Couple

Gordon Walker et al. (1996) found that couples therapy reduced couple distress in parents of children with a chronic illness. In their study, 32 couples were randomly assigned to an intervention or wait-list control group. The intervention consisted of 10 sessions of emotionally focused therapy (EFT) for couples. EFT is a manualized treatment protocol, which has as a central focus on communication, intimacy, affect, and repairing attachment relationships. The protocol was modified slightly to specifically address the issues faced by couples who are caring for a chronically ill child. The treatment group reported significant decreases in couple distress, which was significantly lower than couple distress reported in the control group at both posttreatment and 5-month follow-up. In addition, the treatment couples demonstrated less negative communication at posttreatment and follow-up, as well as greater intimacy at follow-up compared with control couples. Results from another study indicated that a brief educational workshop designed to improve problem-solving skills and communication among parents of children with CF was effective in reducing couple distress, increasing self-esteem, and improving family functioning (Schroder, Casadaban, & Davis, 1988). Taken together, these data suggest that couples therapy is an effective method of treating the negative effects of childhood illness on the couple's relationship.

Family therapy also has been found to be a successful treatment modality for families with a chronically ill child. Data indicate that family therapy may be particularly effective as a form of primary prevention and early intervention. Kupst (1992) randomly assigned families who had a child newly diagnosed with leukemia to one of two intervention groups or to a standard-care control group. Mothers in the intervention groups showed better adjustment to the emotional and physical demands of caring for their ill children during the initial disease-treatment phase than mothers in the control group. At both the 1- and 6-year follow-up assessments, all families appeared to have similar levels of coping. These results suggest that family therapy is an effective early-intervention strategy that promotes positive adjustment in the earliest phases of a specific childhood illness. Thus, it seems that it would be useful to include family intervention strategies to help educate families about their child's specific chronic illness and to teach mastery of illness-related coping skills (Kupst & Schulman, 1988).

Interventions Targeted at the Child

Individual therapy is recommended for children who are having difficulty adapting to a chronic illness. Studies have shown that these children are a greater risk for psychosocial and adjustment problems (Burlew et al., 1989; Drotar, 1997; Wallander & Thompson, 1995). Goals of therapy should include educating the child about her or his illness, as well as teaching stress-management techniques to promote healthy coping skills and create a buffer against stress (Delamater, 1992; Perrin & MacLean, 1988; Perrin, MacLean, Gortmaker, & Asher, 1992; Wallander & Thompson, 1995). Individual therapy may help to reduce stress for the chronically ill child and thus may have an indirect positive impact on the health status of him or her. Intervention with a chronically ill child should be individually tailored to the needs of the child and his or her family and should take into account the child's specific chronic illness. White, Kolman, Wexler, Polin, and Winter (1984) found that the recurrent ketoacidosis of diabetic children stabilized to no more than one hospitalization per year in 17 of 30 families who received individualized interventions (e.g., combinations of individual, family, and psychoeducational group sessions).

In cases where the child's adaptation to the illness results in behavior problems, behavioral parent training may be a useful treatment, in addition to individual therapy for the child. Parent training, in which parents are taught how to use behavioral strategies to increase positive behaviors and reduce negative behaviors, has been shown to be an effective form of treatment for a variety of child behavior problems, including noncompliance and aggressive behavior (see Kazdin, 1993). Therefore, it is reasonable to assume that these strategies would also be effective in teaching parents of chronically ill children how to deal with their child's behavior problems.

Children with chronic illness are first and foremost children and thus experience the full range of developmental challenges common to all children. Parents of chronically ill children need to make the same types of decisions regarding discipline, education, social activities, and so on, as do parents of healthy children. These decisions are sometimes more difficult for parents of chronically ill children because they are complicated by feelings of guilt and a desire to keep their child's life free of stress. In particular, parents may not discipline their child around normal developmental behaviors to avoid conflict with the child. The resulting lax discipline may lead to significant behavioral problems. Developmental guidance and problem-solving-skills training may be an effective tool to help parents make appropriate decisions related to developmental issues.

Other Types of Interventions

Finally, there are data that indicate that group therapy or support groups may be effective in reducing the stress associated with having a child with a chronic illness. Satin, La Greca, Zigo, and Skyler (1989) evaluated the efficacy of group intervention or group intervention plus a 1-week parental simulation of their adolescent's daily diabetes management compared with a control group. They found that both treatment groups produced significant improvements in metabolic control for diabetic adolescents, as well as increased self-esteem compared with diabetic adolescents in the control group. However, there were no differences between groups concerning the adolescents' and parents' perceptions of family functioning. Other types of group experience for children with chronic illness have included social skills training and summer camps, which have been effective in improving self-esteem and adjustment and reducing behavioral problems (Eiser, 1992; Varni, Katz, Colegrove, & Dolgin, 1993). Thus, it appears that group therapy for parents and children in families with a child with a chronic illness may provide crucial social support that helps both the couple and the child cope with and adapt to the illness.

To summarize, a variety of treatment approaches, including couples therapy, individual child therapy, parent training, developmental guidance, and group therapy, may be effective in minimizing the impact of the child's illness on both the child and the couple, depending on each person's needs. Again, this highlights the importance of ongoing assessment of the couple's and child's functioning to determine who should be treated, using what types of intervention strategies and at what points in time.

We now revisit the cases presented at the beginning of the chapter to illustrate how, in one case, a multidimensional treatment approach was needed to address the multiple child and couple problems and, in the other case, where the family had a great deal of social support, only a brief couples intervention was required. In the first case, the diagnostic evaluation indicated that Maria, Raphael's mother, was clinically depressed and that the couple also was experiencing significant distress. Raphael scored in the clinical range on the Externalizing scale of the CBCL, indicating that his behavior problems also required attention. Therefore, a multidimensional intervention approach was adopted that included individual treatment for

Maria and Raphael, as well as couple and family therapy. Because of practical considerations, it was decided to treat Maria's depression pharmacologically, and a consulting psychiatrist placed her on the appropriate dose of an antidepressant medication. Maria and Carlos were referred for weekly couples therapy, with the goals of improving communication, negotiating division of responsibility in caring for Raphael, and increasing intimacy by spending more time together, through respite care, and doing activities they enjoyed.

While Maria and Carlos met with a couple's therapist at the hospital, Raphael participated in weekly individual therapy with the therapist from the pediatric psychology service due to his difficulties adapting to his cancer and escalating behavioral problems. The therapist taught Raphael more effective coping skills, including stress management, relaxation techniques, and pain management, which he practiced with Raphael in vivo at his oncology outpatient and inpatient visits. The therapist also encouraged Raphael to participate in the art therapy group with the other children at the oncology clinic, to increase positive peer relationships for social support and social skills.

Raphael's family also was referred to biweekly short-term therapy, which included Raphael's siblings during several sessions. Sessions focused on educating the family about Raphael's diagnosis, including the course, treatment, and prognosis of his cancer. Additionally, the family therapist focused on helping Raphael's parents treat Raphael as a normal 6-year-old child. They were taught behavioral management skills to reduce Raphael's behavioral problems, including frequent temper tantrums, and there was discussion about helping Raphael separate from his mother and feel comfortable about returning to school. Raphael's parents were also encouraged to attend a support group for families coping with cancer that was held one evening a month at the hospital.

At the end of the first year of Raphael's cancer treatment, the functioning of individual family members had improved dramatically. Maria was no longer clinically depressed, and she and Carlos were fighting less at home. Carlos had reduced his overtime hours to spend more time with his wife and children and to participate in caring for Raphael during his inpatient visits to the hospital. As a result, Maria was able to spend more time with Raphael's siblings at home during the evenings and felt more supported by Carlos in caring for Raphael. Maria and Carlos stated they enjoyed attending the couples sessions because it allowed them time to spend together and communicate their fears and anxiety about Raphael's prognosis. Maria had also developed close friendships with other parents from the oncology clinic, who would watch her children on occasion for respite and listened and understood her struggles with Raphael's illness. Raphael's behavior-management program implemented by his therapist and parents helped to reduce the frequency of his tantrums and fights with siblings, and he began attending school more regularly. Raphael began displaying more smiles and laughter and participated in the group art therapy without having to have his mother present. Maria also began helping Raphael use the pain-management techniques taught to him, which were effective in helping him cope with invasive medical treatment. Although the family continued to struggle with Raphael's cancer, their coping skills had improved with treatment.

In the case example of Jason, early intervention by a therapist while Cherisse and Raymond visited their infant son in the neonatal intensive-care unit helped them cope well with the pain of their son's diagnosis of congenital heart disease. However, it appeared that other factors were also important in helping the family cope effectively with Jason's chronic illness. Cherisse and Raymond had a good social system, which included family and friends who helped the family with respite and support. Cherisse and Raymond divided the responsibility of caring for Jason and taking him to the doctor, so that one parent did not bear the sole burden of managing Jason's care. In addition, the family attempted to make Jason's life as normal as possible under the stressful circumstances he often encountered, which helped Jason adapt to his chronic illness. The family spent the precious hours they had together participating in enjoyable activities that facilitated a sense of family cohesion or closeness. It seems that in this case, early intervention (at the time of the child's diagnosis) was all that was needed because ongoing assessment indicated that the child and the couple were coping well with the child's chronic illness.

CONCLUSIONS AND FUTURE DIRECTIONS

There is a large body of literature on the reciprocal relationships between childhood chronic illness and couple functioning. However, it is difficult to derive any conclusions from the extant data because not only have researchers studied the effects of a wide range of childhood illnesses, but even when comparing results from studies on the effects of the same illness, the data are contradictory. Results of some studies indicate that a specific childhood illness has a detrimental effect on the couple relationship, whereas other data indicate no effects, or even positive effects. How does one make sense of these conflicting results to determine what factors predict a positive versus a negative outcome in terms of the functioning of the couple and the child? One problem is that previous research has neglected to include theoretically relevant variables that could help to account for the discrepant findings. Specifically, although many researchers acknowledge that developmental issues have a critical impact on the effects of a child's illness on the parents, few studies have included developmental variables in their models. Instead, researchers have included children ranging in age from preschool to adolescence without considering how differences in cognitive, social, and emotional development would affect how the child and, therefore, how the couple adapts to the illness. Future research in which the child's developmental stage is included as an independent variable would shed light on specific risk factors that may enhance or hinder the parents' adaptation to the illness. For example, the inability of the preschool child to understand the necessity of a painful medical procedure may lead to conflict between the parents as to how to handle their child's resistance, whereas the parents of an adolescent with the same illness may be spared this particular source of conflict because of their child's more developed cognitive capacities. Therefore, it seems critical to include developmental level or chronological age as a variable in future research examining the child illness–couple functioning relationship. Comparing the functioning of parents of children of different developmental levels who suffer from the same illness will shed light on how developmental variables interact with illness variables to either ameliorate or intensify the stressful effects of the child's illness. Family ecological characteristics are another group of variables that may affect the relationship between childhood chronic illness and couple functioning that have been largely neglected in the literature. For example, it seems obvious that specific ecological variables such as number and ages of other children in addition to the ill child would have an impact on the parents' relationship. Therefore, family ecological characteristics also should be included in future research to determine the role of these variables in moderating the relationship between childhood illness and parent functioning. Finally, because converging data suggest that the impact of the child's illness changes over time, future research should include stage of the child's illness as a variable in the chronic childhood illness–couple functioning relationship.

It seems clear, therefore, that to shed light on the complex, reciprocal relationship between childhood chronic illness and couple functioning, research designs testing multifactorial models are needed. Specifically, it is critical to develop multivariate research designs in which illness-related variables (severity, chronicity, stage of illness), as well as developmental variables and family ecological variables, are used to predict couple (parental) functioning. These models also could be used to examine whether developmental variables and family ecology variables serve as mediators or moderators in the relationship between childhood illness and couple functioning. Furthermore, because the impact of the illness changes over time, longitudinal, prospective research designs are needed. Assessing child and parent functioning, as well as family ecology variables across the various stages of the child's illness, would enable researchers to begin to disentangle the direction of effects in the reciprocal relationship between childhood chronic illness and couple functioning. Once the various factors that enhance coping with a particular illness are identified, then it will be possible to design interventions specifically targeted to the needs of parents and children at different developmental stages to reduce the risk of negative effects and increase the likelihood of positive effects for both parents and children.

REFERENCES

Achenbach, T. M. (1991). *Manual for the Child Behavior Checklist/4–18 and 1991 profile.* Burlington: University of Vermont, Department of Psychiatry.

Achenbach, T. M. (1992). *Manual for the Child Behavior Checklist/2–3.* Burlington: University of Vermont.

Achenbach, T. M., Edelbrock, C., & Howell, C. T. (1987). Empirically based assessment of the behavioral/emotional problems of 2- and 3-year-old children. *Journal of Abnormal Child Psychology, 15,* 629–650.

Allen, M. S. (1993). A comparative study of the marital relationships of parents of chronically ill and nonchronically ill children. *Dissertation Abstracts International, 53*(70), 2558A. (University Microfilms No. 31-7607).

Askildsen, E. C., Watten, R. G., & Faleide, A. O. (1993). Are parents of asthmatic children different from other parents? *Psychotherapy and Psychosomatics, 60,* 91–99.

Barbarin, O. A., Hughes, D., & Chesler, M. A. (1985). Stress, coping, and marital functioning among parents of children with cancer. *Journal of Marriage and the Family, 47,* 473–480.

Beck, A., Ward, C., Mendelson, M., Mock, J., & Erbaugh, J. (1961). An inventory for measuring depression. *Archives General Psychiatry, 4,* 53–63.

Boyce, W. T., Chesney, M., Alkon, A., Tschann, J. M., Adams, S., Chesterman, B., Cohen, F., Kaiser, P., Folkman, S., & Wara, D. (1995). Psychobiologic reactivity to stress and childhood respiratory illnesses: Results of two prospective studies. *Psychosomatic Medicine, 57,* 411–422.

Burlew, A. K., Evans, R., & Oler, C. (1989). The impact of a child with sickle cell disease on family dynamics. In C. F. Whitten & J. F Bertles (Eds.), *Annals of the New York Academy of Sciences: Vol. 565. Sickle cell disease* (pp. 161–171). New York: New York Academy of Sciences.

Cappelli, M., McGrath, P. J., Daniels, T., Manion, I., & Schillinger, J. (1994). Marital quality of parents of children with spina bifida: A case-comparison study. *Developmental and Behavioral Pediatrics, 15,* 320–326.

Chang, P. N. (1991). Psychosocial needs of long-term childhood cancer survivors: A review of literature. *Pediatrician, 18,* 20–24.

Crain, A. J., Sussman, M. B., & Weil, W., Jr. (1966). Effects of a diabetic child on marital integration and related measures of family functioning. *Journal of Health and Human Behavior, 7,* 122–127.

Cummings, E. M., & Davies, P. (1994). *Children and marital conflict: The impact of family dispute and resolution.* New York: Guilford Press.

Dahlquist, L. M., Czyzewski, D. I., & Jones, C. L. (1995). Parents of children with cancer: A longitudinal study of emotional distress, coping style, and marital adjustment two and twenty months after diagnosis. *Journal of Pediatric Psychology, 21,* 541–554.

Delamater, A. M. (1992). Stress, coping, and metabolic control among youngsters with diabetes. In A. M. La Greca, L. J. Siegel, J. L. Wallander, & C. E. Walker (Eds.), *Stress and coping in childhood* (pp. 191–211). New York: Guilford Press.

Denning, C. R., Gluckson, M. M., & Mohr, I. (1976). Psychological and social aspects of cystic fibrosis. In J. A. Mangos & R. C. Talamo (Eds.), *Cystic fibrosis: Projections into the future* (pp. 127–151). New York: Stratton.

Derogatis, L. R. (1983). *SCL–90–R administration, scoring and procedures manual—II for the revised version*. Towson, MD: Clinical Psychometric Research.

Drotar, D. (1997). Relating parent and family functioning to the psychological adjustment of children with chronic health conditions: What have we learned? What do we need to know? *Journal of Pediatric Psychology, 22*(2), 149–165.

Eiser, C. (1992). Psychological effects of chronic disease. In S. Chess & M. E. Hertzig (Eds.), *Annual progress in child psychiatry and child development 1991* (pp. 434–450). New York: Brunner/Mazel.

Evans, R., Burlew, A. K., & Oler, C. (1988). Children with sickle cell anemia: Parental relations, parent–child relations, and child behavior. *Social Work, 33*(2), 127–130.

Garralda, M. E. (1994). Chronic physical illness and emotional disorder in childhood: Where the brain's not involved, there may still be problems. *British Journal of Psychiatry, 164*, 8–10.

Goodman, J. E., Gidron, Y., & McGrath, P. J. (1994). Pain proneness in children: Toward a new conceptual framework. In R. C. Grzesiak & D. S. Ciccone (Eds.), *Psychological vulnerability to chronic pain* (pp. 90–115). New York: Springer.

Gordon Walker, J. G., Johnson, S. M., Manion, I. G., & Cloutier, P. F. (1996). Emotionally focused marital intervention for couples with chronically ill children. *Journal of Consulting and Clinical Psychology, 64*, 1029–1036.

Gordon Walker, J. G., Manion, I. G., Cloutier, P. F., & Johnson, S. M. (1992). Measuring marital distress in couples with chronically ill children: The Dyadic Adjustment Scale. *Journal of Pediatric Psychology, 17*, 345–357.

Graham, A. V., Reeb, K., Levitt, C., Fine, M., & Medalie, J. H. (1982). Care of a troubled family and their child with sickle cell anemia. *The Journal of Family Practice, 15*, 23–32.

Harris, E. S., Canning, R. D., & Kelleher, K. J. (1996). A comparison of measures of adjustment, symptoms, and impairment among children with chronic medical conditions. *Journal of the American Academy of Child and Adolescent Psychiatry, 35*, 1025–1032.

Hauenstein, E. J. (1990). The experience of distress in parents of chronically ill children: Potential or likely outcome? *Journal of Clinical Child Psychology, 19*, 356–364.

Heffron, W. A., Bommelaere, K., & Maters, R. (1973). Group discussions with parents of leukemic children. *Pediatrics, 52*, 831–840.

Ievers, C. E., & Drotar, D. (1996). Family and parental functioning in cystic fibrosis. *Developmental and Behavioral Pediatrics, 17*, 48–55.

Jemerin, J. M., & Boyce, W. T. (1990). Psychobiological differences in childhood stress response: II. Cardiovascular markers of vulnerability. *Journal of Developmental and Behavioral Pediatrics, 11*, 140–150.

Kazak, A. E. (1989). Families of chronically ill children: A systems and social ecological model of adaptation and challenge. *Journal of Consulting and Clinical Psychology, 57,* 25–30.

Kazak, A. E., Reber, M., & Snitzer, L. (1988). Childhood chronic disease and family functioning: A study of phenylketonuria. *Pediatrics, 81,* 224–230.

Kazdin, A. E. (1993). Changes in behavioral problems and prosocial functioning in child treatment. *Journal of Child and Family Studies, 2,* 5–22.

Koocher, G. P., & O'Malley, J. E. (1981). *The Damocles syndrome: Psychosocial consequences of surviving childhood cancer.* New York: McGraw-Hill.

Kupst, M. J. (1992). Long-term family coping with acute lymphoblastic leukemia in childhood. In A. M. La Greca, L. J. Siegel, J. L. Wallander, & C. E. Walker (Eds.), *Stress and coping in childhood* (pp. 242–261). New York: Guilford Press.

Kupst, M. J., & Schulman, J. L. (1988). Long-term coping with pediatric leukemia: A six-year follow-up study. *Journal of Pediatric Psychology, 13,* 7–23.

Lansky, S., Cairns, N. U., Hassanein, R. A., Wehr, J., & Lowman, J. T. (1978). Childhood cancer: Parental discord and divorce. *Pediatrics, 62,* 184–188.

Mahlmann, J. J. (1994). Chronically ill children and marital adjustment in military families. *Dissertation Abstracts International, 55*(6), 1694A. (University Microfilms No. 34-73345).

Martin, P. (1975). Marital breakdown in families of patients with spina bifida cystica. *Developmental Medicine and Child Neurology, 17,* 757–764.

Michael, B. E., & Copeland, D. R. (1987). Psychosocial issues in childhood cancer: An ecological framework for research. *The American Journal of Pediatric Hematology Oncology, 9,* 73–83.

Midence, K. (1994). The effects of chronic illness on children and their families: An overview. *Genetic, Social, and General Psychology Monographs, 120,* 311–326.

Mrazek, D. A. (1991). Chronic pediatric illness and multiple hospitalizations. In M. Lewis, (Ed.), *Child and adolescent psychiatry: A comprehensive textbook* (pp. 1041–1050). Baltimore: Williams & Wilkins.

Mrazek, D. A., Klinnert, M. D., Mrazek, P., & Macey, T. (1991). Early asthma onset: Consideration of parenting issues. *Journal of the American Academy of Child and Adolescent Psychiatry, 30,* 277–282.

Nishiura, E., & Whitten, C. F. (1980). Psychosocial problems in families of children with sickle cell anemia. *Urban Health, 9*(8), 32–35.

Northey, S., Griffin, W. A., & Krainz, S. (1998). A partial test of the psychosomatic family model: Marital interaction patterns in asthma and nonasthma families. *Journal of Family Psychology, 12,* 220–233.

Nulsen, A. M. (1990). An exploration of the parental and spousal experiences of fathers/husbands in families of children with chronic illness. *Dissertation Abstracts International, 50,* 5549B. (University Microfilms No. 28-50246).

Patterson, J. M., Budd, J., Goetz, D., & Warwick, W. J. (1993). Family correlates of 10-year pulmonary health trends in cystic fibrosis. *Pediatrics, 91,* 383–389.

Perrin, J. M. (1986). Chronically ill children: An overview. *Topics in Early Childhood Special Education, 5*(4), 1–11.

Perrin, J. M., & MacLean Jr., W. E. (1988). Children with chronic illness: The prevention of dysfunction. *Pediatric Clinics of North America, 35*, 1325–1337.

Perrin, J. M., MacLean Jr., W. E., Gortmaker, S. L., & Asher, K. N. (1992). Improving the psychological status of children with asthma: A randomized controlled trial. *Journal of Developmental and Behavioral Pediatrics, 13*, 241–247.

Quittner, A. L., DiGirolamo, A. M., Michel, M., & Eigen, H. (1992). Parental response to cystic fibrosis: A contextual analysis of the diagnosis phase. *Journal of Pediatric Psychology, 17*, 683–704.

Quittner, A. L., Espelage, D. L., Opipari, A. C., Carter, B., Eid, M., & Eigen, H. (1998). Role strain in couples with and without a child with a chronic illness: Associations with marital satisfaction, intimacy, and daily mood. *Health Psychology, 17*, 112–124.

Quittner, A. L., Opipari, L. C., Regoli, M. J., Jacobsen, J., & Eigen, H. (1992). The impact of caregiving and role strain on family life: Comparisons between mothers of children with CF and matched controls. *Rehabilitation Psychology, 37*, 289–304.

Radloff, L. S. (1977). The Center for Epidemiological Studies—Depression Scale: A self-report depression scale for research in the general population. *Applied Psychological Measures, 1*, 385–401.

Reynolds, J. M., Garralda, M. E., Jameson, R. A., & Postlethwaite, R. J. (1988). How parents and families cope with chronic renal failure. *Archives of Disease in Childhood, 63*, 821–826.

Sabbeth, B. F., & Leventhal, J. M. (1984). Marital adjustment to chronic childhood illness: A critique of the literature. *Pediatrics, 73*, 762–768.

Satin, W., La Greca, A. M., Zigo, M. A., & Skyler, J. S. (1989). Diabetes in adolescence: Effects of multifamily group intervention and parent simulation of diabetes. *Journal of Pediatric Psychology, 14*, 259–275.

Schroder, K. H., Casadaban, A. B., & Davis, B. (1988). Interpersonal skills training for parents of children with cystic fibrosis. *Family Systems Medicine, 6*, 51–68.

Sheeran, T., Marvin, R. S., & Pianta, R. C. (1997). Mothers' resolution of their child's diagnosis and self-reported measures of parenting stress, marital relations, and social support. *Journal of Pediatric Psychology, 22*, 197–212.

Spanier, G. B. (1976). Measuring dyadic adjustment: New scales for assessing the quality of marriage and similar dyads. *Journal of Marriage and the Family, 38*, 15–28.

Spaulding, B. R., & Morgan, S. B. (1986). Spina bifida children and their parents: A population prone to family dysfunction? *Journal of Pediatric Psychology, 11*, 359–374.

Taanila, A., Kokkonen, J., & Jarvelin, M. (1996). The long-term effects of children's early-onset disability on marital relationships. *Developmental Medicine and Child Neurology, 38*, 567–577.

Tansella, C. Z. (1995). Psychosocial factors and chronic illness in childhood. *European Psychiatry, 10,* 297–305.

Tew, B., Payne, H., & Laurence, K. M. (1974). Must a family with a handicapped child be a handicapped family? *Developmental Medicine and Child Neurology, 16,* 95–98.

Thompson, R. J., Jr., & Gustafson, K. E. (1996). *Adaptation to chronic childhood illness.* Washington, DC: American Psychological Association.

Turk, J. (1964). Impact of cystic fibrosis on family functioning. *Pediatrics, 34,* 67–71.

Vance, J. C., Fazan, L. E., Satterwhite, B., & Pless, I. B. (1980). Effects of nephrotic syndrome on the family: A controlled study. *Pediatrics, 65,* 948–955.

Varni, J. W., Katz, E. R., Colegrove, R., Jr., & Dolgin, M. (1993). The impact of social skills training on the adjustment of children with newly diagnosed cancer. *Journal of Pediatric Psychology, 18,* 751–768.

Varni, J. W., Rapoff, M. A., Waldron, S. A., Gragg, R. A., Bernstein, B. H., & Lindsley, C. B. (1996). Effects of perceived stress on pediatric chronic pain. *Journal of Behavioral Medicine, 19,* 515–528.

Varni, J. W., Wilcox, K. T., & Hanson, V. (1988). Mediating effects of family social support on child psychological adjustment in juvenile rheumatoid arthritis. *Health Psychology, 7,* 421–431.

Wallander, J. L., & Thompson, R. (1995). Psychosocial adjustment of children with chronic physical conditions. In M. C. Roberts (Ed.), *Handbook of pediatric psychology* (2nd ed., pp. 124–141). New York: Guilford Press.

Wallander, J. L., & Varni, J. W. (1992). Adjustment in children with chronic physical disorders: Programmatic research on a disability-stress-coping model. In A. M. La Greca, L. J., Siegel, J. L. Wallander, & C. E. Walker (Eds.), *Stress and coping in child health* (pp. 279–298). New York: Guilford Press.

White, K., Kolman, M. L., Wexler, P., Polin, G., & Winter, R. J. (1984). Unstable diabetes and unstable families: A psychosocial evaluation of diabetic children with recurrent ketoacidosis. *Pediatrics, 73,* 749–755.

Whyte, D. A. (1992). A family nursing approach to the care of a child with a chronic illness. *Journal of Advanced Nursing, 17,* 317–327.

Zimand, E., & Wood, B. (1986). Implications of contrasting patterns of divorce in families of children with gastrointestinal disorders. *Family Systems Medicine, 4,* 385–397.

AUTHOR INDEX

Numbers in italics refer to listings in the reference sections.

Brekke, M. L., 312, *334*
Bremer, B. A., 141, *162*
Bremer, D. A., 277, *303*
Bremer, K. L., 141, *162*
Brennan, P. L., 283, 292, *300, 301*
Brenner, G. F., 112, 115, *131*
Brezinka, V., 55, *63*
Brezinski, A., 230, *235*
Briddell, D. W., 289, *300*
Bright, J., 88, *98*
Broffman, T. E., 283, *306*
Bromet, E., 281, *306*
Bronfenbrenner, U., 293, *300*
Brown, B., 141, *166*
Brown, C., 74, *99*
Brown, E., 294, *306*
Brown, G., 183, *190*
Brown, G. K., 112, 118, *128*
Brown, L. L., 139, 141, 144, *163*
Brown, M. A., 50, *63*, 227, *235*
Brown, P. C., 24, 30, *37*
Brown, R., *333*
Brown, S., 111, *128*
Brown, S. A., 288, 293, *300*
Brown, W. A., 179, *188*
Browne, G., 141, *166*
Brügner, G., 21, *41*
Brush, M. U., 220, *237*
Buchwald, D. S., 75, *102*
Buck, C., *62*
Buckelew, S. P., *133*
Budd, J., 350, *363*
Buescher, K. L., *131*
Buis, M., 78, *101*
Bulcroft, R. A., *214*
Bungay, G., *235*
Burchfiel, C. M., 314, *333*
Burgess, A., *190*
Burgess, C., 139, 142, *162, 168*
Burke, J. D., *214*
Burleson, M. H., 115, *133*
Burlew, A. K., 348, 350, 356, *361, 362*
Burman, B., 3, 4, *11*, 14, 36, *37*, 75, *97*,
    113, *128*, 142, *162*
Burnam, M. A., *69*
Burnett, C. K., 49, 58, *63, 67*
Burnett, K. F., 27, 34, *38*, 46, *68*

Burney, R., 91, *100*
Burnley, I. H., 80, *97*
Burns, D. M., 312, *336*
Burrows, B., 314, *335*
Burrows, G. D., 223, *237*
Burrows, L., 115, *133*
Burzette, R., *334*
Bushman, B. J., 290, *300*
Buske-Kirschbaum, A., *41*
Butler, W. J., *333*
Byrne, T. J., 251, *266*

Cacioppo, J. T., 16, 21, *39, 40, 42*
Caddy, G. R., *300*
Caetano, R., 274, *305*
Cahalan, D., 274, 296, *300*
Cairns, D., 197, *211*
Cairns, N. U., 344, *363*
Caldwell, D. S., *130*
Califf, R. M., *69*
Callahan. L. F., 106, 107, 109, *128*,
    133
Callan, V. J., 246, 252, *263, 264*
Camarano, L., 254, *267*
Camerino, M., 23, *42*
Cameron, A. E., 114, *130*
Cameron, C. L., *169*
Campbell, T. L., 320, *333*
Canar, W. J., 230, 231, *235*
Canning, R. D., 354, *362*
Cannon, C., 78, *103*
Cannon, W. B., 19, *37*
Caplan, R. D., 141, *169*
Cappelli, M., 341, 346, *361*
Caputi, M., *99*
Carballo-Dieguez, A., 177, *190*
Cardella, C., *101*
Cardin, S., 53, *67*
Carey, M. P., 205, *211*
Carlson, S. L., *164*
Carlsson, M., 144, *162*
Carney, R. M., 46, 50, *63*
Carnicke Jr., C. L. M., *163*
Carsrensen, L. L., *40*
Carstensen, H., 220
Carter, B., *364*

Erbaugh, J., 229, *235*, 353, *361*

Eriksen, W., 52, *64*

Esacson, R., 139, *162*

Eshkol, A., *69*

Eshleman, S., *303*

Eskola, J., 144, *164*

Espelage, D. L., *364*

Esposito, V., *99*

Esselstyn, C. B., *168*

Estes, N. C., *169*

Ethier, K. A., 125, *130*

Evans, J. C., 55, *67*

Evans, P., 77, *99*

Evans, R., 348, 350, *361, 362*

Evert, D. L., 274, *301*

Ewart, C. K., 24, 27, 28, 30, 32, 34, 37,
38, 51, *64*

Eysenck, H. J., 229, *235*

Eysenck, S. B. G., 229, *235*

Fahey, J. L., *164*

Falconer, J. J., 19, *40*

Faleide, A. O., 351, *361*

Falger, P. R. J., 52, *65*

Falke, R. L., 142, 153, *163*

Fallowfield, L. J., 139, 141, *164*

Fals-Stewart, W., 285, *307*

Farkas, G., 289, *301*

Farrell, P. M., 74, *100*

Faucett, J., 199, *212*

Fawzy, F. I., 155, 157, *164*

Fawzy, N. W., *164*

Fazan, L. E., 341, *365*

Fehm-Wolfsdorf, G., 25, 31, 34, 36, 37,
38, *39*

Feinauer, L. L., 227, *237*

Feinleib, M., 52, 53, *65, 68*

Feinstein, L. G., 142, 153, *163*

Feldman, M. W., 314, *336*

Felten, D. L., 17, *37*, 144, *164*

Felten, S. Y., *164*

Feng, Z. Z., *99*

Fentiman, I. S., *166*

Ferrando, S., 177, *190*

Ferris, J., 274, *308*

Fetting, J., *163*

Fiducia, D., *101*

Fiedler, J., *336*

Fife, B. L., 153, *164*

Fife, M., 141, *168*

Fifield, J., 107, 113, 123, *127, 132*

Fine, M., 351, *362*

Fingerhut, L. A., 313, *334*

Finlayson, A., 53, *65*

Finney, J. W., 283, *306*

Finney, W. J., 292, *301*

Fireman, B. H., 123, *133*

First, M. B., 292, *308*

Fisher, J. D., 175, *189*

Fisher, L. D., 39, *64, 236*

Fisher, W. A., 175, *189*

Fiske, V., 53, *65*, 116, 124, *129*

Fitzgerald, H. E., 276, *301*

Fitzpatrick, M. A., 36, *41*

Fitzpatrick, R., 108, 110, 112, 113, *129,
131*

FitzSimmons, S., 81, *102*

Fleetham, J. A., 90, *102*

Fleischer, D., *166*

Fleming, B., 229, *237*

Fleming, M., 295, *301*

Flor, H., 30, *38*, 193, 194, 195, 196, 197,
198, *212*

Floreen, A, 197, *211*

Floyd, F. J., 283, 287, 294, *307, 308*

Floyd, R. L., 313, *334*

Flynn, C., *190*

Foeldenyi, M., 220, *237*

Folkman, S., 142, 158, *164*, 176, *188, 361*

Folks, D. G., 54, *65*

Follick, M. J., 194, *211*

Fong, G. T., 275, *304*

Fontana, A. F., 48, 49, *65*

Ford, D. E., *67*

Fordyce, W. E., 192, 196, 197, 208, *212*

Forehand, R., 179, *188*

Forthofer, M. S., 280, *303*

Foster, A., 53, *67*

Fountain, D., 270, *302*

Fowler, R., *212*

Fox, E. E., 221, *235*

Foxall, M. J., 110, *129*

Francis, D. P., 186, *190*

Gordon Walker, J. G., 341, 352, 353, 355, 362
Gorlin, R., 68
Gorman, D. M., 285, 302
Gorsuch, R., 190
Gortmaker, S. L., 364
Gotay, C.C., 139, 142, 164
Gottlieb, B. H., 124, 130, 259, 265
Gottman, J. M., 16, 26, 28, 29, 31, 35, 38, 40, 51, 66, 228, 235, 287, 302
Gottschalk, L. A., 139, 164
Grady, K. E., 109, 112, 130, 132
Gragg, R. A., 365
Graham, A. V., 351, 362
Graham, S., 314, 334, 336
Grant, B. F., 273, 302
Grassi, L., 140, 141, 142, 143, 157, 164
Greden, J. F., 64
Greene, J. G., 319, 336
Greenfeld, D., 245, 265
Greenfield, S., 69, 103
Greenfield, T., 274, 305
Greer, H. S., 140, 167
Greer, S., 139, 144, 157, 165, 167, 168
Greig, P., 101
Greil, A. L., 251, 265
Griffin, W. A., 338, 363
Grim, C., 38
Groeger, A. M., 74, 99
Groenman, N. H., 196, 213
Gross, M., 273, 301
Grossman, L. M., 288, 304
Groth, T., 25, 31, 37, 38, 39
Grothaus, L. C., 335
Grover, D., 238
Grover, G. N., 235
Gruder, C. L., 316, 321, 322, 325, 334
Gruen, R. J., 142, 164
Grunberg, N. E., 17, 18, 22, 28, 37
Grundfest-Broniatowski, S., 168
Grzywacz, J. G., 281, 302
Guck, T. P., 202, 212
Guilleminault, C., 73, 80, 89, 99
Gunn, R. C., 319, 334
Guo, T., 88, 99
Gustafson, K. E., 338, 342, 345, 346, 347, 365

Guthrie, S., 307
Guyre, P. M., 18, 41
Gwaltney, J. M., Jr., 77, 98

Haber, J. R., 285, 287, 302
Habib, S., 82, 100
Hackett, T. P., 48, 51, 65, 70
Hackl, K. L., 177, 188
Hahlweg, K., 25, 31, 32, 36, 37, 38, 39, 41
Hahn, L., 220, 234
Halbreich, U., 221, 235
Halford, W. K., 145, 148, 156, 159, 165, 168, 280, 281, 291, 297, 302
Hall, R. L., 295, 302
Hall, S. H., 316, 334
Halldorsdottir, S., 140, 165
Hallman, J., 221, 222, 236
Hallwig, J. M., 194, 213
Halman, L. J., 247, 249, 250, 263
Halonen, M., 336
Hamilton, M., 183, 189
Hammarback, S., 218, 234
Hamovitch, M., 141, 163
Hamrin, E., 140, 144, 162, 165
Haney, T., 69
Haney, T. L., 69
Hannan, M. T., 107, 130
Hanson, B. S., 50, 53, 65
Hanson, E. I., 78, 99
Hanson, R. W., 199, 212
Hanson, V., 351, 365
Haponik, E. F., 99
Harford, T. C., 302
Hargrove, J. T., 218, 220, 236
Harkapaa, K., 202, 213
Harmon, L., 177, 189
Harper, R. G., 89, 98
Harris, E. S., 354, 362
Harris, S. D., 163
Harris, T. R., 285, 303
Harrison, P. A., 292, 302
Harrison, W. M., 221, 236
Hart, W. G., 223, 236
Harvey, C., 277, 301
Harvey, S. M., 289, 302
Harwood, H., 270, 302

Horwitz, R. I., 48, 49, 66
Horwitz, S. M., 66
Hoskins, C. N., 140, 143, *165*
House, J. S., 14, 36, 39, 47, 66, 113, *130,*
    142, 165, 226, *236*
Houston, N., 46, 54, 68
Houston Miller, N., *64,* 68
Howatt, W. F., *333*
Howell, C. T., 354, *361*
Howell, D. C., 144, *164*
Huang, L. F., 99
Hughes, C., 54, 66
Hughes, D., 341, *361*
Hughes, J., 139, *166*
Hughes, M., *303*
Hughson, A. V. M., 140, *166*
Hull, J. G., 275, 282, 289, *302*
Hunink, M. G., 62, 66
Hurri, H., 202, *213*
Hurt, S. W., 221, *236*
Hurwitz, I., 317, *335, 336*
Hyppa, M. T., 203, *215*

Iasiello-Vailas, L., 49, *64*
Ickovics, J. R., 125, *130*
Ievers, C. E., 342, *362*
Iles, S., *235*
Ingham, J. G., 275, *305*
Inn, A., 293, *300*
Institute of Medicine, 272, 273, 274, 276,
    291, 293, 294, 295, 297, *302*
Invernizzi, G., *190*
Ironson, G., *169*
Irvine, D., 141, *166*
Irving, L. M., *169*
Isacsson, S., 50, 53, *65*
Isoaho, R., 78, *99*
Ito, T. A., 275, *303*

Jackson, J. K., 277, *303, 304*
Jackson, M. M., 174, *188*
Jacob, M. C., 201, *213,* 261, *265*
Jacob, T., 277, 278, 281, 284, 285, 286,
    287, 288, 293, 296, 298, *302, 309*
Jacobs, D. R., 313, *336*

Jacobs, G., *190*
Jacobs, S. B., 78, *103*
Jacobsen, J., 353, *364*
Jacobsen, P. B., 149, *163*
Jacobson, N. S., 92, 99, *100,* 205, *211,*
    212, 243, 255, 257, *264, 265*
Jacobus, S., *333*
Jaffe, A. S., 46, *63*
Jalowiec, A., 88, 98
Jameson, R. A., 341, *364*
Jamner, L. D., *42*
Janis, I. L., 320, 322, 325, *334*
Janoff-Bulman, R., 142, *169*
Janson, C., 86, 99
Janzon, L., 50, 53, *65*
Jarvelin, M., 341, *364*
Jarvik, M. E., 312, *334*
Jarvikoski, A., 202, *213*
Jarvinen, M., *164*
Jayson, M. V., 110, *129*
Jemerin, J. W., 351, *362*
Jenkins, C. D., 52, 53, *64*
Jenner, F. A., 222, *238*
Jennings, J. R., 47, 66
Jensen, M. P., 194, 196, 197, 201, 202,
    208, *212, 214, 215*
Jerrells, T. R., 144, *166*
Jinich, S., 186, *189*
Jobst, S., *41*
Jochimsen, P. R., 140, *162*
Johnson, J. C., *133*
Johnson, J. S., 27, 31, *41*
Johnson, K., 295, *301*
Johnson, S. M., 341, 352, *362*
Johnson, V., 296, *309*
Johnson, V. E., 159, *167*
Johnston, J. J., 314, *335*
Johnston, L. D., 270, *300*
Jones, A., 92, 97
Jones, C. L., 349, *361*
Jones, J. E., 218, *235*
Jones, J. W., 52, *64*
Jones, N. F., 86, *100*
Jones, N. J., 62
Jones, P. K., 111, *129*
Jorgenson, J., 221, *236*
Josephs, R. A., 275, *308*

Jouriles, E. N., 290, *302*
Juliano, M. A., 143, *169*
Jung, S. O., 221, *235*

Kabat-Zinn, J., 91, *100*
Kahn, M., 68
Kain, C., 184, *189*
Kaiser, A., 25, 31, 37, 38, *39*
Kaiser, H. E., 99
Kaiser, P., *361*
Kalichman, S. C., 173, 175, 177, 178, 183, 185, 186, *188*, *189*
Kamarck, T. W., 47, 66, 314, *335*
Kan, L., 144, *165*
Kannel, W. B., 45, 52, 55, *65*, 66
Kantero, R. L., 220, *238*
Kantor, G. K., 290, *303*
Kaplan, B. H., *336*
Kaplan, G. A., 285, *308*
Kaplan, J. R., 20, 38, 44, *64*
Kaplan, M., *102*
Kaplan, N. M., 17, *39*
Kaplan, R. M., 108, *129*
Kaplan De-Nour, A., 139, *162*
Kaprio, J., 142, *166*
Karacan, I., 89, *100*
Karatas, M., 89, *100*
Karch, A. M., 54, *63*
Karney, B. R., 37, *39*
Karno, M., *214*
Kashima, Y., 252, *264*
Kashiwagi, T., 221, *236*
Kaspers, F., *41*
Katon, W., 197, *215*
Katz, E. R., 357, *365*
Katz, P. P., 107, 110, *130*
Kavanaugh, T., *62*
Kay, D. R., 110, *130*
Kazak, A. E., 341, 348, 354, *363*
Kazdin, A. E., 356, *363*
Keefe, F. J., 120, *130*, *131*, 201, *215*
Kegeles, S., *189*
Keistinen, T., 78, *99*
Kelleher, K. J., 354, *362*
Keller, J. B., *333*
Keller, S. E., 23, *42*

Kelley, K. W., 17, *39*
Kellick, K. A., 107, *130*
Kelly, A., 156, *165*
Kelly, J. A., 175, 177, 185, *188*, *189*
Kelly, K. M., 283, *300*
Kemeny, M. E., *164*
Kemeny, M. M., 139, 143, *166*
Kemeny, N., 155, *166*
Kemmann, E., 246, *265*
Kenady, D. E., *163*
Kendler, K. S., *303*
Kendrick, J. S., 313, *334*
Kennedy, S., *39*, *236*
Kern, M. J., 45, *65*
Kernis, M. H., 226, *237*
Kerns, R. D., 48, *65*, 196, 197, 198, 199, 200, 202, 204, 205, *212*, *213*, *215*, 230, 231, *236*
Kesaniemi, A., 142, *166*
Kessel, N., 222, *235*
Kessler, M., 287, *300*
Kessler, R. C., 14, 17, *37*, *38*, 64, 274, 280, *303*
Ketcham, A. S., *163*
Keye, W. R., 228, *236*
Keyes, S., 261, *263*
Kiecolt-Glaser, J. K., 5, *11*, 16, 21, 22, 23, 25, 26, 30, 31, 32, 35, *39*, *40*, 42, 144, *162*, 226, *236*
Kinney, R. K., 192, *214*
Kinsman, R. A., 86, *100*
Kintner, E., 92, *100*
Kirkendol, R., *334*
Kirschbaum, C., 16, 18, 19, *40*, *41*
Kitagawa, H., *167*
Kittel, F., 55, *63*
Kivela, S. L., 78, *99*
Klassen, A. D., 282, 285, 289, *303*, *309*
Klein, D., *102*
Klein, K., 179, *188*
Klein, M. D., 66
Klein, R. F., 46, *65*
Kleinman, A., 192, *214*
Kleinman, J. C., 313, *334*
Klesges, R. C., 316, 322, *334*, *335*
Klinger, M., 276, *301*
Klinnert, M. D., 72, 96, *101*, 350, *363*

Lee, M. S., 143, *166*
Lee, W. W., 314, *335*
Legault, S., *166*
Lehman, D. R., *52*, *64*, 123, *129*
Lehmann, J., *212*
Lehman, J. M., *169*
Lehrer, P. M., 75, 90, 96, *100*
Leiblum, S. R., 243, 246, 253, 255, *265*
Leigh, B. C., 289, *304*
Leigh, J. P., 113, *133*
Leitko, T. A., 251, *265*
Lenhard, R. E., 137, *167*
Lenhart, R. S., 92, *100*
Leonard, K. E., 270, 278, 279, 280, 281,
        283, 287, 290, 291, 296, 298, *303*,
        304, *307*
Lerman, C., 142, 143, *164*
Lerner, D. J., 55, 66
Lesko, L. M., 149, *163*
Levenson, R. W., 16, 26, 28, 29, 31, 35,
        38, *40*, 51, 66, 288, *304*
Leventhal, J. M., 341, 342, *364*
Levin, J. B., 249, 251, 261, *265*
Levine, J., 199, *212*
Levine, S., 52, *64*, 65
Levine, S. B., 81, 98, 111, *129*
Levine, S. R., 74, *100*
Levinger, G., 279, *304*
Levitt, C., 351, *362*
Levitt, E. E., 222, *236*
Levy, D., 55, 67
Levy, G., *101*
Lew, H. T., *64*
Liang, M. H., 109, 124, *129*, *130*, *131*
Lichtenstein, E., 53, 67, 311, 312, 314,
        315, 316, 320, 323, *333*, *335*
Lichter, A. S., 140, *168*
Lichtman, R. R., 142, *169*
Liebens, F., 73, *102*
Liefooghe, R., 82, *100*
Liepman, M. R., 283, *306*
Light, K. C., *42*
Lillo, E., 192, *214*
Lindegard, B., 75, *101*
Lindell, L., 50, 65
Lindsley, C. B., *365*
Linehan, M. M., 95, *101*

Linney, J. D., 282, *307*
Lipworth, L., 91, *100*
Litt, M. D., 142, *166*, 250, *265*
Littlefield, C., 89, *101*
Liu, T. J., 275, *308*
Livermore, G., 270, *302*
Livnat, S., *164*
Lloyd, E., 105, *130*
Lobel, M., 246, 247, *264*, 317, *333*
Lobo, R. A., 244, *266*
Locke, B. Z., *214*
Locke, H. J., *40*
Loeser, J. D., 191, 202, *213*
Logue, C. M., 218, *236*
Loh, E., *101*
Lomas, P., *102*
London, M., 295, *301*
Longabaugh, R., 292, *306*
Lopez, M. C., 152, *163*
LoPiccolo, J., 152, *166*
Lorentzen, L. J., 193, *215*
Lorig, K., 120, 121, *131*, 142, *167*
Lorig, K. R., *131*
Lousberg, R., 196, *213*
Love, N., *169*
Love, S. B., *166*
Lowenthal, M. F., 113, *131*
Lowman, J. T., 344, *363*
Lubeck, D., 121, *131*
Lubin, B., 222, *236*
Lucas, L. A., 220, *234*
Luepker, R. V., 313, *336*
Lurie, Z., 52, *64*
Lushene, P., *190*
Lusk, E. J., 139, 141, 144, *163*
Lyons, R. F., 3, *11*

MacCallum, R. C., *40*
MacDonald, T. K., 275, *304*
Macey, T., 72, *101*, 350, *363*
Macintyre, S., 77, *101*
Mackenzie, T. B., 221, *236*
MacLean Jr., W. E., 341, 356, *364*
MacLeod, J. D., 277, *305*
Madden, K. S., *164*
Maeder, J., 54, 63

Maguire, G. P., 139, *164*
Mahler, H. I. M., 49, 66
Mahlmann, J. J., 341, *363*
Mahlstedt, P. P., 246, 248, 249, *265*
Maiman, L. A., 313, *336*
Maisiak, R., 111, *128*
Maisto, S. A., *285*, 291, 293, 304
Majerovitz, S. D., 110, 111, 113, 119, 122, *131*, *132*
Malarkey, W. B., 16, 25, 30, 31, 32, *39*, 40
Malatesta, V. J., 289, *305*
Maldonado, N., 178, 179, *189*
Malec, J. F., 141, *170*
Maliszewski, M., 193, *211*
Malkoff, S., 39, *236*
Malott, J. M., 322, 323, *335*
Manfredi, C., 78, *101*
Manion, I., 341, *361*
Manion, I. G., 341, 352, *362*
Manley, H., 108, *131*
Manne, S. L., 114, 115, 116, 123, *131*, 155, 156, 158, 160, *166*
Manolio, T. A., 99
Mantell, J., 141, *163*
Manuck, S., 47, 66
Manuck, S. B., 20, 38, *41*, 44, *64*
Manwell, L., 295, *301*
Mao, H., *40*
Mao, K., 252, *264*
Marano, M. A., 72, *97*
Marcari-Hinson, M. M., 68
Marden, T., *190*
Margolese, R. G., *166*
Margolin, G., 3, 4, *11*, 14, 36, *37*, 51, 67, 75, *97*, 113, *128*, 142, *162*, 257, *265*
Margolis, G., 143, 154, *166*
Marietta, C. A., 144, *166*
Mark, D., 69
Markman, H. J., 36, *41*, 51, 67, 156, *165*
Marks, G., 178, 179, *189*, *190*
Marks, G. B., 86, *101*
Marks, N. F., 281, *302*
Marlatt, G. A., 275, *285*, 285, 301, *305*
Marteinsdottir, G., 220, *238*
Martin, P., 341, 342, 346, *363*
Martinez, F. D., 314, *335*, *336*

Martinez-Sanchez, M. A., 153, *167*
Martins-Richards, J., 107, *130*
Maruta, T., 194, *213*
Marvin, R. S., 341, *364*
Mason, H., 179, *189*
Mason, H. R. C., *190*
Mason, J. W., 19, *42*
Masters, R., 344, *362*
Masters, W. H., 159, *167*
Matt, K. S., 115, *133*
Matthews, K. A., 15, 21, 26, *40*, *42*
Maurer, J., *101*
Maxwell, M. H., 38
Mayer, T. G., 192, *214*
Mayou, R., 53, 54, 67
Mazor, M. D., 246, *265*
Mazzuca, S. A., 121, *131*
McArdle, C. S., 140, *166*
McBride, C. M., 313, 314, 318, *335*
McClure, J. H., 221, *236*
McConnaughy, E. A., 292, *305*
McConnaughy, K., *104*
McCourt, W., 294, *306*
McCracken, L. M., 91, *101*, 109, *131*
McCrady, B. S., 270, 277, 279, 281, 286, 291, 294, 297, *305*, *307*, 308, 313, 327, *335*
McCrae, R. R., 222, *235*
McCurry, S. M., 92, *101*
McDaniel, L. K., 109, *127*, *128*
McDaniels, S., 227, 228, *236*
McDermott, N., 48, *63*
McDermott, S., 110, *129*
McDonald, W., *62*
McEwan, K. L., 250, *265*
McEwen, J., 53, 65
McFadden, E. R., 72, *101*
McGee, D., 45, 53, 66, 68
McGlynn, E. A., *103*
McGonagle, K. A., *303*
McGrade, J. L., 251, *266*
McGrath, P. C., *163*
McGrath, P. J., 341, 350, *361*, *362*
McIlroy, M. B., 44, 68
McIntyre, K., 53, 67, 315, *335*
McIntyre-Kingsolver, K., 323, *335*
McKay, J., *285*, 304

Mueser, K. T., 91, *97*, 294, *300*, 326, *333*
Mullen, P. D., 313, 317, 318, *334, 336*
Müller, W., 21, *41*
Mumford, E., 47, *67*
Munck, A., 18, *41*
Munford, A., 50, *63*
Munro, B. H., 78, *103*
Murabito, J. M., 55, *67*
Murawski, B. J., *130*
Murphy, G. P., 137, 138, *167*
Murphy, S., 110, *129*, 175, *190*
Murray, C. J., *66*
Murray, R. P., 314, 319, *335*
Murray, T., 136, *166*
Muse, K. N., 219, *237*
Myers, D., 68, 232, *237*
Myers, J. K., *214*
Myrtek, M., 21, *41, 42*

Nachtigall, R. D., 245, 246, *263, 266*
Nakamura, S., *167*
Nasser, S., 73, *101*
Nathan, P. E., 288, *302*
National Heart, Lung, and Blood Institue, 72, 87, *101*
National Institute on Alcohol Abuse and Alcoholism, 274, 291, *306*
Neale, J. M., 77, *103*
Nee, J., 221, *235, 236*
Neidig, P. H., 290, *307*
Nelson, C. H., *303*
Nelson, D. V., 141, *164*
Nelson, E. C., *103*
Nelson, H. F., 294, *305, 327, 335*
Nelson, J. C., *335*
Neufeld, H. N., *69*
Neuhaus, J., 254, *267*
Nevid, J. S., 324, 332, *335*
Newlin, D. B., 288, *304*
Newman, A. B., *99*
Newman, J., 288, *304*
Newman, K. B., *103*
Newman, R. I., 202, *213*
Newman, S., 108, 112, 113, 116, 124, 126, *129, 131*

Newman, S. P., 110, *131*
Newton, C. R., 250, *266*
Newton, T., *40*
Nezlek, J., 226, *237*
Nguyen, J., *102*
Niaura, R., 46, *65*
Nicassio, P. M., 112, 120, *128, 131, 132*, 203, *214*
Nicholls, P., *307*
Nides, M., 87, *102*
Nirenberg, T. D., 283, *306*
Nishijima, H., *167*
Nishimoto, R., 141, *163*
Nishiura, E., 341, 348, *363*
Nocturnal Oxygen Therapy Trial Group, 88, *102*
Noel, N., 294, *305, 327, 335*
Noguchi, M., 143, *167*
Noller, P., 36, *41*
Nonmura, A., *167*
Norfleet, M., 193, *214*
Noriega, V., *163*
Northey, S., 338, *363*
Northouse, L. L., 139, 143, *167*
Norton, L., *165*
Notarius, C. I., 27, 31, *41*, 51, *67*
Nulsen, A. M., 341, 347, *363*
Nuttal, R. L., 317, *335, 336*
Nyborg, K. F., 324, 332, *335*

Oberst, M., 139, *167*
O'Brien, T. B., 116, *131*
O'Brien, T. R., 186, *190*
Obrist, P. A., 20, *41*
Ockene, B. S., *66*
Ockene, I. S., 317, *335, 336*
Ockene, J. K., 317, *335, 336*
Ockenfels, M. C., 18, *41*
O'Connor, G. T., 84, *102*
O'Farrell, T. J., 281, 283, *285*, 287, 293, 304, *306, 307, 308*
Office of Technology Assessment, 243, 245, 261, *266*
Ogrocki, P., *39*
O'Hara, P., 314, *335*
Ohman, R., 220, *234*

Ohta, N., *167*
Oldridge, N. B., *62*
O'Leary, A., 120, *131*, 142, *167*
O'Leary, K. D., 51, *63*, 197, *211*, 290, *302*,
    307
Olenick, N. L., 298, *307*
Oler, C., 348, 350, *361*, *362*
Olschowki, J., *164*
O'Malley, J. E., 341, *363*
O'Malley, P. M., 270, *300*
Omne-Ponten, M., 139, *167*
O'Neill, H. K., 316, 322, *334*, *335*
Opipari, A. C., *364*
Opipari, L. C., 353, *364*
Oppedisano, G., *164*
Oppenheimer, E., *307*
Orford, J., 277, *307*
Orleans, C. T., 314, 316, 317, 318, *333*,
    336
Orr, E., 142, *167*
Orth-Gomer, K., 47, 53, *67*
Osborn, M., *235*
Osborne, D., 194, *213*
Oscar-Berman, M., 274, *301*
Osgarby, S. M., 280, 281, 291, 297, *302*
Osowiecki, D. M., *164*
Osterweis, M., 192, *214*
Ostrow, D., 186, *189*

Padian, N. S., 186, *190*
Palmblad, J., 144, *167*
Palmer, A. G., 139, *167*
Pan, H. D., 290, *307*
Paolino, T. J., 277, 279, *307*
Papadopoulos, C., 53, 54, *67*
Papillo, J. F., 19, 20, *41*
Parker, D. P., 218, *237*
Parker, E. M., *166*
Parker, J. C., 120, 124, *131*, *133*
Parker, J. O., *62*
Parlee, M. B., 229, *237*
Parmies, R. J., 154, *170*
Pascale, L., 53, *68*
Pasch, L. A., 242, 248, 249, 251, 253,
    254, 259, 261, 264, 266, 267
Pasino, J., 197, *211*

Paskey, S., 179, *190*
Passingham, C., *235*
Patrick, L., 197, 209, *214*
Patterson, C. J., 261, *264*
Patterson, G. A., 88, *102*
Patterson, G. R., 30, *39*
Patterson, J. M., 320, *333*, 350, *363*
Pattinson, T., 252, *264*
Patton, S., 82, *102*
Paul, J., *189*
Paulsen, J., 197, *214*
Paulson, R. J., 244, *266*
Payne, A., 199, 202, 204, 205, *213*
Payne, B., 193, *214*
Payne, H., 341, *365*
Peacock, L. J., 289, *305*
Pearl, D., 25, 30, *40*
Pearlin, L. I., 111, *132*
Pearson, D. C., *336*
Pelcovits, M. A., 285, *304*
Penman, D., *163*
Penninx, B. W. J. H., 112, *132*
Pensiero, L., 140, *168*
Pepe, M., 81, *102*
Pepe, M. V., 251, *266*
Pergami, A., 175, *190*
Perloff, D., *38*
Perodeau, G. M., 281, 283, *307*
Perrin, E., *103*
Perrin, J. M., 338, 341, 356, *364*
Peter, T. J., 285, *302*
Peterson, C., 142, *168*
Peterson, L., 123, *128*
Peterson, L. S., 243, *263*
Petrini, B., 144, *167*
Pettingale, K. W., 139, 142, 144, *162*, *165*,
    168
Pfeiffer, C., 113, 123, *127*
Phillips, L. R., *131*
Pianta, R. C., 341, *364*
Piasetsky, S., *163*
Picard, R. S., 74, *99*
Picciano, J., 175, *189*
Piccinino, L. J., 243, *263*
Pickering, R., *302*
Pickering, T., 51, *67*
Pierce, G. R., 139, *168*

Riccio, M., *190*
Rice, D., 4, *11*
Rich, M. W., *63*
Richard, A., *97*
Richardson, J. L., 178, 179, *189*, *190*
Rickels, K., 201, *211*
Ries, L. A. G., 73, *104*
Rimer, B. K., 313, *334*
Rimm, D. C., *300*
Riskind, J. H., 183, *190*
Rivera-Tovar, A. D., 226, *236*, *237*
Robbins, C., 47, 66, 142, *165*, 226, *236*
Roberts, C. F., 290, *307*
Roberts, J., 141, *166*
Roberts, L. J., 270, 280, 281, 282, 283,
    290, 291, 296, 298, *304*, *307*
Roberts, M. C., 287, *308*
Robertson, P., 261, *263*
Robins, L. N., *214*
Robinson, D. S., *163*
Robinson, E., *130*
Robinson, M. E., 203, *216*
Rock, A. F., 201, *211*
Roehrich, L., 289, *302*
Roffman, R., 175, *189*
Rogers, M. P., *130*, *131*
Rogers, S. J., 279, 280, *300*
Rogers, W., *69*
Rogers, W. H., *103*
Rohsenow, D., 275, *305*
Roivonen, H., *164*
Roland, M., 201, *214*
Rolland, J. S., 3, *11*
Romano, J. M., 192, 194, 196, 197, 198,
    201, 202, 209, *212*, *214*, *215*
Romelsjo, A., 285, *308*
Rompa, D., 175, 185, *189*
Rompf, J., *64*
Rook, K., 123, *132*
Room, R., 274, *308*
Roosa, M. W., 286, *301*
Rosen, M. J., 75, *103*
Rosen, R. C., 289, *301*
Rosenberg, H. M., 73, *104*
Rosenberg, H. S., 248, *264*
Rosenberg, R., 197, *212*, *215*

Rosenberg, R. L., 48, *65*
Rosenfeld, M., 81, *102*
Rosengren, A., 47, *67*
Rosenstein, B. J., 74, *102*
Rosinsky, M., 316, *334*
Roski, J., 316, *336*
Rosner, B., 314, *334*
Ross, C. E., 113, *132*
Rossignol, A. M., 221, *236*
Rosti, G., 140, 141, 143, 157, *164*
Roth, S., 115, *133*
Roth-Roemer, S., 113, *132*
Rothbard, J. C., 270, 279, *304*
Rothenberg, K. H., 179, *190*
Rothman, K. J., 219, *237*
Rotunda, R. J., 293, 294, *307*, *308*
Rovario, S., 54, *68*
Rowat, K., 195, 199, *214*
Rowe, J., 123, *127*
Rowland, J. H., 148, *168*
Roy, R., 193, 199, *214*
Roy-Byrne, P. P., 217, 218, 220, *235*, *237*
Rozenberg, S., 73, *102*
Rubens, R. D., *166*
Ruberman, W., 47, *68*
Rubin, A., 143, *166*
Rubinow, D. R., 217, 218, 220, *235*, *237*
Rudy, E. B., 54, *68*
Rudy, T. E., 193, 200, *212*, *213*, 230, *236*
Ruiz, M., 178, *189*
Ruiz, M. S., *190*
Rupp, S. L., 225, *238*
Russell, J. W., 223, *236*
Russell, O., 47, 54, *69*
Russo, J., 197, *215*
Rutter, C., 156, *168*
Ruuskanen, O., *164*
Rychtarik, R. G., 277, *308*
Ryser, R., 227, *237*
Rytokoski, U., 203, *215*

Saarijavi, S., 203, *214*, *215*
Sabbeth, B. F., 341, 342, *364*
Saini, J., *63*
Saito, Y., *167*
Sakai, C., 197, *215*

Steptoe, A., *42*, 222, *238*
Stern, M. J., 53, *68*
Stern, R. C., 74, 81, *98*, *100*
Stevens, P. A., 319, *336*
Stevenson, L. W., *101*
Stewart, A. L., 69, 86, *103*
Stewart, D., *238*
Stickle, T. R., 255, 263, 294, 300, 326, *333*
Stone, A. A., *41*, 77, *103*
Stoney, C. M., 15, 21, 26, *40*, *42*
Stour, C. J., *39*
Stout, A. L., 225, 227, *238*
Stout, C., *104*
Stout, R., 294, 305, 327, *335*
Straus, M. A., 256, 267, 290, *303*
Strecher, W. J., 327, *335*
Streiner, D., *238*
Strickle, T. R., 91, *97*
Strom, S. E., 201, *212*
Stuart, R. B., 91, *103*
Sudore, R., 254, *267*
Sullivan, M., 197, *215*
Sullivan, M. J., 3, *11*
Sullivan, S. E., 313, *334*
Summers, K., 30, *42*
Sung, H. Y., 4, *11*
Superko, H. R., *64*
Surgeon General, 44, *68*, 313, *336*
Sussman, M. B., 341, *361*
Sutton, G., 313, *336*
Sutton, J. R., *62*
Sveinsdottir, H., 220, *238*
Swafford, J., *130*
Swanson, D. W., 194, *213*
Swanson, M., 314, *336*
Syme, S. L., 47, *63*
Szklo, M., 47, *63*

Taanila, A., 341, 342, 347, *364*
Taillefer, S., *166*
Tal, M., *64*
Tam, T. W., 274, *305*
Tang, C. S., 140, *169*
Tanner, M. A., 141, *170*
Tansella, C. Z., 351, *365*

Tarlov, A. R., 86, *103*
Tartar, R. E., 276, *309*
Tasker, F., 261, *264*
Taussig, L. M., *336*
Taylor, A. G., 193, 194, *215*
Taylor, C. B., 24, 27, 28, 30, 34, 38, 46, 50, 51, 59, *64*, 67, 68, 232, *237*
Taylor, J., 192, *215*
Taylor, J. E., *130*
Taylor, K. L., 155, *166*
Taylor, K. T., 156, *166*
Taylor, P. J., 250, *265*
Taylor, R. W., 220, *237*
Taylor, S. E., 142, 153, *163*, *169*
Teasdale, J. D., 142, *161*
Teiramaa, E., 75, *103*
Telch, C. F., 142, 157, *169*
Telch, M. J., 142, 157, *169*
Telford, L., *103*
Templin, T., 139, *167*
Tennant, C., 54, *66*
Tennen, H., 113, 123, *127*, 249, 250, 265, *267*
TeVelde, A., *63*
teVelde, E. R., 218, *238*
Tew, B., 341, 349, *365*, 345, 346
Thayaparan, B., 125, *130*
Theodos, V., 249, *265*
Thom, T. J., 55, *69*
Thomas, M., *167*
Thomas, R. J., *64*
Thompson, D. R., 53, *69*, 226, *238*
Thompson, R., 350, *365*
Thompson, R. J., Jr., 338, 342, 345, 346, 347, 354, 356, *365*
Thomton, J. C., 23, *42*
Threatt, B. A., 141, *169*
Tibblin, G., 45, *69*
Timko, C., 142, *169*
Timmons, K., *130*
Tollestrup, K., 78, *99*
Tolor, A., 251, *266*
Tonascia, J., 47, *63*
Tonigan, J. S., 292, 295, 300, 305, *306*
Tosteson, A. N., *66*
Tota-Faucette, M. E., 201, *215*
Tovar-Guzman, V., 73, *100*

SUBJECT INDEX

clinical significance of relationship, 136, 142–144

coping strategies, 141–142, 144, 148–149, 157–159

couple-based intervention. *See* Cancer Coping for Couples

epidemiology, 136, 137–138

existential issues, 140, 146–147, 159

long-term adjustment, 140–141

medical decision making, 154–155

medical treatment, 138

mortality, 137–138

practitioner preparation for intervention in, 161

psychological aspects of care, 136

response to diagnosis, 138–140

treatment, 141

See also specific anatomic site

Cancer Coping for Couples

assessment, 147–154

development of coping skills, 157–159

development of partner support, 155–157

existential issues, 159

future prospects, 160–161

goals, 160

initial interview, 148–149

patient selection, 145

relapse prevention, 159–160

sexual issues, 159

therapeutic course, 144–147

Cardiac arrhythmia, 44

Cardiovascular function

assessment, 19–20

communication training effects, 34–35

during dyadic interaction, 30

effects of negative intimate interactions, 5–6

gender differences, 5–6, 21, 35

stress reactivity, 19, 20, 21

See also specific cardiovascular pathology

Caregiver stress

child chronic illness, 341, 342–343, 349–350

chronic pain patient, 193, 195

cystic fibrosis, 82

HIV/AIDS, 176–177

partner with rheumatoid arthritis, 110, 111–112

Catecholamines, 17

measurement, 18

Cellular immune response, 22

Child chronic illness, 5, 10–11

assessment, 352–354

asthma, 350–351

cancer, 343–345

cystic fibrosis, 342–343, 350

developmental considerations, 337–338

diabetes, 346–347

duration effects, 349

economic impact, 338

effects of couple functioning on, 350–352

effects on parents' relationship, 338–341

epidemiology, 338

intervention, 354–359

parent guilt, 342

parenting style, 356–357

positive effects on family functioning, 340–341, 345

research base, 348–349, 359–360

research opportunities, 360

severity of illness, 349

sickle-cell anemia, 347–348, 350

spina bifida, 345–346

Childhood abuse, 186

Cholesterol levels, 45

Chronic obstructive pulmonary disease, 72–73

anger reactions in, 79, 90

assessment, 83, 84

couples therapy, 90

medical intervention, 87, 88, 89

Chronic obstructive pulmonary disease
(*continued*)
relationship correlates, 78–79
sexual activity and, 78–79
treatment adherence, 87
Cognitive-behavioral theory and therapy
chronic pain conceptualization,
199
chronic pain treatment, 204–205
infertility intervention, 254–255
marital, 56
partner with rheumatic disease,
120–121
premenstrual syndrome intervention,
230–232
Common cold, 77
Communication training, 34–35, 36–37
couple-based cancer intervention,
155–157
premenstrual syndrome intervention,
231–232
respiratory disease intervention,
91
Conflicted interactions. *See* Negative
interactions
Contextual approach to treatment,
124–127
alcohol use among couples,
270–271
Coronary heart disease, 6
adherence to treatment, 49
clinical features, 44
couple conflict and hypertension,
51
depression and, 46
epidemiology, 43, 54–55
help-seeking behavior, 48
hostility and, 20–21, 52
recovery and rehabilitation, 46, 47,
48, 49, 50, 51, 53–54
relationship linkages, 6, 47–55
relationship support intervention,
55–62
research opportunities, 62

risk factors, 20–21, 44–47
women's issues, 54–55
Cost of care
alcohol problems, 269–270
asthma, 72
child chronic illness, 338
HIV/AIDS, 186
rheumatoid arthritis, 106
smoking-related illness, 312
Couples intervention
alcohol problem, 293–294,
297–298
cancer intervention. *See* Cancer
Coping for Couples
chronic pain, 202–207, 208–210
infertility treatment, 254–255
parents of child with chronic illness,
355–356
patient with respiratory disorder,
90–95
premenstrual syndrome, 230–233
rationale, 119–120
rheumatoid arthritis, 118–124
smoking cessation, 312–313, 315,
326–333
Cultural sensitivity
in HIV assessment, 182–183
infertility treatment, 261
Cystic fibrosis, 350
in child, parental relationship and,
342–343
clinical features, 74, 342
epidemiology, 74, 338, 342
medical intervention, 90
prognosis, 74
relationship correlates, 81–82

Demand–withdraw interaction sequence,
16
Depression
after myocardial infarction, 46, 50
assessment, 117–118, 229, 353
asthma and, 86

cancer and, 140–141
chronic pain and, 192, 194–195
heart disease risk and, 46, 50–51
HIV assessment, 183–184
premenstrual syndrome and,
    221–222, 229
quality of relationship and, 51, 113
rheumatoid arthritis and, 109–110,
    117–118
Diabetes, juvenile, 346–347

Ecological approach, 7
Educational interventions
    alcohol abuse, 293–294
    cancer treatment, 154–155
    chronic pain, 204
    myocardial infarction recovery, 52
    sexual activity during recovery, 54
Emphysema. *See* Chronic obstructive
    pulmonary disease
Employment, rheumatoid arthritis and,
    109
Endocrine function, in premenstrual
    syndrome, 219–220
Epidemiology
    alcohol problems, 273–274
    cancer, 136, 137–138
    child chronic illness, 338
    chronic illness, 4
    coronary heart disease, 43, 54–55
    HIV/AIDS, 172
    infertility, 243
    lung cancer, 73
    premenstrual syndrome, 218,
        225–226
    respiratory disorders, 72, 73–75
    rheumatic disease, 105
    rheumatoid arthritis, 106
    tuberculosis, 74–75
Epinephrine, 31
Epstein–Barr virus, 31
Expectancy effects in alcohol
    consumption, 275, 289

Family systems
    chronic pain conceptualization,
        199–200
    models of alcohol-complicated
        relationships, 278
    research, 3
Fertility problems, 9
    assessment, 255–256, 262
    assisted reproductive technologies,
        243–244, 252–253
    decision-making aids, 262–263
    definition of infertility, 243
    differences among couples in
        relationship quality, 247–248
    epidemiology, 243
    gender differences in response to,
        249, 250
    gender differences in treatment
        decision-making, 251–252
    importance of couple's participation
        in treatment, 253–254
    individual distress in, 250–251
    interactional style of couples with,
        241–242, 248–250
    male factor, 245
    population diversity and, 261
    preventing relationship problems,
        254–260
    psychological theory, 260–261
    research needs, 261–262
    significance of psychological issues,
        253
    as source of relationship problems,
        246–250
    stress of decision-making, 244–246,
        251–253
    use of donor oocyte or sperm,
        244–245
Fibromyalgia. *See* Rheumatic disease

Gay and lesbian couples, fertility
    problems, 261

childhood abuse issues, 186
clinical course, 173–174
as couple's disease, 175–176
current treatment strategies, 174
disclosure of diagnosis, 178–179
epidemiology, 172
financial stressors in, 186–187
future orientation, 185
mental health intervention,
    184–187
pathophysiology, 172–173
psychosocial effects, 192
relationship changes in, 174–175,
    187
research needs, 187–188
risk of reinfection, 186
seroconcordant couples, 176–177,
    184–185
serodiscordant couples, 177, 184
sexual relationship in couples with,
    177, 178, 186
stress and coping with, 177–179
substance abuse issues, 185–186
transmission, 171, 172, 175
treatment, 174
tuberculosis and, 75
unique relationship issues, 8
Hostility, hypertension and, 52
Human immunodeficiency virus. *See*
    HIV/AIDS
Humoral immune system, 22
Hypertension. *See* Blood pressure
Hypothalamic–pituitary–adrenal (HPA)
    axis, 13
    health effects of negative dyadic
        interaction, 36
    measurement, 18–19
    normal function, 17–18
    stress response, 17

Illness effects on relationship, 7
    alcohol problems, 9, 270–272, 275,
        279–285, 299

child chronic illness, 338–342,
    348–350
child with cancer, 343–345
child with cystic fibrosis, 342–343
child with diabetes, 346–347
child with sickle-cell anemia,
    347–348
child with spina bifida, 345–346
chronic pain, 196–198
heart disease, 53–54
infertility, 246–248
premenstrual syndrome, 226–228
Immune function
    assessment, 22–23
    defense systems, 22
    during dyadic interaction, 30–31
    gender differences in stress reactivity,
        31
    HIV course, 172–173, 174
    neuroendocrine function in, 17–18
    normal, 22
    psychosocial functioning and, 144
    stress response, 21–22, 23
Infection. *See* Upper respiratory infection;
    specific pathogen
Infertility. *See* Fertility problems
Inhalers, 84–85, 87
Inhibition, alcohol effects on,
    275–276
Integrative couple therapy, 257–258
    acceptance-building strategies, 257,
        258–259
    assessment, 255–256
    chronic pain, 205
    empathic joining in, 257–258
    feedback session, 257–258
    infertility intervention, 255
    therapeutic goals, 92, 205, 255
    therapeutic strategies, 92
Interactional style
    alcohol consumption and, 275,
        286–288
    assessment in cancer intervention,
        148, 149–154

on people with rheumatoid arthritis,
114–116

Negative interactions
alcohol consumption and, 286–288
cardiovascular function during, 30,
31–32
cardiovascular reactivity and, 51–52
communication training effects,
34–35
demand–withdraw sequence, 16
effects on person with rheumatoid
arthritis, 114–115
endocrine response, 30–31, 32
enhanced sensitivity to, 115
immune response, 30–31
physiologic effects of communication
training, 34–35
physiological effects, 5–6
physiological predictors of long-term
relationship outcomes in, 35
premenstrual syndrome and,
227–228
psychophysiological model of health
effects of, 14–16, 35–37
psychophysiological research
findings, 23–29
smoking cessation and, 316, 318,
326, 328

Neuroendocrine function
during dyadic interaction, 30–31
measurement, 18–10
normal physiology, 17–18
stress response, 17, 18–19, 23

Neuroticism
assessment, 229
premenstrual syndrome and, 222

Newlyweds, 30–31, 75

Norepinephrine, 31

Nutrition and diet, premenstrual
syndrome and, 230

Obstructive sleep apnea, 73, 79–80, 82,
89–90, 90–91

Osteoarthritis, 120. *See also* Rheumatic
disease

Overprotectiveness, 52, 53–54

Oxygen therapy, 88

Pain, chronic, 8
acceptance of, as therapeutic goal,
91–92
assessment, 200–202
attitudes and beliefs, 205
conceptual models, 192–193,
198–200
coping-skills-training in rheumatic
disease, 120
couple interventions, 202–207
definition, 191
effects of relationship on, 196–198,
207
effects on relationship, 193–196
epidemiology, 191
gender differences in adjustment to,
194
implications for sexual activity, 194,
205
research findings, 207–208
research opportunities, 207–209,
210–211
subtypes, 191
treatment, 202
unique relationship issues, 8

Pharmacotherapy
respiratory disorders, 87
rheumatoid arthritis, 107

Physical activity
heart disease and, 45
rheumatoid arthritis effects, 108–109
social support effects, 53
See also Sexual activity

Posttraumatic stress disorder in cancer
diagnosis, 139

Pregnancy, smoking during, 313–314

Premenstrual syndrome, 8–9
assessment, 228–230

Premenstrual syndrome (*continued*)
    biopsychosocial model, 222–224
    clinical features, 218
    continuum conceptualization,
        224–225
    couples intervention, 230–233
    dichotomous conceptualization,
        218–219
    effects on relationship, 226–228
    as endocrine disorder, 219–220
    epidemiology, 218, 225–226
    learning theory, 223–224
    medical management, 230,
        233–234
    personality correlates, 222
    psychological factors in, 221–224
    relationship quality and, 226, 233
    relationship status and, 225–226
    research opportunities, 234
    symptom perception among women
        with, 223
    symptom severity, 220–221, 227
Prolactin, 17, 31
Prostate cancer, 137, 154
Psychosocial functioning
    assessment, 57–58
    assessment of respiratory disease
        patient, 84–86
    cancer outcomes and, 143–144
    child assessment, 353–354
    chronic pain-associated problems,
        192
    couple assessment, 352–353
    heart disease risk factors, 45–47
    HIV assessment, 182–184
    infertility effects on individual,
        250–251
    influence of partner on chronic pain
        patient, 197
    in premenstrual syndrome,
        221–224
    pulmonary function and, 76
    relationship quality as protective
        factor, 250–251

response to cancer diagnosis,
    138–140
rheumatoid arthritis effects,
    109–110
Psychosocial intervention, 5
    acceptance as therapeutic goal,
        91–92
    alcohol problem, 293–296
    cancer, 7. *See* Cancer Coping for
        Couples
    child chronic illness, 354–359
    chronic pain, 202, 208–211
    communication training, 34–35,
        36–37
    contextual approach, 124–127
    emotional expressiveness training,
        231–232
    HIV/AIDS, 184–187
    illness-specific couples-focused, 5,
        91
    infertility treatment, 254–260
    relationship support for cardiac
        patients, 55–62
    respiratory illness, 6, 90–95
    rheumatoid arthritis, 118–124
    smoking cessation, 10
    See also Couples intervention
Pulmonary function tests, 83

Quality of relationship
    alcohol consumption and, 276–277,
        280–286, 296–297
    assessment, 57–58, 85–86, 93–94,
        229, 352–353
    asthma and, 75–76, 93–94
    cardiac event recovery and, 50–52
    cardiovascular reactivity and, 51
    chronic obstructive pulmonary
        disease and, 78–79
    chronic pain effects, 193–194,
        196–198
    cystic fibrosis and, 81–82
    depression and, 51

effects of child chronic illness,
342–343, 344, 345–346, 347–348
evidence of health linkage, 14–15
as health variable, 4
illness effects on relationships, 53–54
individual distress and, 250–251
infertility-related problems, 246–250
lung cancer and, 81
obstructive sleep apnea and, 80
organ transplantation and, 89
premenstrual syndrome and, 226,
233
psychophysiological models of health
interaction, 14–16, 95–96
psychophysiological predictors, 35
psychophysiological research
findings, 23–29
quality of social support and, 14–16
respiratory disease and, 82–83,
85–86, 96–97
respiratory infection and, 77–78
response to HIV diagnosis, 174–175
rheumatoid arthritis and, 113–114
as target of intervention, 55–56

Recovery and rehabilitation
cardiac event, 46, 47, 48, 53–54,
55–62
contact between partners and, 49
depression and, 46
effects on relationship in, 53–54
marital status and, 48
negative effects of family or partner,
52
patient education, 52
sexual activity in, 54
social support in, 47
Relationship Support Program, 55–62
Respiratory disease, 6
behavioral–psychological assessment,
84–86
couples therapy, 90–95
health–relationship linkage, 96–97

integrative model of
health–relationship system, 95–96
intermittent disorders, 96
medical assessment, 83–84
medical intervention, 87–90
premorbid relationship events and,
82–83
research needs, 82, 97
risk factors, 95–96
treatment adherence, 84–85
types of, 71. *See also specific type*
Rheumatic disease, 6–7
clinical features, 105
epidemiology, 105
types of, 105
See also Rheumatoid arthritis
Rheumatoid arthritis
assessment, 117–118
buffering effect of relationship,
112–114
clinical features, 106
contextual approach to treatment,
124–127
couple intervention, 118–124
couple level-coping, 116–117
depression and, 109–110, 117–118
epidemiology, 106
gender differences, 107, 112
impact on partner, 110
impact on relationship of, 111–112
lifestyle changes related to,
108–109
medical treatment, 107–108
negative effects of relationships,
114–116
research needs, 127
self-help groups, 123
sensitivity to interpersonal stressors,
115
social and economic costs, 106

Satisfaction in relationship. *See* Quality of
relationship

infertility intervention decision making, 244–246, 251–253

neuroendocrine response, 17, 18–19, 30–31

psychophysiological model of health–relationship interaction, 14–16

psychophysiological research findings, 23–29, 36

pulmonary function and, 76–77

relationship as source of, 14

research needs, 37

respiratory infection risk and, 77–78

Substance abuse
  among HIV/AIDS patients, 185–186
  See also Alcohol problems

Sympathetic nervous system, 17, 18

Sympathetic–adrenal–medullary (SAM) system, 13, 36
  measurement, 19

normal function, 17–18

stress response, 17

T lymphocytes, 22
  HIV course, 172, 173–174

Tuberculosis
  assessment, 83
  clinical features, 74
  epidemiology, 74–75
  medical intervention, 87
  relationship correlates, 82

Type A personality, 20–21, 52
  heart disease risk and, 46

Upper respiratory infection, 72, 96
  relationship correlates, 77–78

Violent behavior
  alcohol consumption and, 290–291

ABOUT THE EDITORS

Karen B. Schmaling is an associate professor in the Department of Psychiatry and Behavioral Sciences and training director of the Clinical Psychology Internship Program at the University of Washington School of Medicine. She received her doctorate in clinical psychology from the University of Washington in 1988. In addition to pursuing research on asthma and chronic fatigue syndrome, funded by the National Institutes of Health, she is an active clinician and teacher, working with patients and trainees in inpatient and outpatient psychiatric and medical settings.

Tamara Goldman Sher is an assistant professor in the Department of Psychology at the Illinois Institute of Technology. She received her doctorate in clinical psychology from the University of North Carolina at Chapel Hill in 1989. Following completion of her degree, she served as the director of the Behavioral Medicine and Couples program at Rush-Presbyterian-St. Luke's Medical Center in Chicago, where her interest in the relationship between intimacy and health first took form. Today, Dr. Sher is actively pursuing research on couples and illness, including a project recently funded by the National Institutes of Health on a couples intervention for cardiac risk reduction. In addition to her other teaching duties, Dr. Sher lectures extensively on the topic of couples and health to both lay and professional audiences.